Language Development from Theory to Practice

Khara L. Pence
University of Virginia

Laura M. Justice
University of Virginia

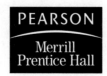

PEARSON

Merrill
Prentice Hall

Upper Saddle River, New Jersey,
Columbus, Ohio

Library of Congress Cataloging-in-Publication Data

Pence, Khara L.
   Language development from theory to practice / Khara Pence, Laura M.
Justice.
      p. cm.
   ISBN 0-13-170813-9
   1. Language acquisition.   I. Justice, Laura M.,   II. Title.
   P118.P396 2008
   401'.93—dc22

2006029134

**Vice President and Executive
   Publisher:** Jeffery W. Johnston
Executive Editor: Ann Castel Davis
Editorial Assistant: Penny Burleson
Development Editor: Heather Doyle Fraser
Production Editor: Sheryl Glicker Langner
Production Coordination: Techbooks
Design Coordinator: Diane C. Lorenzo

Cover Design: Ali Mohrman
Cover Image: Corbis
Photo Coordinator: Lori Whitley
Production Manager: Laura Messerly
Director of Marketing: David Gesell
Marketing Manager: Autumn Purdy
Marketing Coordinator: Brian Mounts

This book was set in Helvetica by Techbooks. It was printed and bound by Edwards Brothers.
The cover was printed by Phoenix Color Corporation.

Chapter Opening Photo Credits: Krista Greco/Merrill, p. 2; AP Wide World Photos, p. 40;
Mike Good © Dorling Kindersley, p.72; © Roger Ressmeyer/Corbis, p. 110; © Dex Images,
Inc./Corbis, p. 146; Geri Engberg/Geri Engberg Photography, p. 182; Anthony
Magnacca/Merrill, p. 220; David Young-Wolff/PhotoEdit Inc., p. 252; David Levy/Getty
Images Inc. – Stone Allstock, p. 286; Laura Bolesta/Merrill, p. 316

Pearson Education Ltd
Pearson Education Singapore Pte. Ltd.
Pearson Education Canada, Ltd.
Pearson Education–Japan

Pearson Education Australia Pty, Limited
Pearson Education North Asia Ltd.
Pearson Educación de Mexico, S.A. de C.V.
Pearson Education Malaysia, Pte. Ltd.

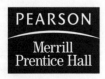

10 9 8
ISBN: 0-13-170813-9
ISBN: 978-0-13-170813-6

To Doug, for the fun you bring to my life
—K.P.

To Ian and Adelaide, who make me laugh every single day and who never waver in their support of my writing and my work
—L.J.

PREFACE

The field of language development is an incredibly exciting area of study for college and university students in diverse disciplines, including allied health (e.g., speech–language pathology, audiology), liberal arts (e.g., linguistics, psychology), and education (e.g., elementary education, special education). For students in many preprofessional training programs, a basic course in language development is required at the undergraduate or graduate level. Yet, instructors teaching courses in language development commonly say that the language development textbooks currently available do not address several important criteria:

- Integration of theory and practice, including discussion of how theories of language development influence state-of-the-art educational and clinical practices with children

- Discussion of individual differences in language development, including those of children who are developing language in diverse cultures or developing language atypically (e.g., children with disabilities)

- Descriptions of techniques educators, therapists, and researchers use to measure children's language achievements, including computer software

- Examination of language development from a multidisciplinary perspective, including its relevance to theory and practice in different disciplines

Language Development from Theory to Practice was designed to meet and exceed these criteria. This text provides a survey of key topics in language development, including research methods, theoretical perspectives, major language milestones from birth to adolescence, and language diversity and language disorders. The research base and theoretical foundation this text provides is designed to prepare students for advanced study in subjects associated with language development, such as language disorders, psycholinguistics, instruction of English as a second or foreign language, developmental psychology, and so forth.

ORGANIZATION OF THE TEXT

Language Development from Theory to Practice includes 10 chapters. Chapters 1–4 provide a basis for understanding language development. Specifically, in Chapter 1, we define language and explain how language relates to the areas of speech, hearing, and communication. We also introduce the three domains of language—content, form, and use—and describe the features of language that make it so

v

remarkable. Chapter 1 concludes with an introduction to language differences and language disorders. In Chapter 2, we describe the kinds of people who study language development and their reasons for doing so. We introduce some of the major approaches to studying language development as well as some major language development theories. The theories and approaches we introduce are referenced subsequently in several places in the text. We conclude Chapter 2 by describing how theories of language development influence practice in several areas. In Chapter 3, we introduce the "building blocks" of language: semantic, morphological, syntactic, phonological, and pragmatic development. Chapter 4 covers the neuroanatomy and neurophysiology of language. We describe the major structures of the brain, explain how the brain processes and produces language, and discuss sensitive periods in neuroanatomical and neurophysiological development.

Chapters 5–8 provide a developmental account of language acquisition for four age groups (infancy—Chapter 5; toddlerhood—Chapter 6; preschool age—Chapter 7; and school age and beyond—Chapter 8). More specifically, in each of these four chapters, we describe the major language development milestones that are achieved during the period in question; examine achievements in language content, form, and use; explain some of the intra- and interindividual differences in language development; and discuss methods researchers and clinicians use to measure language development.

In Chapters 9 and 10, we explore language diversity and language disorders. In Chapter 9, we detail the connection between language and culture, explain how languages evolve and change, describe bilingualism and second language acquisition, and discuss some theories of second language acquisition and their implications for practice. In Chapter 10, we define the term *language disorder,* explain who identifies and treats children with language disorders, discuss the major types of language disorders, and describe how language disorders are identified and treated.

KEY FEATURES OF THE TEXT

Each chapter of the text bridges language development theory and practice by providing students with a theoretical and scientific foundation to the study of language development. We emphasize the relevance of the material to students' current and future experiences in clinical, educational, and research settings.

Multicultural Considerations

Current perspectives emphasize the importance of taking into account multicultural considerations in understanding language development. This text promotes students' awareness of the way in which culture interacts with language development for children from diverse backgrounds within and beyond the many types of North American communities.

Research Foundations

Current initiatives in the educational, social science, and health communities emphasize the use of evidence-based practices. Such practices emphasize the importance of research results to making educational and clinical decisions. In keeping with this premise, we emphasize in this text the research foundations of the study of language development, and the most current empirical findings are used to describe children's language achievements.

Multidisciplinary Focus

The study of language development is constantly evolving and being influenced by many diverse disciplines; this multidimensional and multidisciplinary foundation attracts many students to the study of language development. We introduce exciting innovations in theory and practice from many diverse areas of research.

Easy-to-Read Format

Language Development from Theory to Practice is presented in a way that promotes student learning. First, the chapters are infused with figures, tables, and photographs to contextualize abstract and complex information. Second, important terms are highlighted for easy learning and reference. Third, discussion questions are integrated throughout to provide students the opportunity to pause and consider important information. All these features create opportunities for students to actively engage with the material in the text.

Pedagogical Elements

The text includes many pedagogical elements:

- Focus Questions to organize each chapter
- Discussion questions interspersed throughout each chapter
- Chapter summaries
- Lists of key resources, including research-based articles, books, and Web sites
- Boxed inserts:
  - *Developmental Timeline:* In this type of box, we present milestones for language development, observable features of these milestones, and the ages by which the milestones are usually reached.
  - *Multicultural Focus:* In this type of box, we introduce cultural differences in language development and describe the observable features of these differences. We also discuss educational and clinical implications with regard to cultural differences.
  - *Research Paradigms:* In this type of box are descriptions of various research paradigms used to inform practitioners' understanding of language development.
  - *Theory to Practice:* In this type of box, we discuss some of the implications of different theoretical perspectives for educational and clinical practice.

Supplemental Materials

Accompanying this text are the following resources:

- An online Instructors' Manual with discussion items, chapter summaries, and a bank of assessment questions

- The Companion Website (www.prenhall.com/pence), which has reflection questions and study items for each chapter as well as additional Web links to sites of interest

- A CD-ROM that contains language samples of children from ages newborn through 13 years, and video clips of research paradigms used to learn about language development

ACKNOWLEDGMENTS

We extend our thanks to our family members, friends, and colleagues who supported us throughout this project. Among these persons are the Pence family, the Powell family, Doug Turnbull, and the Justice family. We are indebted to them for their interest in and support of this text. We also thank our doctoral mentors—Dr. Roberta Golinkoff and Dr. Helen Ezell—for helping both of us, early in our careers, to learn all we could about language acquisition. Both were impeccable guides. Last, but definitely not the least, we thank Elizabeth Bottonari, who gracefully took on the challenge of developing the Instructor's Manual and Companion Website for this text; we are so grateful for her help.

We thank Alice Wiggins for assisting with securing permission to reprint copyrighted materials in this book. Further appreciation goes to our colleagues at the University of Virginia who share in our excitement for language development: Anita Bailie, Angela Beckman, Ryan Bowles, Elizabeth Cottone, Sarah Friel, Anita McGinty, Bob Pianta, Sara Rimm-Kaufman, Lori Skibbe, Amy Sofka, and Maurie Sutton. For helping us gather videos for the CD-ROM accompanying this text, thanks to Wanda Colvin, Heather Emmons, Sarah Friel, Roberta Golinkoff, Susan Massey, and Becca Seston. Likewise, thanks to the families who allowed us to showcase their children's language in the videos.

At Merrill/Prentice Hall, Allyson Sharp and Jeffery Johnston supported this project; Kathy Burk ensured smooth coordination of the writing, editing, and production processes; and Lori Whitley coordinated the photo selections for this text. To them we express our deep gratitude. We are especially grateful, too, for the careful attention of Heather Doyle Fraser, Senior Development Editor at Merrill/Prentice Hall, to all aspects of this project—from the most minute details to the overall organization and design of the text. We also thank Kathy Riley-King, our copy editor, who did a lot more than cross our *t* 's and dot our *i* 's, and Sarvesh Mehrotra, who ensured a high degree of quality during the production process.

Finally, we are indebted to a number of experts who reviewed this manuscript: Eileen Abrahamsen, Old Dominion University; Linda C. Badon, University of Louisiana at Lafayette; Ross A. Flom, Brigham Young University; Susan Johnston, University of Utah; and Shelia M. Kennison, Oklahoma State University.

BRIEF CONTENTS

CONTENTS

5 INFANCY: LET THE LANGUAGE ACHIEVEMENTS BEGIN   146

Note: Every effort has been made to provide accurate and current Internet information in this book. However, the Internet and information posted on it are constantly changing, so it is inevitable that some of the Internet addresses listed in this textbook will change.

Language Development
from Theory to Practice

1

Language Development

An Introduction

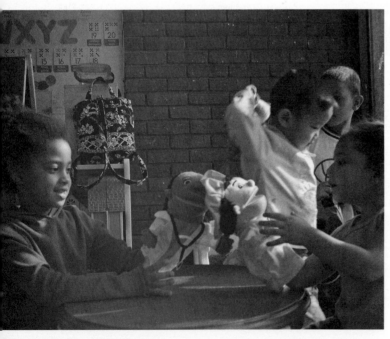

FOCUS QUESTIONS

In this chapter, we answer the following five questions:

1. What is language?
2. How does language relate to speech, hearing, and communication?
3. What are the major domains of language?
4. What are some remarkable features of language?
5. What are language differences and language disorders?

Hundreds of scientists worldwide study the remarkable phenomenon of language development. Each year, these scholars publish the results of numerous studies in scientific journals, considering such questions as the following:

- Does the language a child is learning (e.g., Chinese vs. English) influence the rate of language development?
- How do the ways in which parents interact with their child affect the time at which the child produces his or her first word?
- Do children who show early delays in language development typically catch up with their peers?
- Do children learning sign language develop language in a way similar to that of children learning a spoken language?
- Why do adults have more difficulty learning a new language than children do?

These questions provide the student of language development with a glimpse into many of the interesting topics language scientists focus on in their work around the world. These questions also suggest how important language research is to informing the everyday practices and activities of parents, teachers, psychologists, and other professionals who are invested in helping children achieve their fullest language development potential. That these questions have yet to be fully answered shows that the study of language development is a constantly evolving and complex area of science in which practitioners have many more questions than answers.

In this chapter, we provide a general introduction to the study of language development and consider five major topics. In the first section, we answer the question "What is language?" and present a definition of language that we build on throughout the text. In the second section, we discuss differences among speech, hearing, and communication—three aspects of human development and behavior that are closely related but are nonetheless distinct capacities. In the third section, we cover the five major domains of language, a topic that is introduced here and discussed more fully in Chapter 3. The fourth section includes a discussion of several remarkable features of language, and in the fifth section, we describe differences and disorders of language development—two topics explored more comprehensively in Chapter 9 (language differences) and Chapter 10 (language disorders).

WHAT IS LANGUAGE?

Language Defined

You probably have an intuitive sense of what language is because it is a human behavior you have acquired to a sophisticated level and use regularly for various purposes. In fact, you are using your language abilities as you read and analyze the content of this chapter. However, if you take a moment to define language more explicitly, you may find the task challenging. Ask 10 classmates for a definition of language, and each will likely respond differently. The same outcome would probably occur if you questioned 10 language researchers.

You are also most likely aware that language is a basic and essential human behavior that develops early in life. You probably recognize that language involves words and sentences and both expression (production of language) and comprehension (understanding of language). In addition, you know that language is a process of the brain that helps people communicate their thoughts to other individuals, although you may be somewhat unclear about how language differs from speech and communication.

However, to be as specific as possible about what language is and is not, we first would like you to consider the following definition from N. W. Nelson (1998):

> **Language** is a "socially shared code that uses a conventional system of arbitrary symbols to represent ideas about the world that are meaningful to others who know the same code." (p. 26)

Next, we delineate in more detail the four characteristics of language identified in this definition:

1. *Language Is Socially Shared.* The first important characteristic of language is that it is shared by the members of a community. A *language community* is a group of people who use a common language. In fact, somewhere in the history of the human species, a single language probably emerged within a social community of about 100 hominids (Cartwright, 2000). Some experts contend that language emerged within this community as a type of grooming behavior, essentially an efficient way to share socially useful information (Dunbar, Duncan, & Nettle, 1994). Accordingly, the numerous languages of the world emerged from this single community of language users.

Language communities emerge for many reasons. Some form as a result of geographic circumstances, as in the case of Ukrainian, the language spoken in Ukraine, a country in the western region of the former Soviet Union. Alternatively, a language community may emerge for sociological reasons, as in the case of Hebrew, which many persons of Jewish faith share, or American Sign Language, which persons in the U.S. Deaf community use. A language community can organize for economic reasons as well. For instance, the World Trade Organization (WTO), a global group that coordinates and regulates trade among 148 countries, conducts its activities in English, French, and Spanish.

2. *Language Is a Code That Uses a System of Arbitrary Symbols.* The second characteristic of language is that it features a code using a set of symbols, specifically **morphemes.** Morphemes are the smallest units of language that carry meaning; they are combined to create words. Some words consist of a single morpheme (e.g., *school*), but many words comprise two or more morphemes, such as *schools* (two morphemes—*school* + -*s*) and *preschools* (three morphemes— *pre-* + *school* + -*s*).

The term *code* refers to the translation of one type of information into another type of information. In language, words are created by using morphemes to represent myriad aspects of the world around the language community. For instance, as English speakers, we can represent an internal feeling of happiness by using the single word *happy.* When we use the word *happy* in a conversation with other people to describe our feelings, we use the word to translate our feelings. Although we can share feelings and ideas through other means—such as gestures, facial expression, and posture—words are much more specific and provide a uniquely powerful tool for communicating.

One important characteristic of language code is that the relationship between a word and its **referent** (the aspect of the world to which the word refers) is arbitrary. For example, although English speakers recognize that *happy* refers to a specific feeling, any other word (e.g., *sprit, nopic,* or *grendy*) would do. Likewise, in English, one way to denote plurality is by attaching the morpheme -*s* to words (e.g., *pens, dogs*). Various other ways to denote plurality could also be used because the relationship between the plural morpheme -*s* and its plural marking is arbitrary. In contrast, the code used to organize words into sentences is not arbitrary; rather,

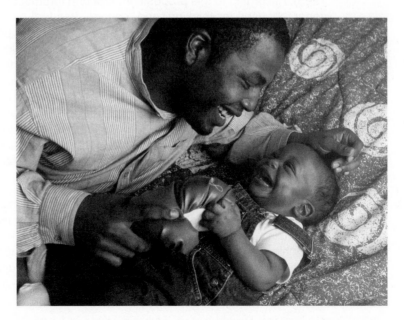

The relationship between a word and its referent is arbitrary. English speakers use the word happy *to represent an internal feeling of happiness, but any word would do.*

(*Photo Source:* © Michael Newman/PhotoEdit Inc.)

specific rules must be followed for organizing thoughts into words and sentences, as discussed next.

3. The *Language Code Is Conventional.* The third characteristic of language is the specific, systematic, and rule-governed conventions it must follow to make it nonrandom. These conventions govern the way a particular linguistic community arranges sounds into words and words into phrases, clauses, and sentences. When speakers of American English produce sounds, phrases, clauses, and sentences, they must abide by a strict set of rules. When speakers violate these rules, other community members are usually aware of the violation. For instance, a young child's comments of "I sweepeded the room" and "I goed with daddy" may be considered cute, but we are also aware that some type of linguistic rule has been violated. Yoda, a character in the *Star Wars* films, speaks an English dialect that follows unique rules. He says such things as "Agree with you the council does" and "The dark side of the force easily does flow." Yoda's language (which some persons call *Yodish*) follows its own set of conventions, even if not those of standard English dialects.

4. *Language Is a Representational Tool.* The fourth characteristic of language is that it is a cognitive tool that provides a "picture of the world that we use for thinking and communicating" (Bickerton, 1995, p. 23). This "picture of the world" includes not only symbolic representations of linguistic concepts (e.g., *big, fly, crazy*) that are organized in a vast network, but also the formal syntactic rules that organize these concepts into orderly, surface-level representations (Bickerton, 1995). According to this proposition, first and foremost language is a representational tool used for thinking, and, second, this tool permits people to communicate these thoughts to other individuals. Language probably emerged in the human species for the latter reason: to provide an efficient and effective means for communication within a community. Some experts suggest that language emerged in the human species because of increases in the size of human communities (e.g., from about 50 members of a group to more than 100 members) and therefore increases in the complexity of social dynamics (Dunbar & Aiello, 1993). With time, the neural circuitry of the human brain responded to the adaptive advantage of using language not only as a social tool but also as an inner representational tool, emerging as a specialized part of the human mind (Cartwright, 2000).

The human brain uses language as a representational tool to store information and to carry out many cognitive processes such as reasoning, hypothesizing, memorizing, planning, and problem solving (Bickerton, 1995). Considering the functioning of a human brain absent of language is nearly impossible because cognition and language become heavily intertwined during development. For instance, suppose you are asked to reason through the following problem-solving task:

A jet leaves Washington, DC, at 2 P.M., traveling south at 450 mph (724 km/h), and another jet leaves Atlanta at 5 P.M., traveling north at 500 mph (805 km/h). Over which city will the two jets pass each other?

DISCUSSION POINT

Try to consider thought without language. Doing so is extremely difficult. How do you distinguish between the two constructs? How can an individual think without language?

You would have difficulty generating an answer without using language as a tool. Although some persons may contend that they think in images and not in words, certain thoughts—such as "My trust in you has been shattered forever by your unfaithfulness"—are impossible to view as images and require language to be invoked as a representational tool (Bickerton, 1995, p. 22).

Language as a Module of Human Cognition

As we consider the definition of language, we need to explore the concept of *modularity.* **Modularity** is a cognitive science theory about how the human mind is organized within the brain structures. Questions about modularity concern whether the human brain contains a set of highly specific modules—regions of the brain developed to process specific types of information—or whether the human brain is itself a generalized module in which all parts work together to process information. A module is therefore a specialized problem-solving device in the brain that responds to information of a restricted type. Because of the specificity of such modules, they are termed **domain specific,** meaning they can process only specific types of information (Cartwright, 2000).

Some language theorists argue that the human brain contains a language-specific module developed solely to process linguistic information. These theorists contend that during human evolution, the neural circuitry of the brain became highly specialized in several regions to handle the task of developing and using language (Cartwright, 2000).

Researchers have long known that specific regions of the brain are associated with specific language abilities. For instance, persons who sustain damage to certain areas of the left frontal lobe, such as during a stroke, often exhibit difficulty with grammaticality that is called **agrammaticism.** These persons may omit grammatical markers and speak with a "telegraphic" quality (e.g., "Tommy go store now"), which suggests that this region of the brain governs aspects of grammar (Grodzinsky, 1990). The results of brain-imaging studies of the workings of undamaged brains also indicate that various regions of the brain correspond to highly specific aspects of language (Bookheimer, 2002), a concept elaborated on in Chapter 4. However, the existence of just one language module is unlikely. Rather, the brain seems to contain "a large number of relatively small but tightly clustered and interconnected modules with unique contributions to language processing" (Bookheimer, 2002, p. 152).

The concept of language modularity is not without its critics (Cartwright, 2000). Some theorists argue that language emerges in response to an individual's culture rather than to any specific internal architecture. Other researchers argue that language is processed by a general neural network that operates on all aspects of language and that the hypothesized language modules lack "neurological reality" (Bickerton, 1995, p. 76). Bickerton, in a well-reasoned critique of modularity theory as it applies to language, showed that the results of research on disorered language due to developmental disability (e.g., mental retardation) and brain injury have failed to support the modularity concept. For instance, Bickerton reviewed studies of persons with damage to a specific area of the brain purportedly linked to aggramaticism, noting that these individuals showed diverse patterns of syntactic impairment. Because the same module was likely damaged in these individuals, the expectation would be little variability in their impairment. Undoubtedly, researchers in the next several decades will better elucidate how language is represented in the neural architecture of the brain.

HOW DOES LANGUAGE RELATE TO SPEECH, HEARING, AND COMMUNICATION?

Language, speech, hearing, and communication together represent basic and interrelated human abilities. Although simple forms of communication such as gesturing do not necessarily require language, speech, and hearing, more advanced forms of communication—particularly talking and listening—require them.

Often, the terms *language, speech,* and *communication* are used synonymously, but in fact they describe substantially different processes. The term *language* was previously defined as the rule-governed, code-based tool that a person uses to represent thoughts and ideas. Once these ideas and thoughts are formulated, they can be communicated to other people through speech or manual use of a sign system; otherwise, individuals can choose to keep these thoughts and ideas to themselves (**inner language**) or can write them down (**written language**).

Speech describes the neuromuscular process by which humans turn language into a sound signal that is transmitted through the air (or another medium such as a telephone line) to a receiver. **Hearing** is the sensory system that allows speech to enter into and be processed by the human brain. **Communication** is the process of sharing information among individuals. A spoken conversation between two persons involves language, hearing, and speech; in contrast, communication between two persons in an Internet chat room involves only language.

DISCUSSION POINT

Speech, hearing, communication, and language are distinct processes, although the terms are often used interchangeably. Before reading further, consider your definition for each, focusing on what differentiates the four processes.

Speech

Speech is the voluntary neuromuscular behavior that allows humans to express language and is essential for spoken communication. In spoken communication, after people formulate ideas in the brain by using language, they must then transmit the message by using speech. Speech involves the precise activation of muscles in four systems: **respiration, phonation, resonation,** and **articulation** (Duffy, 1995). These four systems represent the remarkable coordination of a breath of air that is inspired into and then expired from the lungs (respiration); then travels up through the trachea, or windpipe (also part of respiration); over the vocal cords (phonation); and into the oral and nasal cavities (resonation). The breath of air is then manipulated by the oral articulators—including tongue, teeth, and jaw (articulation)—to come out as a series of speech sounds that are combined into words, phrases, and sentences. Figure 1.1 illustrates these systems.

Consider that the systems used for speech—respiration, phonation, resonation, and articulation—did not evolve for this purpose. Rather, speech superimposed itself on systems already in place. The structures of the respiratory, phonatory, resonatory, and articulatory systems developed early in the evolutionary history of

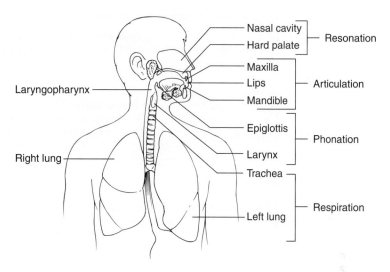

FIGURE 1.1
Systems involved with speech production.

Source: Justice, Laura M., *Communication Sciences and Disorders: An Introduction,* 1st Edition, © 2006. Reprinted with permission of Pearson Education, Inc., Upper Saddle River, NJ.

the human species as critical, functional mechanisms involved with breathing, eating, and drinking. In fact, the capacity for speech was developed in the human species "at the expense of vegetative functions such as chewing and swallowing" (Lieberman, 1991, p. 73). When and how humans first began to use speech is the subject of considerable popular, philosophical, and scientific debate; estimates range from 2 million years ago with *Homo erectus* to only 35,000 years ago with *Homo sapiens* (Cartwright, 2000). Nevertheless, experts generally agree that speech became the mode for language expression because of its advantages over other modalities (e.g., gesturing or grunting). Speech enables communication in the dark, around corners, from relatively far distances, and even when people are busy with their hands (Borden, Harris, & Raphael, 1994). In addition, speech allows an individual to communicate with a larger number of persons, which became necessary as the group size of early humans increased from small bands of hunter–gatherers of a dozen or so individuals to larger organized communities of more than 100 members (Cartwright, 2000). Finally, and possibly most important, speech provides the medium for sharing language.

Model of Speech Production

A **model** is a way to represent an unknown event on the basis of the best current evidence governing the event. Models of speech production provide a theoretical description of how an individual can move from a cognitive representation ("I forgot to bring paper. . . . I'll have to borrow a piece. . . . I see she has an extra one in her notebook") to a clearly articulated spoken product ("May I borrow a piece of paper?").

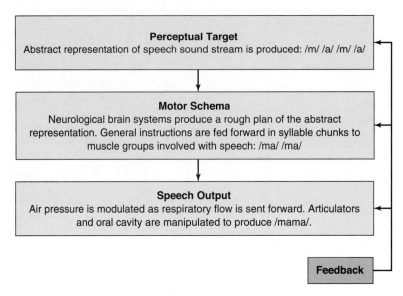

FIGURE 1.2
Model of speech production.

Source: Justice, Laura M., *Communication Sciences and Disorders: An Introduction,* 1st Edition, © 2006.
Reprinted by permission of Pearson Education, Inc., Upper Saddle River, NJ. (Adapted from Borden,
Harris, and Raphael, 1994.)

Figure 1.2 presents a basic model of speech production based on current understanding of this complex process. According to this model, speech production
has three stages (Borden et al., 1994). The first stage is a perceptual event: The
speech production process is initiated with a mental, abstract representation of the
speech stream to be produced. This abstract representation is the language code,
which provides a *perceptual target* of what is to be produced by speech. At the
perceptual level, the code is represented by the phoneme. A **phoneme** is the
smallest unit of sound that can signal a difference in meaning, and in the production of syllables and words, a series of phonemes are strung together. For instance, the word *big* comprises three phonemes, whereas the word *buy* comprises
two. In written form, phonemic representations are usually bounded by slashes;
thus, *big* is written as /b/ /ɪ/ /g/, and *buy* is written as /b/ /aɪ/. Conventionally,
phonemes are represented by the symbols of the International Phonetic Alphabet
(IPA; see Figure 1.3).

The next stage of speech production is development of a *motor schema* to represent the perceptual language-based representation. The motor schema is a
rough motor plan based on the abstract representation of the perceptual target.
The rough plan organizes the phonemes into syllable chunks; for instance, for an
infant wanting to call her mother, *mama* is represented as two syllables to be exe-
cuted: /ma/ /ma/. The rough plan is sent forward to the major muscle groups involved with speech production, including those in the respiratory system, which

CONSONANTS (PULMONIC)

© 2005 IPA

	Bilabial	Labiodental	Dental	Alveolar	Postalveolar	Retroflex	Palatal	Velar	Uvular	Pharyngeal	Glottal
Plosive	p b			t d		ʈ ɖ	c ɟ	k g	q ɢ		ʔ
Nasal	m	ɱ		n		ɳ	ɲ	ŋ	N		
Trill	ʙ			r					ʀ		
Tap or Flap		ⱱ		ɾ		ɽ					
Fricative	ɸ β	f v	θ ð	s z	ʃ ʒ	ʂ ʐ	ç ʝ	x ɣ	χ ʁ	ħ ʕ	h ɦ
Lateral fricative				ɬ ɮ							
Approximant		ʋ		ɹ		ɻ	j	ɰ			
Lateral approximant				l		ɭ	ʎ	ʟ			

Where symbols appear in pairs, the one to the right represents a voiced consonant. Shaded areas denote articulations judged impossible.

CONSONANTS (NON PULMONIC)

Clicks		Voiced implosives		Ejectives	
ʘ	Bilabial	ɓ	Bilabial	ʼ	Examples:
ǀ	Dental	ɗ	Dental/alveolar	pʼ	Bilabial
ǃ	(Post)alveolar	ʄ	Palatal	tʼ	Dental/alveolar
ǂ	Palatoalveolar	ɠ	Velar	kʼ	Velar
ǁ	Alveolar lateral	ʛ	Uvular	sʼ	Alveolar fricative

SUPRASEGMENTALS

ˈ	Primary stress
ˌ	Secondary stress
	ˌfoʊnəˈtɪʃən
ː	Long eː
ˑ	Half-long eˑ
̆	Extrashort ĕ
ǀ	Minor (foot) group
‖	Major (intonation) group
.	Syllable break ɹi.ækt
‿	Linking (absence of a break)

TONES AND WORD ACCENTS

LEVEL			CONTOUR		
e̋ or ˥	Extra high	ě or ˈ	Rising
é ˦	High	ê ˈ	Falling
ē ˧	Mid	e᷄ ˈ	High rising
è ˨	Low	e᷅ ˈ	Low rising
ȅ ˩	Extra low	e᷈ ˈ	Rising–falling, etc.
↓	Downstep	↗	Global rise
↑	Upstep	↘	Global fall

VOWELS

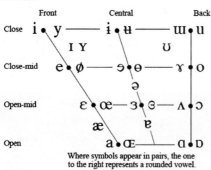

Where symbols appear in pairs, the one to the right represents a rounded vowel.

OTHER SYMBOLS

ʍ	Voiceless labial–velar fricative	ɕ ʑ	Alveolo–palatal fricatives
w	Voiced labial–velar approximant	ɺ	Voiced alveolar lateral flap
ɥ	Voiced labial–palatal approximant	ɧ	Simultaneous ʃ and x
ʜ	Voiceless epiglottal fricative		
ʢ	Voiced epiglottal fricative	Affricates and double articulations can be represented by two symbols joined by a tie bar if necessary.
ʡ	Epiglottal plosive	k͡p t͡s

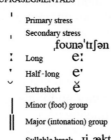

DIACRITICS

Diacritics may be placed above a symbol with a descender, e.g., ŋ̊

̥	Voiceless	n̥ d̥	̤	Breathy voiced	b̤ a̤	̪	Dental	t̪ d̪
̬	Voiced	s̬ t̬	̰	Creaky voiced	b̰ a̰	̺	Apical	t̺ d̺
ʰ	Aspirated	tʰ dʰ	̼	Linguolabial	t̼ d̼	̻	Laminal	t̻ d̻
̹	More rounded	ɔ̹	ʷ	Labialized	tʷ dʷ	̃	Nasalized	ẽ
̜	Less rounded	ɔ̜	ʲ	Palatalized	tʲ dʲ	ⁿ	Nasal release	dⁿ
̟	Advanced	u̟	ˠ	Velarized	tˠ dˠ	ˡ	Lateral release	dˡ
̠	Retracted	e̠	ˤ	Pharyngealized	tˤ dˤ	̚	No audible release	d̚
̈	Centralized	ë	~	Velarized or pharyngealized	ɫ			
̽	Midcentralized	e̽	̝	Raised	e̝	(ɹ̝ = voiced alveolar fricative)
̩	Syllabic	n̩	̞	Lowered	e̞	(β̞ = voiced bilabial approximant)
̯	Nonsyllabic	e̯	̘	Advanced Tongue Root	e̘		
˞	Rhoticity	ɚ a˞	̙	Retracted Tongue Root	e̙		

FIGURE 1.3
International Phonetic Alphabet.

Source: From *The International Phonetic Alphabet (Revised to 1993, Updated 1996),* by The International Phonetic Association, 1996, Thessaloniki, Greece: Author. Copyright 1996 by The International Phonetic Association. Reprinted with permission. http://www.arts.gla.ac.uk/IPA/ipa.html

initiate and modulate the flow of air; those around the larynx, which contains the vocal folds; and those of the oral cavity, which govern the movement of the tongue and the positioning of the upper and lower jaw and lips.

Sending forward the motor schema stimulates the production of speech, or *speech output*. The airflow, vocal fold vibration, and oral cavity movements are all finely manipulated to carry out the motor schema and to create speech.

Ongoing **feedback** relays information about speech output back to the origination of the perceptual target and motor schema. This feedback monitors the flow of speech by relaying information about timing, delivery, and precision. On most occasions, the speaker is unaware of this ongoing feedback, yet it provides information about what is to come next at the perceptual and motor levels. Occasionally, feedback occurs at a conscious level, such as when a person is aware that he or she is stumbling over words and thus speaks more deliberately.

Relationship of Speech to Language

Speech is the voluntary and complex neuromotor behavior that humans use to share language. Language does not depend on speech because people can share language by other means, such as writing, reading, and signing, or we can keep it to ourselves as a tool for thinking. However, speech depends wholly on language because language gives speech its meaning. Without language, speech is just a series of meaningless grunts and groans. Persons with significant speech disorders, such as those occurring in some instances of cerebral palsy (a motor-based disorder present at birth), may be able to produce little or no speech, or they may

Humans can share language through many means, such as writing, reading, and manually communicating (e.g., sign language).

(*Photo Source:* Mark Lewis/Getty Images Inc.—Stone Allstock.)

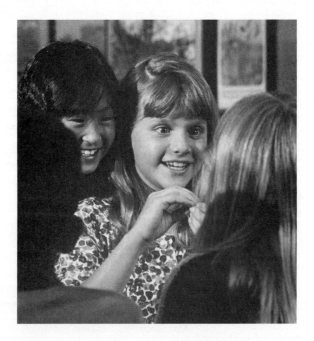

produce unintelligible speech. These persons cannot use speech to translate their thoughts to other people.

DISCUSSION POINT

Speech and language are independent processes, as illustrated by the case of Dr. Hawking. Can you think of other illustrations of the independence of speech and language?

Speech and language are independent processes; thus, some persons can have a speech disorder yet have excellent language skills. For example, Stephen Hawking (a well-known theoretical physicist at Cambridge University) has a profound speech disorder resulting from amyotrophic lateral sclerosis (ALS). ALS is a disease of the motor neurons that often results in a progressive loss of motor functioning, which has a significant impact on speech production. Although Dr. Hawking lost his ability to produce speech conventionally, his language skills remain intact, and he uses an alternative communication device, a speech synthesizer, to communicate with others.

Hearing

When people produce speech to share language for communication, not only a sender (the speaker), but also a receiver (the listener) is necessary. The receiver's task is to receive and comprehend the information the speaker conveys, and hearing is essential to both *reception* and *comprehension* of spoken language. Hearing, or **audition,** is the perception of sound, and it includes both general auditory perception and speech perception.

Sound Fundamentals

So that you understand hearing and how it relates to language and speech, you should have a general sense of **acoustics,** or the study of sound (Borden et al., 1994). The transmission and reception of speech involves four acoustic events: creation of a sound source, vibration of air particles, reception by the ear, and comprehension by the brain (Champlin, 2000):

1. *Creation of a Sound Source.* A sound source sets in motion a series of events. The sound source creates a disturbance—or set of vibrations—in the surrounding air particles. When you bring your hands together to clap, doing so sets the air particles near the sound source into a complex vibratory pattern. Likewise, when you produce the word *coffee,* this too sets the air particles near the sound source (in this case, just in front of your mouth) into a complex pattern of vibration.

2. *Vibration of Air Particles.* Fundamentally, sound is the movement or vibration of air particles. The air particles, set in motion by the sound source, move back and forth through the air (or another medium, such as water). How *fast* the particles move back and forth is the sound **frequency,** or pitch. How *far apart* the particles move when they are going back and forth creates **intensity,** or the loudness of the sound. When you clap your hands or say a word, you set the air particles around the sound source into a vibratory pattern, and the way by which the particles move carries information about frequency (pitch) and intensity (loudness). This information is represented in the movements of air particles between the sender and the receiver.

3. *Reception by the Ear.* The ear is specially designed to channel information carried by the air-particle vibrations into the human body. The ear is a complex structure with three chambers. The outer chamber (the outer ear) captures the sound and channels it to the middle chamber (the middle ear). The middle chamber then forwards the acoustic information to the inner chamber (the inner ear), which contains the cochlea. From the cochlea, the auditory information travels up the auditory nerve to the auditory regions of the brain.

4. *Comprehension by the Brain.* The auditory centers of the brain—located in the left hemisphere—translate the auditory information sent through the ear and along the auditory nerve. If the information that arrives at the brain involves speech sounds, the speech and language centers of the brain help in the comprehension process. If the information that arrives at the brain is not a speech sound (e.g., a clap of the hands or the hum of a fan), the speech and language centers are not involved. Sound information is differentiated by the human brain as speech versus nonspeech; in fact, the human ear and the brain are designed to be "remarkably responsive" to processing the sounds of speech (Borden et al., 1994, p. 176).

Speech Perception

Speech perception refers to how the brain processes speech and language. Speech perception is different from **auditory perception,** which is a more general term describing how the brain processes any type of auditory information. Processing a clap of the hands or the hum of a fan involves auditory perception, but processing the word *coffee* requires speech perception. The brain differentiates between general auditory information and speech sounds, processing speech differently than other auditory stimuli.

Speech perception involves specialized processors in the brain that have evolved specifically to respond to human speech and language. Infants enter the world with biologically endowed processing mechanisms geared toward the perception of speech, and, with exposure to a specific language (or languages), the perceptual mechanism is calibrated to reflect this language. Calibration of the speech perception mechanism is aided by a few capacities of the young child. First, young children show a preference for auditory rather than visual information; this phenomenon is called *auditory overshadowing* (Sloutsky & Napolitano, 2003), a principle of early development suggesting that young children have a bias toward attending to auditory information in their environment. Second, young children—mostly infants—show a striking ability to process and analyze speech as a particular type of auditory stimuli. From an early age, infants "engage in a detailed analysis of the distributional properties of sounds contained in the language they hear," which helps calibrate their speech perception abilities for their native language or languages (Tsao, Liu, & Kuhl, 2004, p. 1068).

At the most basic level, speech perception involves processing phonemic information, such as the four phonemes contained in the word *coffee* (/k/ /a/ /f/ /i/). Sometimes, analogies are made between how the brain processes a series of phonemes in a spoken word and how a reader reads a series of letters in a written word, as if speech perception involves the sequential one-on-one pro-cessing of individual speech sounds. This analogy is incorrect. When humans produce phonemes, the phonemes overlap with one another in a process called **coarticulation.** For instance, the initial /k/ in *coffee* and the initial /k/ in *coop* are produced differently because the initial /k/ in each word carries information about the subsequent vowels, which differ. The /k/ in *coffee* is influenced by the subsequent *ah* sound, whereas the /k/ in *coop* is influenced by the subsequent *oo* sound. As a result, the /k/ in *coop* is produced with rounded lips in anticipation of the *oo* sound. Coarticulation is the term that describes this "smearing," or overlapping, of phonemes in the production of strings of speech sounds. The articulators (lips, tongue, etc.) coarticulate speech sounds because doing so is much more efficient than producing just one sound at a time, and the speech-processing mechanisms of the brain have evolved to process the rapidly occurring and coarticulated speech sounds.

Communication

Communication is the process of sharing information among two or more persons, or, more specifically, "the transmission of thoughts or feelings from the mind of a speaker to the mind of a listener" (Borden et al., 1994, p. 174). For communication to occur, it must involve a sender (speaker) and a receiver (listener). Typically in communication, only one person is the sender, although this situation is not always the case, such as when a group of administrators prepares a written memo or when a trio sings a song. In addition, although communication may at times involve only one receiver, it can also involve numerous receivers, such as when a speaker gives a speech to an audience of thousands or an author writes a book that millions of people read.

Regardless of the number of senders and receivers, communication involves four basic processes: formulation, transmission, reception, and comprehension. The **sender** formulates and then transmits the information he or she would like to convey, and the **receiver** takes in and then comprehends the information. *Formulation* is the process of pulling together your thoughts or ideas for sharing with another person. *Transmission* is the process of conveying these ideas to another person, often by speaking but alternatively by signing, gesturing, or writ-ing. *Reception* is the process of receiving the information from another person, and *comprehension* is the process of making sense of the message.

Symbolic communication, also called **referential communication,** occurs when an individual communicates about a specific entity (an object or event), and the relationship between the entity and its referent (e.g., a word) is arbitrary (Leavens, Russell, & Hopkins, 2005). For instance, the 1-year-old who says "bottle" to request something to drink is communicating symbolically because the relationship be-tween the word *bottle* and its referent is arbitrary. Symbolic communication also "knows no limitations of space or time" (Bickerton, 1995, p. 15).

However, some communication is not symbolic and is thus constrained to a particular space and time. **Preintentional communication** is communication in which other people assume the relationship between a communicative behavior and its referent. For example, the purring of a cat and the crying of an infant both represent preintentional communication. The cat and the baby are communicating, but the actual referent or goal of the communication must be inferred by the communicative partner. The infant's cry could mean "I am really hungry" or "This blanket is too hot." Likewise, **intentional communication** is relatively more precise in its intent, but the relationship between the communicative behavior and its referent is not arbitrary. Rather, it relies on the shared spatial position among the sender, the recipient, and the referent (Leavens et al., 2005). This type of communication is also called **iconic communication** because of the transparent (or iconic) relationship between the message and its referent (Bickerton, 1995). For instance, when an infant points to a bottle or a chimpanzee gestures toward a banana, the act is intentional, iconic communication.

Whether communicating intentionally or symbolically, people share information for three basic purposes: to request ("May I have some cake?"), to reject ("I don't want this cake"), and to comment ("This cake is delicious"). Requesting, rejecting, and commenting need not use language, as any adult interacting with an 8-month-old infant can attest. Infants at this age can request, reject, and comment using an array of nonlinguistic yet intentional means, including crying, laughing, gesturing, smiling, and cooing. However, as infants develop as language users, they begin to use language and speech as a means to disseminate their needs and wants more precisely. By 1 year of age, toddlers use language for all three purposes, even if their vocabulary is not yet well developed ("Bottle?" "Bottle!" "Bottle.").

The combination of speaking and listening is a common mode of communication called **oral communication.** However, communication need not be spoken or heard. A person can reject by turning away, a baby can comment by smiling, and a dog can request by panting at the door. What is particularly unique about *human* communication, though, is the use of *language* and *speech* in the communication process. In much of this text, we emphasize the development and use of language as a tool for uniquely human, sophisticated communication.

Model of Communication

Figure 1.4 provides a model of communication that includes three essential components: (a) a sender to formulate and transmit a message, (b) a receiver to receive and comprehend the message, and (c) a shared symbolic means for communication. Figure 1.5 shows the roles of language, speech, and hearing in formulation, transmission, reception, and comprehension during communication.

In addition to these basic processes is another aspect of communication: *feedback* (see Figure 1.4). Feedback is information provided by the receiver to the sender. In effective communication, feedback is provided continually by the receiver, and the sender responds to this feedback to maintain the ongoing effectiveness of the communication process. The feedback system is what makes communication *active* and *dynamic*. It is active because both sender and receiver must be fully engaged. It is dynamic because the receiver is constantly sending feedback that the sender interprets and uses to modulate the flow of communication.

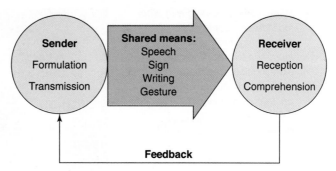

FIGURE 1.4
Model of communication.

Source: Justice, Laura M., *Communication Sciences and Disorders: An Introduction,* 1st Edition, © 2006.
Reprinted by Permission of Pearson Education, Inc., Upper Saddle River, NJ.

A receiver can provide feedback in numerous ways. **Linguistic feedback** includes speaking, such as saying "I totally agree," "I hear what you are saying," or "Wait; I don't get it." It also includes vocalizing, such as saying "mm-hmm" or "uh-oh." **Nonlinguistic feedback,** or **extralinguistic feedback,** refers to the use of eye contact, facial expression, posture, and proximity. This type of feedback may

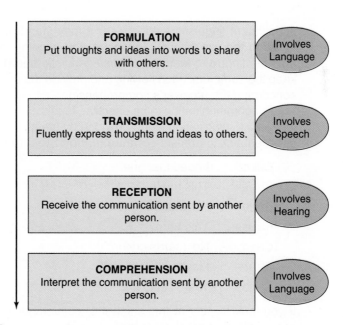

FIGURE 1.5
Roles of language, speech, and hearing in communication.

Source: Justice, Laura M., *Communication Sciences and Disorders: An Introduction,* 1st Edition, © 2006.
Reprinted by Permission of Pearson Education, Inc., Upper Saddle River, NJ.

When communicating with other individuals, people often supplement their speech and language with nonlinguistic, *or* extralinguistic, feedback*, such as eye contact, facial expression, posture, and proximity.*

(*Photo Source:* Charles Gupton/ Corbis/Bettmann.)

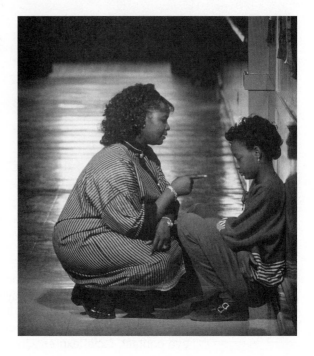

supplement linguistic feedback, or it may stand alone. **Paralinguistic feedback** refers to the use of pitch, loudness, and pausing, all of which are superimposed over the linguistic feedback. These linguistic and nonlinguistic forms of feedback keep the communication flowing and provide the speaker with valuable information concerning the receiver's comprehension.

For communication to be effective, feedback from the receiver is just as important as the information being provided by the sender. The sender and the receiver use feedback to prevent **communication breakdowns** from occurring:

CHILD: I need that one.

FATHER: This one?

CHILD: No, that one.

FATHER: This here?

CHILD: No. (*starts crying*)

FATHER: Maybe it's this one?

CHILD: Yeah, I said that one.

If you look closely at this snippet of conversation, you should be able to find a communication breakdown that seems to occur because of inadequacies of both the sender and the receiver. The child appears not to have the language abilities to produce sufficiently explicit information about what he or she desires, and the father does not provide adequate feedback to clarify the lack of specificity.

TABLE 1.1
Seven purposes of communication

Purpose	Description	Example
Instrumental	Used to ask for something	"Will you pass me the butter, please?"
Regulatory	Used to give directions and to direct others	"Go ahead and sit down over there."
Interactional	Used to interact and converse with others in a social way	"How was the game last night?"
Personal	Used to express a state of mind or feelings about something	"There is no way I passed that test!"
Heuristic	Used to find out information and to inquire	"Do you know how much this book is?"
Imaginative	Used to tell stories and to role-play	"OK, let's practice what you're going to say when you call her."
Informative	Used to provide an organized description of an event or object	"So, we got to the hotel, and they had no record of our reservation. Then, they tell me they have no rooms left at all. . . ."

Source: Based on *Learning How to Mean: Explorations in the Development of Language Development,* by M. A. Halliday, 1975, London: Arnold; and "Presentation of Communication Evaluation Information," by C. Simon and C. L. Holway, in *Communication Skills and Classroom Success* (pp. 151–199), edited by C. Simon, 1991, Eau Claire, WI: Thinking Publications.

Eventually the father repairs the breakdown, which is called a **conversational repair.** Minor communication breakdowns occur in every conversation but are easily recognized and repaired if the sender is closely monitoring the receiver's feedback and the receiver is providing ongoing feedback. More serious communication breakdowns occur when receivers do not provide appropriate types or amounts of feedback or when senders do not attend to the feedback.

Purpose of Communication

The primary purpose for communication is to provide and solicit information. Humans communicate to provide information about their feelings and to obtain information from other people. Individuals communicate to share information about trivial and exciting events and to describe their needs and desires. Table 1.1 provides one system used to differentiate the major purposes of communication. All these purposes are vitally important to developing and maintaining social relationships with other people and for meeting personal basic needs and desires.

WHAT ARE THE MAJOR DOMAINS OF LANGUAGE?

Content, Form, and Use

Language is a single dimension of human behavior that consists of three interrelated domains: content, form, and use (Lahey, 1988). Consider the following utterances by 3-year-old Adelaide: "I beating you up the stairs." "I wonned!" "I am so fast." These utterances provide an array of analytical possibilities for characterizing Adelaide's language. First, you can consider their *content*. **Content** refers to the meaning of language—the words used and the meaning behind them. We humans convey content through our vocabulary system, or **lexicon,** as we select and organize words to express our ideas or to understand what other individuals are saying. You can consider the content of Adelaide's utterances in a variety of ways: She uses 12 words; of these, she repeats 1 word (*I*) several times, for a total of 10 different words. The words *beating, wonned,* and *fast* create lexical ties across the utterances because they conceptually work together to denote that a race of some type is occurring. The words she uses and the concepts she expresses through these words are fairly concrete. She does not use figurative or idiomatic words, nor does she use abstract language. The focus is clearly on the here and now. Language that focuses on the immediate context is **contextualized,** and typically the content of highly contextualized language is concrete and supported by cues within the environment (e.g., gestures, facial expressions). Thus, in this particular example, the context in which Adelaide speaks provides important information that supplements the content of the language. In contrast, imagine that Adelaide was telling the story of this race over the telephone to her grandmother. She would need to be much more precise to convey the content. When we share language with little reliance on the context for conveying content, it is **decontextualized.**

Second, you can consider the *form* of Adelaide's utterances. **Form** is how words, sentences, and sounds are organized and arranged to convey content. When you consider form, you examine such things as sentence structure, clause and phrase usage, parts of speech, verb and noun structures, word prefixes and suffixes, and the organization of sounds into words. For instance, in examining the form of Adelaide's utterances, note that she uses three simple sentences, the first of which contains a prepositional phrase (*up the stairs*). She uses various parts of speech, including nouns (*stairs*), pronouns (*I*), articles (*the*), prepositions (*up*), verbs (*running*), and adverbs (*so*). Adelaide also uses a number of speech sounds, including a variety of vocalic sounds (i.e., vowels) and several consonantal sounds (i.e., consonants; e.g., /b/, /w/, /f/).

DISCUSSION POINT

In the example of Adelaide's language, she said the word *wonned.* What are some possible explanations for this error?

In considering form, you must take a closer look at how sentences are structured. Examination of Adelaide's sentence structures reveals that each sentence contains a subject, which in all cases is the personal pronoun *I*. Each sentence also contains a predicate, or verb, structure. In her three short utterances, she uses three different verb structures. In the first sentence, *I beating you up the stairs,* she uses the transitive verb *beating,* which requires an object (i.e., *you*). Note that while she has inflected the verb *beat* with the present progressive marker *-ing* to show that the actions are occurring continuously at the present, she has also omitted the auxiliary verb *am.* In the second sentence, Adelaide uses the verb *wonned.* In this case, she produced the irregular past tense form of *win* but added the past tense marker *-ed.* This verb is an intransitive verb, which does not require an object, and none is provided. In the third sentence, the verb structure comprises a *be* verb (*am*) that serves as the main verb in the sentence and requires a subject complement (*so fast*).

Third, you can consider the *use* of language. **Use** pertains to how people draw on language functionally to meet personal and social needs. When you examine this domain of language, you are asking about the intentions behind the utterances and how well the utterances achieve these intentions. Thus, you examine individual utterances to consider their intent. One possible scheme is Halliday's seven communication functions (see Table 1.1). For the analysis of Adelaide's language use, you can conclude that the intentions behind her utterances are primarily interactional (language used to interact socially) and personal (language used to express a state of mind).

Examination of use also involves consideration of how well language achieves these intentions—for example, whether an individual can maintain a topic through several turns in a conversation, can regulate the participation of other people (e.g., through eye contact, facial expressions, pausing), and can adjust language given the particular demands of the communicative situation and the listener's needs. Because analysis of use requires understanding of the context in which language is occurring, fully considering use by looking at a written transcript of language is difficult. For example, you have no way to know from the transcript of Adelaide's utterances whether she is meeting the contextual needs of the situation and whether she is effectively regulating her language use to achieve her intentions.

Components of Content, Form, and Use

Content, form, and use thus compose a three-domain system used to represent and organize the major dimensions of language. A five-component system can provide a slightly more refined description of the components of each of the three domains. The five components are semantics, syntax, morphology, phonology, and pragmatics. The components of semantics and pragmatics are synonymous with the domains of content and use, respectively, and syntax, morphology, and phonology are three components of form. Following is a brief description of each component (these topics are considered in more depth in Chapter 3):

1.   Semantics (content) refers to the rules of language governing the meaning of individual words and word combinations. When people produce a given word (e.g., *cat*) or phrase (*black cat*), they express a certain meaning. Semantics thus involves consideration of the meaning of various words and phrases. For instance, you know that a *culprit* is someone who has done something wrong; the word *run* has many meanings, whereas the word *stapler* has only one meaning; the phrase *bent over backwards* has both a figurative and a literal meaning; and the words *papaya, banana,* and *kiwi* go together conceptually. If a person is asked to produce the first word that comes to mind when he or she is given the prompt "vehicle," the semantic relationship among words provokes the person to respond "car" (or, alternatively, "truck" or "tractor"). Knowledge of semantics tells you that something is wrong with the sentence *Colorless green ideas sleep furiously,* a sentence produced by the linguist Noam Chomsky to differentiate the meaning expressed by words (semantics) from the grammar used to organize them into a sentence (Pinker, 1994).

2. Syntax (form) refers to the rules of language governing the internal organization of sentences. Knowledge of the rules governing syntax allows readers to readily turn the simple statement *He did it* into the question *Did he do it?* and to embed one simple sentence (e.g., *Andre is angry*) in another (e.g., *Andre is not coming*) to produce a complex sentence (e.g., *Andre, who is angry, is not coming*). Syntax is what permits a child to produce a seemingly endless sentence by linking a series of simple sentences: *This is Thomas and he is so mad at Lady and Lady goes off the siding and here comes Percy and Thomas gets out of the way and Percy is coming so fast.* In short, whereas semantics provides the meaning to utterances, syntax provides the structure. Consideration of Chomsky's proposition that *Colorless green ideas sleep furiously* illustrates the difference between semantics and syntax, in which a sentence is devoid of meaning but conforms to sophisticated syntactic rules.

3. Morphology (form) pertains to the rules of language governing the internal organization of words. Previously, *morpheme* was defined as the smallest unit of language that carries meaning; many words contain two or more morphemes. Words are "morphed" (manipulated) in a variety of ways to change their meaning. For instance, prefixes can be added to words to change their meaning—for example, the addition of the morpheme *pre-* to words to create *preschool, predisposition, preview,* and *pretest.* Also, suffixes are used to add grammatical information to words (i.e., to indicate basic grammatical categories such as tense or plurality). These types of suffixes are called *grammatical morphemes.* Grammatical morphemes include the plural *-s* (*cat–cat<u>s</u>*), the possessive *'s* (*mom–mom'<u>s</u>*), the past tense *-ed* (*walk–walk<u>ed</u>*), and the present progressive *-ing* (*do–do<u>ing</u>*), to name a few. Morphology is an important linguistic tool that allows not only precision to be added to language (e.g., "Tamika walk" vs. "Tamika had walked") but also vocabulary to be expanded exponentially in that a relatively small core of words (base vocabulary) can be morphed into a much larger pool of word families (e.g., *school, schools, schooling, schooled, preschool*).

4. Phonology (form) refers to the rules of language governing the sounds used to make syllables and words. Every language has a relatively small number of meaningful sounds, or *phonemes.* **General American English** (GAE; also called *Standard American English*) has about 39 phonemes (give or take a few, depending on the dialect), as shown in Table 1.2. GAE relies on the combination of 15 vowels and 24 consonants to create about 100,000 words. Some languages use more phonemes; others use fewer.

Allophones are the subtle variations of phonemes that occur as a result of contextual influences on how phonemes are produced in different words. For instance, the two /p/ phonemes in *pop* are produced differently, given the position of each in the word. The initial /p/ is aspirated, meaning that it is produced with a small puff of air. In contrast, the final /p/ is unaspirated. (The final /p/ can be aspirated but typically is not.) The two /p/ sounds in *pop* are allophonic variations of a single phoneme, and many phonemes have several allophones. In addition, each language has rules governing how sounds are organized in words, called

TABLE 1.2

Vowels and consonants of General American English

Consonant symbol	Example	Consonant symbol	Example
b	_b_at	r	_r_ose
p	_p_at	s	_s_un
d	_d_ip	ʃ	_sh_ine
t	_t_ip	t	_t_oast
g	_g_ive	ʧ	_ch_urch
h	_h_ot	ɵ	_th_ink
j	_y_es	ð	_th_at
k	_c_at	v	_v_et
l	_l_ot	w	_w_ash
m	_m_ine	z	_z_ag
n	_n_ose	ʒ	trea_s_ure
ŋ	ri_ng_	ʤ	_j_ail

Vowel symbol	Example	Articulatory features
i	f_ee_t	high, front, unrounded
ɪ	f_i_t	high, front, unrounded
e	m_a_ke	mid, front, unrounded
ɛ	b_e_t	mid, front, unrounded
æ	c_a_t	low, front, unrounded
a	f_a_ther	low, front, unrounded
u	bl_ue_	high, back, rounded
ʊ	h_oo_f	high, back, rounded
ɔ	b_ou_ght	mid, back, rounded
o	g_o_	mid, back, rounded
a	b_o_x	low, back, unrounded
ʌ	b_u_g	mid, central, unrounded
ə	_a_round	mid, central, unrounded
ɝ	b_ir_d	mid, central, unrounded
ɚ	fath_er_	mid, central, unrounded

Source: Justice, Laura M., _Communication Sciences and Disorders: An Introduction,_ 1st Edition, © 2006. Adapted by permission of Pearson Education, Inc., Upper Saddle River, NJ.

phonotactics. For instance, in English the phoneme /g/ never follows /s/ or /l/ at the beginning or end of a syllable.

5. Pragmatics (use) pertains to the rules of language governing how language is used for social purposes. Pragmatics comprises the set of rules that govern three important aspects of the social use of language: (a) using language for different functions or intentions (communication intentions), (b) organizing language for discourse (conversation; Lahey, 1988), and (c) knowing what to say and when and how to say it (social conventions). In using language for social purposes, pragmatic rules govern linguistic, extralinguistic, and paralinguistic aspects of communication, such as word choice, turn taking, posture, gestures, facial expression, eye contact, proximity, pitch, loudness, and pauses.

WHAT ARE SOME REMARKABLE FEATURES OF LANGUAGE?

Language is one of the most extraordinary capacities of the human species, and extremely rapid language acquisition by young children is one of the most remarkable aspects of early development. Given the thousands of scientific studies exploring the extraordinariness of language, including how children go about learning the languages of their communities, you might assume that nothing is left to learn about language development. Such an assumption could not be further from the truth; in fact, experts contend that "the acquisition of a child's first language is one of the mysteries of human life" (Lieberman, 1991, p. 127).

Why is language such a mystery? In part, its mysteriousness relates to several "remarkable features of language" that work together to make it a particularly complicated area of study, albeit one that continues to capture the attention of numerous scholars around the world. In this section, we consider five of these remarkable features of language: acquisition rate, universality, species specificity, semanticity, and productivity.

Acquisition Rate

Faced with the task of explaining how children develop their remarkable skills with language, scholars have often noted that the sheer **acquisition rate** of language makes it difficult to study. For instance, consider the following interaction between a mother and her 30-month-old daughter:

TAJIKA:	Thomas the very useful engine is in the siding.
MOTHER:	He's in the what?
TAJIKA:	The siding. This is the siding.
MOTHER:	Oh, that's the siding?

This brief interaction shows the extraordinary capacity of young children to learn and use new words at a stunning rate. *Siding* is a part of a train track that runs off the main course. In this vignette, Tajika has placed her miniature Thomas the Tank Engine on the siding. Her mother did not know the meaning of *siding,* but Tajika clearly did.

Erica Hoff, a scientist who studies early language development, stated that language development "reveals the genius in all children. . . . [I]t is remarkable that 3-year-olds who can't tie their shoes or cross the street alone have vocabularies of thousands of words and can produce sentences with relative clauses" (Hoff-Ginsberg, 1997, p. 3). Her observation points out that although at birth children understand and use no words, within a year they begin to understand and use several words, and by about 24 months they have a vocabulary of several hundred words and are combining them into short sentences. Whereas the 1-year-old can say only "mama" to request something to drink, the 3-year-old can say, "Mom, Daddy said I could have some chocolate milk and I think I'll have it in the pink sippie cup."

DISCUSSION POINT

In this section, we consider the concept of critical period as it applies to language deveopment. What are some other areas of development in which the concept of critical period applies?

What should be evident is that (a) children develop language at a remarkably rapid rate, and (b) each child apparently has a "powerful array of learning procedures at his or her disposal" (Hoff, 2004, p. 923). Also evident is that the first 5–7 years of life are a **critical period** (sometimes referred to as a *sensitive period*) for language development, meaning that a window of opportunity exists during which language develops most rapidly and with the greatest ease. The critical period for language was demonstrated by one team of researchers who studied the English language ability of native Chinese- and Korean-speaking individuals who were between 3 and 39 years of age when they arrived in the United States (J. S. Johnson & Newport, 1989). The persons who learned English as a second language before age 7 years had the most sophisticated English language abilities, whereas those who learned English after age 17 had the least sophisticated abilities. The critical period in the human species for language development is similar to the critical periods seen in other species for acquisition of behaviors considered essential for survival. For instance, songbirds show a critical period for song learning, although considerable differences in the ways in which songbirds acquire songs occur among the more than 4,000 songbird species (e.g., some songbirds require early exposure to songs for song learning, whereas others can develop song in isolation; Brenowitz & Beecher, 2005). Because only one species of *Homo sapiens* exists, the critical period of language development applies to all children everywhere.

Universality

Language is ubiquitous among the communities of the world. Every human culture has one language, and sometimes many languages, and all are equally complex. The **universality** of language, as Steven Pinker wrote in *The Language Instinct* (1994), fills linguists with awe, and is the first reason to suspect that language is not just any cultural invention but the product of a special human instinct. . . . Cultural inventions vary widely in their sophistication from society to society. . . . [L]anguage, however, ruins this correlation. There are Stone Age societies, but there is no such thing as a Stone Age language (p. 26).

The universality concept as applied to language suggests that all persons around the world apply the same cognitive infrastructure to the task of learning language and that this cognitive infrastructure is particularly suited to the task of developing symbolic representations for objects and actions (Bickerton, 1995). Although world languages clearly vary in their syntactic organization (e.g., some languages do not have auxiliary verbs, whereas others do; see Tomasello, 2003), the cognitive infrastructure is the same for all languages. Therefore, the way in which children learn language and the time points at which they achieve certain milestones appear to be fairly invariant among global language communities.

Species Specificity

Language is strictly a human capacity. No other animals share this aptitude; thus human language shows **species specificity.** Although many nonhuman species can communicate, their communication abilities are wholly iconic (Bickerton, 1995). Remember, iconic communication systems are those for which a transparent relationship exists between *what* is being communicated and *how* it is being communicated. All nonhuman communication systems are more or less iconic, but little is iconic about human language.

In addition to being iconic, animal communication systems differ from human communication systems in their combinatorial properties (Bickerton, 1995). Human language provides a syntactic framework that permits the combination of ideas into larger propositions; in fact, humans can produce an endless array of novel constructions with the tool of syntax. As Bickerton explained, except for the cotton-top tamarin (which can combine a chirp and a squeak to signal alert and alarm), no other animal has a communication system that provides the means for combining symbols in the way that syntax allows humans to use language.

Semanticity

Human language allows people to represent events that are decontextualized, or removed from the present—to share what happened before this moment or what may happen after this moment. This concept is called **semanticity.** As mentioned previously, human language has no time or space boundaries because the relationship between a referent and the language used to describe it is completely arbitrary. For instance, the word *cup* has no relationship to that which it refers; the relationship is completely arbitrary. As such, a person can say the word *cup* without having a cup present, and other people will know to what the person is referring. Semanticity is the

Although many nonhuman species can communicate, their communication is iconic *in that a transparent relationship exists between what is being communicated and how it is being communicated.*

(*Photo Source:* © Francine Fleischer/ Corbis.)

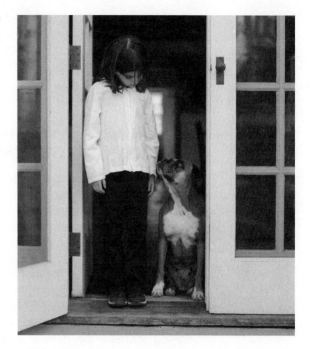

aspect of language that allows people to represent the world (Bickerton, 1995)—a remarkable capacity shared by no other species.

Productivity

Productivity describes the principle of combination—specifically, the combination of a small number of discrete units into seemingly infinite novel creations. Productivity is a phenomenon that applies to other human activities—such as mathematics and music—as well as to language. With a relatively small set of rules governing language, humans can produce an endless number of ideas and new constructions. For instance, humans use only a small set of sounds (speakers of GAE use about 39 or so) and can combine these small units— according to a set of rules that are known intuitively (e.g., /g/ cannot follow /l/ in English)—into an infinite number of words. Likewise, humans use a relatively small number of words and with these can create an infinite variety of new sentences, most of which no one has ever heard. Because of the remarkable principle of productivity, you could, right now, produce a sentence that no other person has ever uttered.

The principle of productivity is inherent to language in its earliest stages of acquisition: Children who are 18 months old and have about 50 words in their vocabulary can combine and recombine this small set of words to produce sentences that neither they nor others have ever heard. This feature of language is unique to humans because the units of nonhuman communication systems cannot be recombined to make new meanings. For instance, night monkeys have 16 communication units. These units cannot be recombined to make more than 16 possible ways to communicate because the principle of productivity does not apply (Bickerton, 1995).

WHAT ARE LANGUAGE DIFFERENCES AND LANGUAGE DISORDERS?

For most children, language development follows a fairly invariant path. Children around the world typically begin to communicate by using words at about the same time (12 months), and they often begin to combine words to form two-word combinations (e.g., *daddy shoe, mommy go*) by around 18 months. From that point, they accrue thousands of words in their productive vocabulary by age 5 years and achieve an adultlike grammar well before puberty. However, although this general developmental trajectory characterizes that of most children, it does not describe them all. In fact, a comparison of any two children of about the same age will reveal considerable differences in the content, form, and use of their language. Such differences are influenced by the language being learned, by gender and temperament, and by the language-learning environment. In addition, some children show mild to severe disorders in language acquisition as a result of innate genetic predispositions, developmental disability, or injury or illness. In Chapters 9 and 10, we provide a more in-depth examination of these topics.

Language Differences

Language difference is a general term used to describe the variability among language users. Two children of exactly the same age will likely show a range of differences if their language abilities are compared. For example, they may differ in the number of words they understand, the length of their sentences, the types of words they use, and the way they share language with other people during conversation. Sometimes, the differences between two individuals are subtle. However, in other instances the differences may be more significant and may even compromise communication. For instance, consider the following descriptions of young children in the United States:

- Lamika, a 5-year-old girl, speaks a dialect of African American Vernacular English. She attends a day care center in which all the other children and her teachers speak GAE.

- Angela, a 3-year-old child with hearing loss, communicates by using Signed Exact English. She attends a special preschool for children with hearing loss, and most of her peers sign with American Sign Language.

- Jack, a 2-year-old child, is simultaneously learning Spanish and English. His family speaks both languages at home. In his preschool, which includes mostly monolingual Spanish-speaking children, he speaks primarily Spanish but sometimes uses the grammar of English.

- Mimi, a 3-year-old child adopted from China at age 18 months, uses fewer vocabulary words and produces shorter sentences than those used by other children in her day care.

These examples reveal how children (as well as adults) who live in culturally and linguistically diverse communities show variability in their language. In this section, we discuss several major influences on language development that help explain differences among individuals—specifically, dialect, bilingualism, gender, genetic predisposition, and language-learning environment.

Dialect

DISCUSSION POINT

What English dialect do you speak? What dialects do your friends speak? To what extent do these differences affect your communication with one another?

Dialects are the natural variations of a language that evolve within specific cultural or geographic boundaries. These variations affect form, content, and use. Given the many speakers of English around the world, the fact that numerous English dialects exist is not surprising. In the United States, common dialects include Appalachian English, African American Vernacular English, and Spanish-Influenced English. Each of these dialects may show subtle to more significant variations in form, content, and use from those of the GAE dialect. This finding is also true of the dialects of English spoken around the world, including those of Great Britain, Australia, and New Zealand.

Every language includes a range of dialectal variations, and the number of dialects for a given language increases when users of a language are spread across a large geographic region, when significant geographic barriers isolate one community from other communities, or when social barriers are present within a language community. Multicultural Focus: *African American Vernacular English* provides an in-depth look at the African American Vernacular English dialect.

Bilingualism

Although many children in the United States learn a single language (**monolingualism**), others acquire two or more languages (**bilingualism**). Bilingualism is the norm in many countries, such as Belgium, where many citizens speak both French and Dutch. Children raised bilingually often show language differences not seen in children who are raised monolingually, such as interchanges between the syntax and the vocabulary of the two languages they are learning. This phenomenon is referred to as **code switching** (Muñoz, Gillam, Peña, & Gulley-Faehnle, 2003). For instance, a child who is bilingual in Spanish and English may produce a sentence in Spanish that includes an English phrase, or an English sentence that reflects Spanish syntax.

Children who learn multiple languages can do so simultaneously or sequentially. With *simultaneous bilingualism,* children acquire their two languages concurrently. With *sequential bilingualism,* children develop one language initially, then acquire a second language later. Sequential bilingualism is relatively common for Hispanic children in the United States who learn Spanish at home but then develop English in preschool or elementary school. The English skills of a sequential

MULTICULTURAL FOCUS

African American Vernacular English

The English language has many dialects. The term dialect refers to the natural variations in form, content, and use within a single language. In the United States, African American Vernacular English (AAVE) is a prominent dialect used not only by some African American individuals but also by persons of various ethnicities and races, including Hispanic and non-Hispanic Caucasians (Poplack, 1978). An individual's use of AAVE is typically influenced by the amount of contact that person has with AAVE-speaking peers rather than his or her ethnic or racial heritage, a point that holds true for any English dialect. For instance, in one study of Puerto Rican sixth graders in Philadelphia, Poplack found that Puerto Rican boys were more likely to speak AAVE than other dialects in their community, including General American English (GAE) and Puerto Rican Spanish.

Sociolinguists, who study variability in languages as a function of social influences, have provided rich descriptions of some of the most prominent features of AAVE that distinguish it from GAE (e.g., W. Labov, 1972; Washington & Craig, 1994). Some features of AAVE involve the form of language, including phonology (e.g., reduction of final consonant clusters, such as /mos/ in AAVE vs. /most/ in GAE) and grammar (e.g., omission of the copula verb, such as "that hers" in AAVE vs. "that is hers" in GAE; Charity, Scarborough, & Griffin, 2004). Additional features of AAVE involve the content and use of language.

As with all other English dialects, AAVE is a systematic, rule-governed system with its own rules and conventions that influence form, content, and use. In every way, AAVE is equivalent in its complexity to any other English dialect (Goldstein & Iglesias, 2004). This point is important because some scholars in the past have suggested that AAVE is an "impoverished" version of English (e.g., Bereiter, 1966), a perspective that shows a clear lack of understanding of dialectal variations, including the fact that all languages (and their dialects) are equivalent in complexity. Still, in many language communities around the world, some dialects are valued more than others and carry greater prestige or value.

In the United States, some experts contend that speakers of AAVE face risks in educational achievement because their dialect differs from that used most commonly in schools, sometimes called *School English (SE;* Charity et al., 2004). One reason for this risk may be a mismatch between the AAVE speaker's representation of linguistic features and the features prominent in the dialect of his or her teachers, which often (but not always) is GAE (Charity et al., 2004). Another possibility is that some teachers, particularly those who speak the GAE dialect, may have a negative bias toward pupils who speak AAVE, holding lower expectations and providing less effective instruction to these pupils. However, because some research shows that the level of familiarity with SE among pupils who speak AAVE is associated positively with their reading achievement (Charity et al., 2004), practitioners must improve their understanding of how dialectal variations both aid and circumvent children's success in school.

Spanish–English bilingual in the early stages of development will differ from those of a child who learned both Spanish and English from birth, and both children may show some differences in language form, content, and use from those of monolingual English-speaking children.

DISCUSSION POINT

Fewer children are raised bilingually in the United States than in a number of other countries. Why?

Although the language a child learns has clear influences on his or her language development—for instance, the stories produced by Chinese-speaking children differ in their organizational structure from those of English-speaking children (Wang & Leichtman, 2000)—all languages are approximately equal in complexity (Bickerton, 1995). In other words, although some differences can be seen among children as a function of the language (or languages) they are learning, all languages use the same infrastructure of the human brain and thus are similar in complexity (Bickerton, 1995).

Gender

One relatively well-known fact is that girls have an advantage over boys in language development. Girls usually begin talking earlier than boys do (Karmiloff & Karmiloff-Smith, 2001) and develop their vocabulary at a faster rate than boys do in the second year of life (J. Huttenlocher, Haight, Bryk, Seltzer, & Lyons, 1991). Also, boys are more likely to have significant difficulties with language development, or **language impairment;** in fact, prevalence estimates show a ratio of about 2 or 3 boys to 1 girl (P. S. Dale, Price, Bishop, & Plomin, 2003; Spinath, Price, Dale, & Plomin, 2004). Despite these apparent differences between the genders, Kovas and colleagues (2005) pointed out that **gender differences** in language development are relatively minor, particularly as children move beyond toddlerhood into the preschool years.

Why such gender differences in language development occur is unclear. Experts point to the possibility of both biological and environmental influences (Kovas et al., 2005). For example, parents may talk more often to girls than to boys, which would help speed language development. Alternatively, hormonal factors may contribute to these differences.

Genetic Predisposition

Any preschool teacher is well aware that young children of about the same age show incredible variability in their language development. Some of this variability relates to genetic predisposition. As a complex human trait, language ability is unlikely to reside on a single gene. However, evidence points to the influence of different alleles from a set of genes on all aspects of language development, including syntax, vocabulary, and phonology (Stromswold, 2001). **Twin studies** are one method researchers use to estimate the contribution of genetics to language development, as well as the heritability of language disorders (see Research Paradigms: *Twin Studies*). In twin studies, researchers compare the language abilities of identical (*monozygotic,* or *MZ*) and fraternal (*dizygotic,* or *DZ*) twins; MZ twins are genetically identical, whereas DZ twins share 50% of their genetic material. Twin studies allow researchers to identify the exact contributions of genetic and environmental influences to language development.

RESEARCH PARADIGMS

Twin Studies

Both genetic and environmental influences play significant roles in language development. However, identifying the exact contributions of genetic influences relative to environmental influences can be difficult. One way to estimate the unique influences of genetics versus environment is *twin studies,* or the *twin method* (Kovas et al., 2005). Monozygotic (MZ) twins share 100% of their genetic material, whereas dizygotic (DZ) twins share 50%. When twins—MZ or DZ—grow up in the same household, they are assumed to share 100% of their environmental influences, both prenatally (in the womb) and postnatally (in the home environment; Kovas et al., 2005). Researchers interested in estimating the influence of genetic versus environmental influences on language development collect measures of language from sets of twins, often repeatedly across time. These researchers use a number of sophisticated statistical techniques to determine the genetic heritability of certain language skills by comparing MZ and DZ twins, and they also can isolate environmental influences on language by carefully controlling the amount of variability in language skill that can be attributed to genetic influences.

One of the largest twin studies to date is the Twins Early Development Study (TEDS), conducted in the United Kingdom and supported financially by the UK Medical Research Council (Trouton, Spinath, & Plomin, 2002). This study involved 6,963 sets of twins; 2,351 were MZ twins, 2,322 were same-gender DZ twins, and 2,290 were opposite-gender DZ twins. All the twins were born in the United Kingdom between 1994 and 1996, and their language development was studied at ages 2, 3, and 4 years by using parent questionnaires. Twins born with severe medical or genetic problems or perinatal complications were not included in the sample, nor were twins whose zygoticity could not be determined and those whose parents did not speak English at home (Spinath et al., 2004). Various studies have been conducted by using the data from these twins to examine not only genetic and environmental influences on language development, but also to compare language development for boys versus girls and to estimate the heritability of language impairment. As a result of TEDS, researchers will be able to answer numerous questions in the next decade by using data from these nearly 14,000 children.

How much of human language ability is inherited? The results of one study involving 787 pairs of twins revealed that about 16% of the variability in language ability in 4-year-old children could be attributed to heritability (Kovas et al., 2005). However, language disorders among twins seem to be more strongly influenced by genetic factors than do language disorders among children in the typical population; in fact, about 49% of variability in language ability can be attributed to heritability (Spinath et al., 2004). If one MZ twin has a language impairment, the other twin has about an 85% likelihood of also having the impairment.

Language-Learning Environment

The language-learning environment in which children are reared exerts considerable influence on their language development. Although children bring biologically endowed abilities and propensities to the language-learning task, the neural architecture that supports language acquisition is an "open genetic program" (Cartwright, 2000, p. 195). This term means that the neural architecture is calibrated on the basis of input from the environment, or the "actual evidence" children receive from the environment, concerning the form, content, and use of the language or languages to which they are exposed (Cartwright, 2000). In short, everything the child experiences in his or her environment will help calibrate his or her language-learning apparatus.

DISCUSSION POINT

Hart and Risley's work on language input in the home environment showed differences in the amount of words heard by children in middle-class homes relative to those heard by children in lower class homes. Explain why such differences exist.

The environmental aspects that seem to figure most prominently in the young child's language development are the quantity and quality of language experienced. *Quantity* refers to the sheer amount of language a child experiences. In a classic study by Hart and Risley (1995), the volume of words children heard in their homes was shown to map directly to the size of the children's vocabularies: Children who heard relatively few words had relatively sparse vocabularies, whereas children who heard an abundance of words had large vocabularies.

As important as quantity of experience is to language development, so too is the quality of the child's language-learning experiences. *Quality* refers to the characteristics of the language spoken in the child's caregiving environment: the types of words (e.g., nouns, verbs, adverbs), the construction of sentences (e.g., simple, complex, compound), the intention of sentences (e.g., directives, declaratives, interrogatives), and the organization and specificity of stories (e.g., emotional expression, situational details). Children whose language-learning experiences include exposure to an array of complex sentence forms (e.g., sentences with subordinate clauses, such as *That boy who hit me is not my friend*) in addition to simple sentence forms (e.g., *That boy is not my friend*) will use more complex sentence forms than those used by children not exposed to such syntax (J. Huttenlocher, Vasilyeva, Cymerman, & Levine, 2002). Therefore, the experiences children have with language in their prominent caregiving environments (home, preschool, etc.) explain a considerable amount of the variability seen in children's language development (e.g., Rush, 1999).

Studies of infants reared in mainstream North American communities have revealed one particularly important aspect of the language-learning environment: caregiver **responsiveness.** This term refers to the promptness, contingency, and appropriateness of caregiver responses to children's bids for communication through words or other means (Tamis-LeMonda, Bornstein, & Baumwell, 2001). Experts contend that responsiveness provides a significant aid to children's language development because it reflects the child's current topic of interest and provides sensitive input that promotes semantic and syntactic learning. Higher degrees of caregiver responsiveness during infancy and early toddlerhood are associated with accelerated rates of language development in children: For instance, the results of one study showed that toddlers of highly responsive mothers achieved the 50-word milestone, on average, at age 15 months, whereas children of less responsive mothers were more likely to achieve this milestone at about age 21 months (Tamis-LeMonda et al., 2001). The contribution of caregivers' responsive and sensitive language input to children's language development indicates that quality of language input is just as important as quantity. See Theory to Practice: *Children Who Are Linguistically Reticent in the Classroom* for a description of how the relation between temperament and language has influenced practice in the area of promoting linguistic interactions with children who are reticent.

Language Disorders

Like any complex human trait, the ability to develop language in a timely and effortless manner can be adversely influenced by heritable weaknesses in the language mechanism as well as by the presence of certain developmental disabilities and brain injuries. Children with language impairment show significant difficulties in the development of language, typically achieving language milestones more slowly than other children do and exhibiting long-standing difficulties with various aspects of language form, content, and use. Next, we provide a brief overview of childhood language impairment, a topic addressed in more detail in Chapter 10.

Heritable Language Impairment

Children with a **heritable language impairment** exhibit depressed language abilities, typically with no other concomitant impairment of intellect. Because of its specificity to the functioning of language, this condition is often called **specific language impairment** (SLI), and it affects about 7–10% of children (Beitchman et al., 1989; Tomblin et al., 1997). SLI is the most common type of communication impairment affecting children. It is the most frequent reason for administering early intervention and special education services to toddlers through fourth graders.

Evidence suggests that SLI is a heritable condition, as indicated by both twin studies and family pedigree studies (Lai, Fisher, Hurst, Vargha-Khadem, & Monaco, 2001; Spinath et al., 2004). The results of twin studies reveal a strong likelihood for an MZ twin to have SLI if his or her twin is affected. Family pedigree studies show a strong likelihood for a child to have SLI if a parent is affected.

Developmental Disability

Language impairment often co-occurs with certain developmental disabilities. In such cases, language impairment is considered a secondary disorder because it results secondary to a primary cause. Common causes of a secondary language impairment include intellectual disability and autism spectrum disorder. Intellectual disability is a "condition of arrested or incomplete development of the mind, which

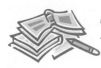

THEORY TO PRACTICE

Children Who Are Linguistically Reticent in the Classroom

The frequency with which children use language as a tool to communicate with other people varies substantially among individual children. To some extent, frequency relates to a child's facility with his or her language, but it also relates to temperament. *Temperament* describes an individual's "innate way of approaching and experiencing the world" (Kristal, 2005, p. 5), and it is a theoretical construct of human behavior that helps researchers understand why some children are bold and energetic, others are sensitive and timid, and some are inflexible (Kristal, 2005). Given that language development requires a child to experience input from the environment to "calibrate" his or her language-learning mechanisms, a reasonable conclusion is that a child's temperament might influence the amount of language input he or she experiences. For instance, the child who is bold may solicit more language from parents and teachers, whereas the child who is reticent and shy may solicit less language.

Theoretical perspectives on the potential interaction of language development and temperament suggest that an *interaction* occurs between these two constructs, or that they influence one another. The results of studies on the possible interaction of language and temperament provide support for this theory. For example, Evans (1996) found that 18 kindergartners who were characterized by teachers as very reticent (e.g., rarely asking for assistance when it is needed, seldom participating in class discussions) performed poorer than their more talkative peers did on a variety of measures of language ability in first grade. What remains unclear is whether some children are less talkative because they have less developed language skills or whether children with less developed language skills are less talkative.

Theory and research on the possibility of a temperament–language interaction have important implications for instruction in the preschool and kindergarten classroom, in which several important goals include fostering children's language skills, promoting socialization among children, and promoting children's ability to use language for a variety of purposes. Teachers may have difficulty helping children who are verbally reticent achieve these goals. One approach that has been tested for increasing children's language use and complexity in the preschool classroom is training teachers to use interaction-promoting responses (Girolametto, Weitzman, & Greenberg, 2003). Examples of interaction-promoting responses include (a) using a variety of questions, (b) inviting children to take turns, and (c) scanning the classroom and inviting uninvolved children to participate. Evidence shows that when teachers use these and other language-promoting techniques in the preschool classroom, the children talk more and use a more complex vocabulary and grammar. Although the effects of these techniques have not been determined specifically for children who are verbally reticent, they provide a promising way to translate theory and research on the temperament–language interaction to inform practice.

is especially characterized by impairment of skills manifested during the developmental period" (American Association on Mental Retardation [AAMR], 2002, p. 103). For intellectual disability to be diagnosed, an individual must also exhibit limitations in adaptive behavior and the activities of daily living, such as difficulties in conceptual skills (communication, functional academics, self-direction, health and safety), social skills (social relationships, leisure), or practical skills (self-care, home living, community participation, work; AAMR, 2002). One of the most common causes of intellectual disability is Down syndrome, which is due to a chromosomal anomaly during the initial stages of fetal development. Whether intellectual disability occurs because of Down syndrome or other causes, it is often accompanied by significant language impairment.

Another type of secondary language impairment is *autism spectrum disorder* (ASD). *ASD* is an umbrella term describing a variety of developmental conditions characterized by significant difficulties in social relationships and communication, by repetitive behaviors, and by overly restricted interests (Lord & Risi, 2000). The autism spectrum includes four types of disabilities: autism, childhood disintegrative disorder, Asperger's syndrome, and pervasive developmental disorder—not otherwise specified (PDD-NOS). These four conditions together affect about 1 in 500 children (Yeargin-Allsopp et al., 2003). Children with any one of the spectrum disorders usually exhibit a mild to profound secondary language impairment, and some children with autism never develop a productive use of language.

Brain Injury

Language impairment can also occur as a function of damage or injury to the mechanisms of the brain involved with language functions. Brain injuries can occur in utero (before birth) and perinatally (during the birthing process), but they can also occur after birth; these injuries are called **acquired brain injuries.** Acquired brain injuries are the leading cause of death and disability among young children (U.S. Department of Health and Human Services, 1999). Brain damage resulting from physical trauma, particularly blunt trauma to the head, is referred to as **traumatic brain injury,** or TBI. Causes of TBI in children include abuse (e.g., shaken baby syndrome), intentional harm (e.g., being hit or shot in the head), accidental poisoning through ingestion of toxic substances (e.g., prescription medications, pesticides), car accidents, and falling. Injuries may be *diffuse,* affecting large areas of the brain, or they may be *focal,* affecting only one specific brain region. The frontal and temporal lobes of the brain, which house the centers for most executive functions (e.g., reasoning, planning, hypothesizing) and language functions, are often damaged in head injuries (National Institute on Deafness and Other Communication Disorders, 2003).

Language impairment resulting from brain injury is influenced by the severity of the injury, the site of damage, and the characteristics of the child before the injury occurred (S. B. Chapman, 1997). Compared with children with less serious injuries, children with more severe injuries have less chance of a full language recovery. Contrary to popular thought, the brain of the young child is not necessarily better able to withstand and heal from injury than the brain of the older child:

Infants, toddlers, and preschoolers show long-lasting cognitive and language impairments following TBI (Aram, 1988). One possible reason for this misperception is that some young children may have a delayed onset of impairment; problems sustained during a brain injury may not be evident until years later, when damaged areas of the brain are applied to certain skills and activities (Goodman & Yude, 1996).

SUMMARY

Language is the socially shared and rule-governed code of arbitrary symbols that humans use as a representational code for thought and communication. The human brain uses language as a representational tool to store information and to carry out many cognitive processes, such as reasoning, hypothesizing, and planning. As a communication tool, language provides a productive and efficient means for sharing information with other people. Some experts consider the human capacity for language to reside in a particular module of the brain; other researchers contend that a more general neural network serves language processes.

Language, speech, hearing, and communication are different albeit interrelated processes. Speech is the voluntary neuromuscular behavior that allows humans to express language and is essential for spoken communication. Hearing is the perception of sound, which includes both general auditory perception and speech perception. Speech perception involves specialized processors in the brain that have evolved specifically to respond to human speech and language. Communication is the act of sharing information among two or more people. Although communication need not involve speech, language, and hearing, the capacity for humans to use these processes to share information makes human communication the most sophisticated among all species.

Language comprises three major domains: content, form, and use. *Content* is the meaning of language, including the specific words people use and the concepts represented by words and groups of words. *Form* is how words, sentences, and sounds are organized and arranged to convey content. Form includes phonology (rules governing the sounds used to make syllables and words), syntax (rules governing the internal organization of sentences), and morphology (rules governing the internal organization of words and syllables). *Use* describes the functions served by language, or how people draw on language functionally to meet personal and social needs.

Five remarkable features of language make it particularly fascinating to both researchers and practitioners. First is the acquisition rate of language; young children exhibit a striking capacity for developing language rapidly and efficiently. Second is the universality of language. Language is ubiquitous among world communities, and every human culture has one or more languages that its members share. The third feature is species specificity. Language is a uniquely human capacity; no other animal species shares this aptitude. The fourth feature is semanticity. Human language allows people to represent events that are decontextualized, or removed from the present, including not only real events of the past or future, but also events and concepts that are wholly imaginary and abstract. The fifth feature is productivity—or the principle of combination—which is how the rule-governed code of language provides its users with a generative code by which they can combine a small number of discrete units (e.g., phonemes, morphemes) into seemingly infinite novel creations.

Comparison of the language achievements of any two persons, whether children or adults, will reveal considerable individual differences in the content, form, and use of language. *Language differences* and *language disorders* are terms that describe this variability in language achievements among individuals. Language differences occur because of the natural variability in language achievement that results from different dialects, bilingualism, gender differences, genetic predisposition, and varied language-learning environments. A language disorder occurs when an individual shows significant difficulties in language achievement; such disorders result from heritable language impairment, developmental disability, and brain injury.

KEY TERMS

acoustics, p. 13
acquired brain injuries, p. 36
acquisition rate, p. 24
agrammaticism, p. 7
allophones, p. 22
articulation, p. 8
audition, p. 13
auditory perception, p. 14
bilingualism, p. 29
coarticulation, p. 15
code switching, p. 29
communication, p. 8
communication breakdowns, p. 18
content, p. 20
contextualized, p. 20
conversational repair, p. 19
critical period, p. 25
decontextualized, p. 20
dialects, p. 29
domain specific, p. 7
extralinguistic feedback, p. 17
feedback, p. 12
form, p. 20
frequency, p. 13
gender differences, p. 31
General American English, p. 22
hearing, p. 8

heritable language impairment, p. 34
iconic communication, p. 16
inner language, p. 8
intensity, p. 13
intentional communication, p. 16
language, p. 4
language difference, p. 28
language impairment, p. 31
lexicon, p. 20
linguistic feedback, p. 17
model, p. 9
modularity, p. 7
monolingualism, p. 29
morphemes, p. 5
morphology, p. 22
nonlinguistic feedback, p. 17
oral communication, p. 16
paralinguistic feedback, p. 18
phonation, p. 8
phoneme, p. 10
phonology, p. 22
phonotactics, p. 24
pragmatics, p. 24
preintentional communication, p. 15
productivity, p. 27
receiver, p. 15
referent, p. 5

referential communication, p. 15
resonation, p. 8
respiration, p. 8
responsiveness, p. 33
semanticity, p. 26
semantics, p. 21
sender, p. 15
species specificity, p. 26
specific language impairment, p. 34

speech, p. 8
speech perception, p. 14
symbolic communication, p. 15
syntax, p. 22
traumatic brain injury, p. 36
twin studies, p. 31
universality, p. 25
use, p. 21
written language, p. 8

For online resources related to chapter content, including audio samples, valuable Web sites, suggested readings, and self-quizzes, please go to the Companion Website at http://www.prenhall.com/pence

2

The Science and Theory of Language Development

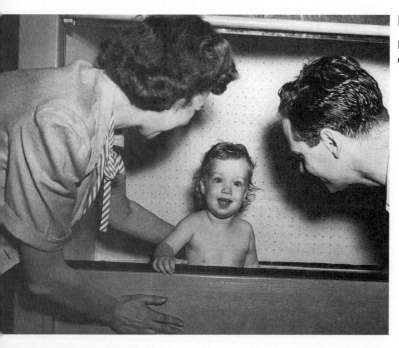

FOCUS QUESTIONS

In this chapter, we answer the following four questions:

1. Who studies language development and why?
2. What are some major approaches to studying language development?
3. What are some major language development theories?
4. How do language development theories influence practice?

In this chapter, we introduce the theory and science of language development. **Theory** refers to descriptive statements that provide "stable explanations" for a given phenomenon (Shavelson & Towne, 2002, p. 3). In essence, a theory is a claim or hypothesis that is repeatedly tested with an array of scientific methods; when the accumulated evidence consistently supports a given theory throughout time, it becomes part of the knowledge base in a particular discipline. In the area of language development, theories provide explanations for how and why children develop their capacity for language across the different domains. For example, one language development theory discussed subsequently in this chapter is that children's environments influence their language achievements.

Theory and science complement each other in intricate ways. Science is the process of generating and testing theories and can be considered the "final court of appeal for the viability of a scientific hypothesis or conjecture" (Shavelson & Towne, 2002, p. 3). Researchers who study language development use the scientific method to examine the adequacy of theories on the "how" and "why" of language development and to generate new theories. Ultimately, the goal of science is to generate "cumulative knowledge by building on, refining, and occasionally replacing, theoretical understanding" (Shavelson & Towne, 2002, p. 3). Therefore, theories provide the foundation for scientific studies, and the outcomes of scientific studies help experts refine and even replace their theories with time. All the concepts and understandings presented in this textbook are based on the accumulated theoretical and scientific knowledge of language development scholars.

WHO STUDIES LANGUAGE DEVELOPMENT AND WHY?

Language has fascinated people for thousands of years. The ancient philosophers Plato and Aristotle questioned the relationships among language, thought, and reality, whereas early linguists such as Dionysius studied the form and structure of language. In the 21st century, experts are still searching for answers to the same questions these ancient philosophers asked. Researchers continue to expand and refine the theoretical understanding of language development and to seek answers to practical questions about how to support children's early and later language achievements.

Scientists who conduct language development research are from many disciplines, including psychology, linguistics, psycholinguistics, anthropology, speech–language pathology, education, and sociology. Each discipline has a different major focus and different research questions with respect to language development (see Table 2.1 for some examples). However, because many disciplines include specializations in language, identifying specific areas of study that are governed by a given discipline is difficult. For example, researchers in each of the previously listed disciplines conduct studies on the relationship between parental language use and children's language growth. Scientists in all these disciplines, as well as others, are making important improvements to existing language development theories.

TABLE 2.1
Scientific disciplines, their foci, and their research questions about language development.

Discipline	Major focus	Sample research questions
(*Developmental*) *psychology*	Human mind and behavior and the changes that occur in humans as they age	What are the effects of experimentally manipulated language input on preschoolers' syntactic skills? (Vasilyeva, Huttenlocher, & Waterfall, 2006)
Linguistics	Aspects of human language, including phonetics, phonology, morphology, syntax, and semantics	To what extent does speech recognition software designed for children need to differ from speech recognition software designed for adults? (Strommen & Frome, 1993)
Psycholinguistics	Psychological and neurobiological factors that enable humans to acquire, use, and understand language	To what extent can electrophysiological studies reveal how infant phonetic representations develop into adult representations? (Phillips, 2001)
(*Linguistic*) *anthropology*	Relationship between language and culture; social use of language; language variation across time and space	To what extent is the information encoded in gesture influenced by how that information is expressed verbally? (Kita & Özyürek, 2003)
Speech–language pathology	Prevention, diagnosis, and treatment of speech and language disorders	To what extent does evidence support the use of commercially available tests of child language for identifying language impairment in children? (Spaulding, Plante, & Farinella, 2006)
Education	Aspects of teaching and learning	To what extent does a comprehensive language and literacy intervention promote language and literacy development in preschool children? (Wasik, Bond, & Hindman, 2006)
Sociology	Aspects of society such as cultural norms, expectations, and contexts	Which demographic factors contributed most to U.S. immigrants' transition to the English language at the beginning of the 20th century? (T. G. Labov, 1998)

DISCUSSION POINT

Why are you study-
ing language devel-
opment? How will
knowing about
childhood language
development help
you in your career?

People study language development for many reasons. Some do so to further basic understanding about language as a human phenomenon. This type of
research is called *theoretical research,* or **basic research:** It focuses primarily
on generating and refining the existing knowledge base. Other people do so to
address specific problems in society and to inform practices relevant to language
development. This type of research is called **applied research:** People typically
conduct applied research to test different approaches and practices that pertain
to real-world settings. Basic and applied research provide important complementary contributions to the study of language development, and many language
scientists conduct both types of research.

Basic Research

Many language development scholars conduct basic research, the outcomes of
which advance fundamental understanding of human learning and development.
In this type of research, experts develop, test, and refine theories about language
development. When the outcomes of basic research consistently confirm a theory,
the theory becomes an accepted explanatory principle—akin to knowledge.

Scientists who conduct basic research on language development do so primarily to improve understanding of this particular phenomenon. Basic research topics
in language development include the ways children learn the meanings of words,
the order in which children acquire the grammatical structures of their native language, and the ages by which children typically produce speech sounds. One
example of basic research is a study by Saylor and Sabbagh (2004), which was
conducted to improve general understanding of how children learn new words.
These researchers studied how different types of information present in the environment influence children's learning of new words. Basic research in language
development, such as Saylor and Sabbagh's work, not only helps build a knowledge
base concerning how children develop their language abilities, but also provides an
important foundation for applied research, which we discuss in the next section of
this chapter. See Multicultural Focus: *Dialect Discrimination* for an example of basic
research on discrimination based on the English dialect an individual speaks.

Although much basic research focuses specifically on developing, testing,
and refining theories, one type concentrates on building connections between
theory and practice. This kind of research, called **use-inspired basic research,**
addresses useful applications of research findings (Stokes, 1997). For example,
use-inspired basic research in language development might involve exploring
how and when children acquire particular language abilities so that this knowledge can be built on to help children lagging in language growth. As another
example of use-inspired basic research, Charity, Scarborough, and Griffin (2004)
studied the language skills of African American kindergartners and considered
how children's familiarity with the English dialect used in their school influenced
their success in reading. These researchers also examined how children's familiarity with the school dialect changed with time. Theoretically, the findings of this
study are informative to understanding not only the relationship between spoken
dialects and reading development but also how children's dialects are influenced

MULTICULTURAL FOCUS

Dialect Discrimination

Sociolinguistic research on the differential treatment of persons because of their language or dialect can make significant contributions to understanding civil rights issues. In a series of four experiments, Purnell, Idsardi, and Baugh (1999) confirmed that speech characteristics alone can precipitate housing discrimination. In this study, a tridialectal experimenter—using Standard American English (SAE), African American Vernacular English (AAVE), and Chicano English (ChE)—conducted telephone interviews to make appointments to discuss apartments for rent in five geographic areas. Results showed that the experimenter secured appointments between 60% and 70% of the time in all regions when he used the SAE dialect. However, when he used the AAVE and ChE dialects, his success rates declined significantly. Furthermore, the experimenter's success rate when he used the AAVE and ChE dialects was related to the local population composition. For example, in a geographic area with a 95% White population, the experimenter confirmed 70% of his appointments by using SAE and only 29% and 22% of appointments when using AAVE and ChE, respectively. Results of other experiments in this study verified that average listeners can discriminate among dialects with as little information as a single word. The results of this study provide compelling evidence that discrimination against individuals on the basis of speech characteristics and in the absence of visual cues is a valid concern in the housing market, and it may occur in other social arenas as well.

DISCUSSION POINT

What other legal or civil rights issues may benefit from sociolinguistic research? How might researchers systematically test the questions you raise?

by their instructional environment. Moreover, these findings have some useful applications to practice because the researchers found that children who were more familiar with the English dialect of the school had better reading outcomes than those of children who were less familiar with it. The findings suggested the need to design and study programs that promote children's familiarity with the school dialect to determine whether such familiarity improves their reading achievement.

Applied Research

More than 200 years ago, philosopher Jean-Jacques Rousseau (1712–1778) offered the following advice to parents about speaking to their children: "Always speak correctly before them, arrange that they enjoy themselves with no one as much as with you, and be sure that imperceptibly their language will be purified on the model of yours without your ever having chided them" (A. Bloom, 1979, p. 71).

Assuredly, Rousseau's advice was based on then-current language development theories, particularly the influence of language models on children's language

Jean-Jacques Rousseau's theory of language development emphasized the role of the environment, especially the language input that parents provide to children.

(*Photo Source:* Corbis/Bettmann.)

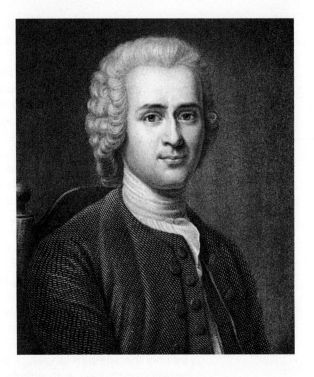

acquisition. As important as theories are to informing everyday practices, though, specific practices require direct testing by science, in the same way that theories need to be tested to build a knowledge base. Applied research contributes to specific societal needs by testing the viability of certain practices and approaches (Stokes, 1997). It typically involves using experimental research designs to examine the causal relationship between a specific approach, program, or practice, and a specific language outcome.

DISCUSSION POINT

Applied research focuses on responding to specific societal needs. What are some additional societal needs that might involve the study of language development?

The results of applied research are important for various reasons. As discussed in Chapter 1, language is a critical tool that members of all world societies use to establish relationships with other people and to negotiate needs and wants. In many societies, language is an essential tool for learning in academic contexts at all levels, from early childhood through adulthood. Persons with poor language skills risk not achieving their full academic potential. In most societies, language is also a tool used in many employment contexts, and persons with poor language skills may face challenges to obtaining and maintaining gainful employment. Scientists who study language development for applied purposes respond to such societal needs by determining why some individuals progress relatively slowly in language development, by learning how to identify persons at risk for or exhibiting disordered language development, and by developing ways to remediate delays and disorders in language when they do occur. The consumers of such research include, among others, teachers, psychologists, pediatricians, special educators, day care providers, social workers, physicians, speech–language pathologists, and teachers of English as a second, or foreign, language.

Scientists who conduct applied research on language development are from the same disciplines as scientists who conduct basic language research. Applied researchers usually test language development practices relevant to three main contexts: homes, clinics, and schools. In studies of the home environment, these researchers examine the effectiveness of specific practices or approaches parents can use to help their children develop language during home activities. For instance, applied researchers may study whether a specific style of parent–child book reading improves children's vocabulary more or less than a different style does (e.g., Whitehurst et al., 1988). In studies of the clinical environment, applied researchers examine the effectiveness of different approaches that clinical professionals, such as speech–language pathologists and clinical psychologists, may use with specific populations of patients. For instance, Thompson, Shapiro, Kiran, and Sobecks (2003) studied the effectiveness of different approaches for improving the sentence comprehension of adults with language disorders due to stroke. In studies of the school environment, applied researchers examine the effectiveness of different approaches that educators may use in the classroom to build children's language skills. For example, Throneburg, Calvert, Sturm, Paramboukas, and Paul (2000) showed that elementary-grade students with language impairment learned more vocabulary words during lessons team taught by a speech–language pathologist and a classroom teacher than during an intervention delivered in a "speech room" by only the speech–language pathologist. As all these examples show, applied research provides particularly valuable information for parents and professionals vested in ensuring the language achievements of children, adolescents, and adults.

WHAT ARE SOME MAJOR APPROACHES TO STUDYING LANGUAGE DEVELOPMENT?

In the previous sections, we discussed why persons in a range of disciplines study language. We also emphasized the integrative relationship between theory and science and how language development theories are developed and refined through both basic and applied research. In this section, we discuss approaches scientists use to study three aspects of language development: speech perception, language production, and language comprehension. In Chapters 5–8, which cover major achievements in language development during the infant, toddler, preschool, and school-age years, respectively, we describe these approaches in more detail.

Approaches to Studying Speech Perception

Goal of Speech Perception Studies

When infants enter the world, they bring with them a keen capacity to attend to speech and other auditory stimuli in the world around them. In Chapter 5, we discuss some theories on how infants begin to parse the stream of speech around them to begin to learn the sounds and words of their native language. *Speech perception* studies help researchers learn about the kinds of language abilities infants have when they are born and how children use their speech perception to learn language.

Methods for Studying Speech Perception

The study of speech perception has improved dramatically during the past few decades as a result of a range of technological advances, one of which is digitization. Researchers who study speech perception typically present auditory stimuli to participants and measure their response to the stimuli. With digital technologies, researchers have an important tool for preserving media, for ensuring high-quality presentations of auditory stimuli, and for allowing fine manipulation of the stimuli. Using specially developed computer software, speech perception researchers can record a specific speech sound and then carefully manipulate it into a series of fine-grained variants to determine how much auditory information an individual needs to hear to recognize the sound. Researchers examining speech perception in infants frequently use digital media to manipulate the speech stream. For instance, Jusczyk, Hirsh-Pasek, and colleagues (1992) developed digitized sentences that had pauses spliced in at "correct" and "incorrect" clause boundaries to identify when infants become sensitive to clause boundaries in running speech.

In addition to benefiting from digital technologies, researchers who study speech perception in very young children have profited from another cutting-edge technology. While infants are still in the womb, scientists can measure the infants' heart rates and kicking rates as a response to different auditory stimuli and examine, for example, the extent to which infants differentiate speech sounds from non-speech sounds (Karmiloff & Karmiloff-Smith, 2001). Although studies of prenatal speech perception are relatively new, a long, rich history of infant speech perception research has substantially improved general understanding of the development of speech perception (see Gerken & Aslin, 2005). Research Paradigms: *Psycholinguistics and the Head-Turn Preference Procedure* provides a description of one type of speech perception study, the *head-turn preference procedure,* and in Chapter 5, we describe another type of speech perception study, the *high-amplitude nonnutritive sucking (HAS) procedure.* Researchers using these procedures take advantage of natural human reflexes (orientation to sound in the case of the head-turn preference procedure and sucking in the case of the HAS procedure) to learn about how people perceive speech.

Speech perception researchers have also long relied on behavioral testing, in which children or adults respond by speaking, pointing, or pressing buttons in response to different speech stimuli. An important complement to behavioral testing is newer brain-imaging technologies, such as magnetic resonance imaging (MRI). These technologies allow researchers to conduct direct, real-time investigations into speech perception by presenting individuals with specific speech sounds and identifying the exact areas of the brain in which speech perception occurs. The researchers can then develop *tonotopic maps* that link the brain areas to the types of auditory stimuli processed (Fitch, Miller, & Tallal, 1997).

Approaches to Studying Language Production

Goal of Language Production Studies

Language production studies help inform practitioners of children's ability to use language expressively. In these studies, researchers examine children's emergent form, content, and use capabilities. Such studies may involve **normative research,** in which experts compile data from individuals on a certain aspect of language

RESEARCH PARADIGMS

Psycholinguistics and the Head-Turn Preference Procedure

Psycholinguistics is a field that lies at the intersection of psychology and linguistics. Psychologists who study language aim to uncover the processes by which humans learn and use language, whereas linguists try to learn more about language form (syntax, phonology, morphology) and content (semantics).

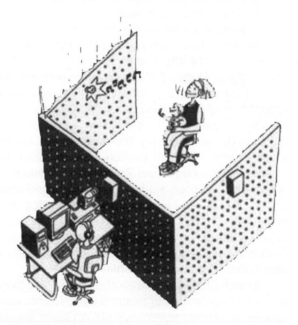

Head-turn preference procedure.

Source: From *Babies Can Un-Ravel Complex Music,* by B. Ilari, L. Polka, and E. Costa-Giomi, 2002, paper presented at the 143rd meeting of the Acoustical Society of America, Pittsburgh, PA. Retrieved from http://www.acoustics.org/press/143rd/Ilari.html. Copyright 2002 by Bertriz Ilari. Reprinted with permission.

One research paradigm that psycholinguists use to investigate language comprehension is the *head-turn preference procedure,* which takes place in a three-sided booth. On the front wall of the booth are a green light and a hole through which the researcher can view the inside of the booth. The left and right sides of the booth each contain a single red light with an audio speaker behind each light. An infant sits on a caregiver's lap in the center of the booth.

The experiment begins when the researcher flashes one or the other red light in the booth to attract the infant's attention. Once the infant is attending, a sound stimulus begins to play through the speaker and continues to play until the infant looks away for a specified amount of time (e.g., 2 seconds). This sequence of events continues as the infant is exposed to different stimuli on the right side and left side of the booth. Because the infant controls the length of time he or she listens to the audio stimuli, researchers conclude that a preference for one of the two sounds indicates that the infant can distinguish between the two sounds. The head-turn preference procedure has revealed that infants learning English prefer the stress patterns of the English language to other stress patterns (Jusczyk, Cutler, & Redanz, 1993), can segment familiar words from passages of speech (Jusczyk & Aslin, 1995), and are sensitive to the phonotactics (acceptable combinations of sounds) of their native language (Mattys, Jusczyk, Luce, & Morgan, 1999).

DISCUSSION POINT

Scholars generally use the head-turn preference procedure to answer basic research questions. Can you think of any use-inspired basic research questions about language development that this procedure might help answer?

development and from these data determine and chart the ages (or grades) by which children typically meet certain milestones. For example, Justice and colleagues (2006) published descriptive data describing the narrative productions of kindergartners through sixth graders, providing the average number of words and the average length of utterances for children's fictional stories at each grade level. Normative data such as these are useful for many professionals who need to know children's typical language production skills at a given age or grade.

One of the most well-known normative studies of early language production was used to develop a communication development checklist: the MacArthur–Bates Communicative Development Inventories (CDI; formerly the MacArthur Communicative Development Inventories). P. S. Dale and Fenson (1996) gathered language production information from more than 1,800 infants and toddlers, and from it developed the CDI. Parents, educators, and clinicians consult the CDI norms to determine how many words typically developing children understand and produce at various ages.

Sander conducted a similarly well-known normative study in 1972 and identified when children typically acquire specific speech sounds, or *phonemes.* Sander's norms (see Figure 2.1) describe the ages by which children can produce particular phonemes, as well as the order in which children master them. Other normative studies have, for the most part, provided similar results, as shown in Table 2.2.

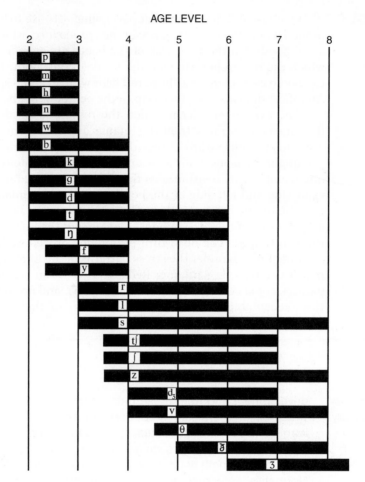

FIGURE 2.1

Sander's (1972) customary ages of production of English consonants.

Source: From "When Are Speech Sounds Learned?" by E. K. Sander, 1972, *Journal of Speech and Hearing Disorders, 37,* p. 62. Copyright 1972 by the American Speech–Language–Hearing Association. Reprinted with permission.

Methods for Studying Language Production

Language production studies are either observational or experimental. In *observational studies,* researchers examine children's language use in naturalistic or semi-structured contexts, usually by using a tape recorder or another audio recording device to capture children's language for a certain period. In naturalistic settings, the researcher does not manipulate the context. For instance, a researcher may observe the language occurring between parents and children for a certain period. One of the most well-known naturalistic observational studies is that of Hart and Risley (1995), who collected monthly audio samples of parents' and children's language in the home environment for more than 2 years. In addition to illuminating

TABLE 2.2

Normative references for English speech sound acquisition from six sources.

Consonant	Arlt & Goodban[a]	Prather et al.[b]	Poole[c]	Sander[d]	Templin[e]	Wellman et al.[f]
				Age (yr)		
/m/	3–0	2	3–6	<2	3	3
/n/	3–0	2	4–6	<2	3	3
/h/	3–0	2	3–6	<2	3	3
/p/	3–0	2	3–6	<2	3	4
/ŋ/	3–0	2	4–6	2	3	*
/f/	3–0	2–4	5–6	2–6	3	3
/j/	—	2–4	4–6	2–6	3–6	4
/k/	3–0	2–4	4–6	2	4	4
/d/	3–0	2–4	4–6	2	4	5
/w/	3–0	2–8	3–6	<2	3	3
/b/	3–0	2–8	3–6	<2	4	3
/t/	3–0	2–8	4–6	2	6	5
/g/	3–0	3	4–6	2	4	4
/s/	4–0	3	7–6	3	4–6	5
/r/	5–0	3–4	7–6	3	4	5
/l/	4–0	3–4	6–6	3	6	4
/ʃ/	6–0	3–8	6–6	3–6	4–6	—
/tʃ/	4–0	3–8	—	3–6	4–6	5
/ð/	5–0	4	6–6	5	7	—
/ʒ/	4–0	4	6–6	6	7	6
/dʒ/	4–0	>4*	—	4	7	6
/θ/	5–0	>4*	7–6	4–6	6	—
/v/	3–6	>4*	6–6	4	6	5
/z/	4–0	>4*	7–6	3–6	7	5
/ʍ/	3–0	>4*	7–6	*	*	—

* = Sound not produced correctly by 75% of subjects at oldest age tested; — = sound not tested or not reported.

Source: From *Reference Manual for Communication Sciences and Disorders* (pp. 285–286), by R. D. Kent, 1994, Austin, TX: PRO-ED. Copyright 1994 by PRO-ED. Reprinted with permission.

[a] Arlt, P. B., & Goodban, M. T. (1976). A comparative study of articulation acquisition as based on a study of 240 normals, aged three to six. *Language, Speech, and Hearing Services in Schools, 7,* 173–180. (Criterion: 75% of children tested for initial, medial, and final word positions)

[b] Prather, E. M., Hedrick, E. L., & Kerin, C. A. (1975). Articulation development in children aged two to four years. *Journal of Speech and Hearing Disorders, 40,* 179–191. (Criterion: 75% of children tested; average for initial and final word positions)

[c] Poole, I. (1934). Genetic development of consonant sounds in speech. *Elementary English Review, 11,* 159–161. (Criterion: 100% of children tested for initial, medial, and final word positions)

[d] Sander, E. K. (1972). When are speech sounds learned? *Journal of Speech and Hearing Disorders, 37,* 55–63. (Criterion: 51%, based on average from Templin [1957] and Wellman, Case, Mengert, and Bradbury [1931])

[e] Templin, M. C. (1957). *Certain language skills in children* (Institute of Child Welfare Monograph Series 26). Minneapolis: University of Minnesota Press. (Criterion: 75% of children tested for initial, medial, and final word positions)

[f] Wellman, B., Case, I., Mengert, I., & Bradbury, D. (1931). Speech sounds of young children. *State University of Iowa Studies in Child Welfare, 5,* 2. (Criterion: 75% of children tested for initial, medial, and final word positions)

the relationship between features of parental language and children's language growth, the results of this study provided useful references for the number and types of words children use as they develop their vocabulary skills.

Alternatively, in semistructured settings, researchers manipulate in some way the environment in which they are observing children's language form, content, and use. Typically, researchers manipulate contexts to elicit the aspects of language they are interested in studying. We previously noted the Justice and colleagues (2006) study, in which the fictional narratives of kindergartners through sixth graders were examined. In this study, researchers were interested in examining characteristics of children's fictional narratives at each of seven grades. Therefore, they set up a condition for eliciting narratives from children by using different types of stimuli (e.g., a sequence of pictures).

In observational studies, researchers typically record children's language for a certain period, after which they transcribe the language and analyze it for specific properties or qualities. Hart and Risley's (1995) study involved transcribing hundreds of hours of parent–child conversation, then analyzing these transcripts for the quantity and types of words used. Although the observational aspect of this research may require only a few minutes or hours, the subsequent transcription and analysis of language can take hundreds to thousands of hours. Some computer software is available to support the analyses, but typically transcription requires listening and relistening to audiotapes and videotapes and manually typing the transcription by hand into the computer programs.

Experimental studies differ from observational studies in that the researcher actively manipulates variables of interest. One classic experimental design used in language production studies is to manipulate the context in which or the conditions

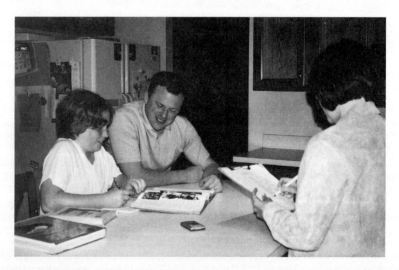

Researchers can observe children interacting with other people in naturalistic settings, make an audio recording of the interaction, transcribe the recording, and then analyze the transcript to learn how children's language develops.

(*Photo Source:* Maria B. Vonada/Merrill.)

under which children experience new words and then examine children's production of these words and how production varies by context. For instance, Saylor and Sabbagh (2004) exposed 3- and 4-year-old children to a series of new words and systematically varied the way in which the children were exposed to the new words. After the children heard the new words, these researchers used a puppet to ask the children questions about each new word and recorded the children's responses to examine how the conditions of exposure influenced the children's learning of the new words. Many experimental studies of language production take place in a research laboratory and follow strict protocols so that researchers can accurately determine the extent to which children can produce specific language structures.

Experimental studies of language production vary widely and are used to examine many aspects of production, including vocabulary, morphology, syntax, phonology, and pragmatics. Researchers are inventive in designing experiments to assess children's production abilities in these various areas. In some studies, researchers may use *pseudowords* (nonsense words) to assess children's morphological skills or vocabulary skills. Pseudowords allow control over children's previous experience with words; because these words are made up, researchers can assume children have no experience with them. A classic pseudoword task used to examine children's morphological skills was designed by Jean Berko (1958; now Jean Berko Gleason), who presented pseudowords to children and asked them to produce plural forms of these words. For example, children might demonstrate their understanding of the English plural morpheme by producing the plural form of *glorp* as *glorps* and the plural form of *dax* as *daxes*. We provide a complete description of this pseudoword task in Chapter 6.

Language production studies may also require children to repeat sentences so that the researchers can determine whether the children have a grasp of certain grammatical structures. For example, an examiner may ask a child to repeat the sentence *She is going to the party.* A child who has not yet mastered the auxiliary verb *is* will likely omit it ("She going to the party") and not produce an exact repetition of the sentence. Researchers may also ask children to correct erroneous sentences as another way to gauge their ability to produce more complex grammatical structures.

Approaches to Studying Language Comprehension

Goal of Language Comprehension Studies

Many times, researchers would like to understand what children know about language, even if they cannot express what they know. **Language comprehension** studies specifically tap into what children understand about language, and with the assistance of some creative research paradigms, experts can measure children's language comprehension even before the children speak their first word.

Methods for Studying Language Comprehension

Language comprehension research requires a different set of tools and techniques than those used in language production studies. In the study of comprehension, researchers try to estimate what children or adults understand rather than produce.

For prelinguistic infants, researchers generally use visual fixation (looking time) on a stimulus as a measure of language comprehension. For example, a researcher can determine whether an infant knows the words *mommy* and *daddy* by placing pictures of the infant's mother and father side by side and asking the infant to look at either "mommy" or "daddy." The researcher must take into account other considerations as well to ensure the validity of the experiment. In Chapter 5, we provide additional details on research paradigms that use visual fixation as a measure of language comprehension.

For older children, researchers can use pointing as a measure of language comprehension instead. For instance, the researcher may present a child with a word or sentence and ask the child to select from an array of pictures the one that matches the word or sentence. This technique is common in standardized language assessments and can be used to study children's comprehension of morphology, such as the plural form ("Point to the picture of two cats"); syntax, such as passive sentences ("Point to the picture showing *The boy was kicked by the girl* "); and vocabulary ("Point to the picture of the compass").

Alternatively, researchers may ask children to act out a series of sentences with toy props. For instance, to assess children's comprehension of the semantic roles *agent* and *recipient,* the researcher could provide the child with a toy dog and a toy cat; say "The dog is pulling the cat's tail"; and instruct the child to act out the scenario with the dog and cat props. Likewise, to test a child's comprehension of passive sentences, a researcher could give the child a set of farm animals and request the child to show the sentence *The horse is being kicked by the cow.*

WHAT ARE SOME MAJOR LANGUAGE DEVELOPMENT THEORIES?

Questions That Should Be Answered by Language Theories

Recall from the beginning of this chapter that theories provide testable explanations concerning children's language development. In large part, language development theories attempt to explain *how* children go about learning their native language, a question of great interest for both theoretical and practical reasons. Researchers are interested in theories to build on knowledge about language development as a uniquely human phenomenon that is remarkable for various reasons (see Chapter 1). Likewise, practitioners are interested in language development to better help children and adults who may have difficulties with such development. Professionals who work with children and adults with language difficulties draw on theory to make informed decisions about the practices and programs they use with these individuals.

Theories about language development are both abundant and varied in focus. Some theories address specific language accomplishments, such as word learning or question formation (e.g., Hirsh-Pasek, Golinkoff, & Hollich, 2000; Hollich, Hirsh-Pasek, & Golinkoff, 2000). Other theories focus on language development at particular ages (c.f. Nippold, 1998) or in the context of specific disabilities. The extent to which a theory helps *in general* to provide an explanation of language development is an important consideration. Some theories are too limited in scope to provide a useful explanation of language development in general, whereas others are so broad that they fail to account for variability in language development when different language domains or achievements across the life span are considered. Next, we present three questions that you may use to consider each theory presented subsequently in this chapter (Hirsh-Pasek & Golinkoff, 1996). We consider an adequate theory to provide some type of explanation for each question:

1. What do infants bring to the task of language learning?
2. What mechanisms drive language acquisition?
3. What types of input support the language-learning system?

What Do Infants Bring to the Task of Language Learning?

Some theorists propose that infants arrive in the world essentially preprogrammed to acquire language. Other theorists argue that infants learn language through their experiences and that they are not born with innate language capabilities. These divergent views fuel what is called the *nature versus nurture* debate. Most language development theories lie somewhere between the *nature* and *nurture* ends of the continuum and contend that some aspects of the language system are innate and other abilities are acquired through individuals' experiences with the culture and people of their communities.

What Mechanisms Drive Language Acquisition?

The question of what mechanisms drive language acquisition addresses the processes by which language develops from infancy forward. For example, some theorists propose that the processes people use to learn language are *domain specific,* or dedicated solely to the tasks of comprehending and producing language. Other theorists contend that people use processes for learning language that are **domain general,** or the same as those used in other situations such as solving problems and perceiving objects and events in the environment. Recall from Chapter 1 our brief discussion on the concept of modularity. *Modularity* is a theoretical account of how the brain is organized for various cognitive processes. A strict modularity perspective includes a domain-specific account of language acquisition, whereas a nonmodularity perspective provides a domain-general account.

What Types of Input Support the Language-Learning System?

DISCUSSION POINT

What are some other fundamental questions that you would use to guide a comparison of language development theories?

The final question asks about the kinds of input that drive language development after birth, as children grow and develop. Some theorists suggest that increasing knowledge of social conventions and a child's desire to interact with others are the most important supports for language development. Other theorists propose that when children simply hear more and more language, they use this "positive evidence" that other people provide to make assumptions about the structure of their native language.

TABLE 2.3

Overview of language development theories.

Theory (proponent)	Nature–nurture continuum	Major tenets	Key concepts
Behaviorist theory (Skinner)	Nurture inspired	Language is like any other human behavior, and it does not reflect any special innate endowment.	Operant conditioning
		Children learn language through operant conditioning and shaping; some verbal behaviors are reinforced and others are suppressed.	Reinforcement
		Complex behaviors (e.g., speaking in complete sentences) are learned as a series of steps in a chain, in which each step stimulates each successive step.	
Social-interactionist theory (Vygotsky)	Nurture inspired	Language emerges through social interaction with peers and adults.	Social plane–psychological plane,
		Language skills move from a social plane to a psychological plane.	Zone of proximal development
		Initially, language and cognition are intertwined processes but become separate capabilities by about age 2 years.	
Cognitive theory (Piaget)	Nurture inspired	Children's cognitive development precedes their language development.	Cognition hypothesis
		Children's speech begins as egocentric because children can view the world only from their own perspective.	Egocentric speech
Intentionality model (Bloom)	Nurture inspired	The tension between the desire to communicate intentions to other people and the effort required to communicate these intentions drives language development.	Intentionality
Competition model (MacWhinney)	Nurture inspired	Repeated exposure to reliable language input strengthens children's "correct" representations of the morphology, phonology, and syntax of their language.	Reliable input, Strengthened representation

Major Language Development Theories

Language development theories can generally be grouped into those that are relatively nurture inspired and those that are nature inspired. *Nurture-inspired theories* are often called *empiricist theories,* and they rest on the notion that humans gain all knowledge through experience. The extreme empiricist position is that an infant arrives in the world as a "blank slate," with no innate language abilities. In contrast, *nature-inspired theories,* also called *nativist theories,*

Theory (proponent)	Nature–nurture continuum	Major tenets	Key concepts
Usage-based theory (Tomasello)	Nurture inspired	Children attend to and understand other people's intentions and then imitate other persons' intentional communicative actions to learn language.	Joint attention, Intention reading
Modularity theory (Fodor)	Nature inspired	Language is organized in highly specific modules in the brain. Language modules perform dedicated functions but can interact with one another to produce combinations of functions.	Localization Encapsulization
Universal grammar (Chomsky)	Nature inspired	Children are born with general grammatical rules and categories common to all languages. Children use input to discover the parameters their language uses to satisfy the general grammatical rules and categories they are born with.	Language acquisition device Parameters
Syntactic bootstrapping (Gleitman)	Nature inspired	Children use their knowledge of syntactic categories to make inferences about the meanings of new words.	Bootstrapping, Syntax
Semantic bootsrapping (Pinker)	Nature inspired	Children use their knowledge of word meanings to make inferences about the syntactic categories to which the words belong.	Bootstrapping, Semantics
Connectionist theories (Rumelhart & McClelland)	Nature or nurture inspired	Language is organized in a network containing nodes and connections. The network of nodes and connections undergoes constant transformation in response to language input.	Nodes Connections

generally hold that much knowledge is innate and genetically transmitted rather than learned by experience. The extreme nativist position is that an individual's underlying language system is in place at birth and that children use this system to extract rules about their native language apart from other cognitive abilities.

See Table 2.3 for an overview of the language development theories we present next. Table 2.4 shows the answers each theory provides for the three questions posed in the preceding section.

TABLE 2.4
Answers to three questions about the nature of language development theories.

Theory	Questions		
	What do infants bring to the task of language learning?	**What mechanisms drive language quisition?**	**What types of input support the language-learning system?**
Behaviorist theory	No mention	Operant conditioning by parents and adults—a domain-general process	Reinforcement of desirable verbal behavior and punishment of undesirable verbal behavior
Social-interactionist theory	General social structure	Social interactions with others—a domain-general process	Linguistic input that is within the child's zone of proximal development
Cognitive theory	General cognitive structure	General cognitive processing abilities—a domain-general process	Understanding events, relations, and phenomena in a nonlinguistic sense
Intentionality model	General social structure	Engaging with other people and objects—a domain-general process	The tension between the desire to engage with other people and the effort required to express elaborate intentional states
Competition model	Ability to attend to and organize linguistic data	Induction and hypothesis testing—domain-general processes	Reliable and frequent input patterns
Usage-based theory	Intention reading, which emerges during infancy	The child's interpretation of the social environment—a domain-general process	Reproducing intentional communicative actions through cultural or imitative learning
Modularity theory	Specialized modules in the brain	Functions performed by dedicated language modules—domain-specific processes	Input that promotes parameter setting of modules and interactions among language modules
Universal grammar	Explicit, domain-specific linguistic knowledge	Discovery of the parameters that a person's language encompasses—domain-specific processes	General linguistic input (even of an impoverished quality)
Syntactic bootstrapping	Syntactic categories	Domain-general processes to understand how language works, domain-specific processes to notice correlations between syntax and meaning	Syntactic input
Semantic bootstrapping	Semantic categories, ability to parse sentences, ability to link words in sentences to semantic categories	Domain-general processes to understand how language works, domain-specific processes to make hypotheses about new words	Semantic input
Connectionist theories	Ability to attend to and organize linguistic data	Pattern detection—a domain-general process	Reliable and frequent input patterns

Nurture-Inspired Theories

DISCUSSION POINT
Describe the link among theory, science, and practice in ABA interventions. How might subscribing to a different language development theory influence language therapy techniques for children with autism?

Skinner's Behaviorist Theory. B. F. Skinner (1904–1990), who appears in the chapter opening photo with his wife and his daughter Deborah, popularized the notion of *behaviorism,* according to which all learning is believed to be the result of **operant conditioning** (Skinner, 1957). In operant conditioning, behaviors are shaped by responses to the behaviors, so that behaviors that are reinforced become strengthened and behaviors that are punished become suppressed. To Skinner, language is not a special behavior; rather, it is a behavior like any other behavior humans can learn. Thus, Skinner's theory of language learning is essentially identical to his general learning theory in that it focuses on observable and measurable aspects of language (the behavior) children produce as they interact with the environment. See Theory to Practice: *Applied Behavior Analysis* for a practical application of Skinner's theory.

According to this language development theory, children arrive at the task of language learning without innate knowledge; rather, environmental stimuli elicit verbal responses, or language, from children. Children then "learn" language as adults reinforce their verbalizations, as in the following example:

THEORY TO PRACTICE

Applied Behavior Analysis

Applied behavior analysis (ABA) is an umbrella term that encompasses several methods stemming from Skinner's behaviorist theory. It is often used as an intervention approach for children with autism. The principles of operant conditioning—stimulus, response, and reinforcement—are common to ABA interventions for autism. In such interventions, an adult or a therapist first makes a request of the child. This request may consist of asking the child to repeat a word or phrase or to fill in the blank of a *cloze* statement (e.g., "I want to eat _____"). The request serves as the stimulus for the behavior that follows. When the child responds by performing the requested behavior, the adult or therapist immediately reinforces the child to promote such linguistic behavior in the future.

ABA interventions can be intensive and time consuming, sometimes requiring training in ABA and several to many hours per week of one-on-one therapy. Some ABA interventions use *discrete trial training* (DTT), which consists of a series of distinct trials that the adult or therapist repeats until the child masters the target skill. Subsequent trials build on these skills to shape more complex skills. To build language skills, DTT moves from eliciting simple behaviors, such as direct imitation, to more advanced behaviors, such as forming *wh-* questions (e.g., "What?" "When?" "Where?"). The results of some research suggest that children with autism who undergo ABA-inspired therapy make significant gains in their academic, intellectual, and language functioning, during both the short term and the long term (Lovaas, 1987; McEachin, Smith, & Lovaas, 1993). However, this approach to language intervention is not without controversy (Heflin & Simpson, 1998).

Eight-month-old Margo would shriek loudly when she was hungry and wanted to be fed. Margo's mother would grab Margo's bottle and say; "You want your bottle? Baaaaah-ttle." On one occasion, Margo imitated her mother by saying "ba." Margo's mother was so excited at Margo's attempt that she laughed and smiled as she fed Margo her bottle, reinforcing Margo's use of this "word." Margo then began to say "ba" when she wanted her bottle and Margo's mother would get her bottle more quickly than when Margo would simply shriek. Because Margo's mother rewarded her quickly with a bottle each time she uttered "ba," Margo eventually stopped shrieking and continued to say "ba" when she was hungry. Margo's mother eventually began to accept only close approximations of the word *bottle,* including "ba-ba" and later "ba-bble" before she would hurry to get a bottle.

DISCUSSION POINT

Skinner equates language to other human behaviors such as learning to walk. How are learning to talk and learning to walk similar? How do they differ?

You may wonder how children ever learn to speak in complete sentences if reinforcement is the key to learning, but Skinner's theory of verbal behavior accounts for complex linguistic behavior as well. Complex behavior consists of a series, or chain, of behaviors, in which each step in the process stimulates each successive behavior. In the case of even complex verbal behavior, operant conditioning is the mechanism that drives language learning.

Vygotsky's Social-Interactionist Theory. In the early 20th century, Soviet psychologist Lev Vygotsky (1896–1934) stressed the importance of social interaction for children's language development. He argued that all human knowledge exists first on a *social plane* and then on a *psychological plane.* More simply, Vygotsky contended that all concepts are introduced first in the context of social interaction (the social plane), then, with time, these concepts are internalized to the psychological plane. Social interaction between an infant and other more capable peers (parents, siblings, teachers, etc.) is a critical mechanism for children's language acquisition. Vygotsky viewed language as a uniquely human ability that exists independent of general cognition starting at about age 2 years: Prior to this time, general cognition and language are intertwined, but, at about age 2 years, these two processes begin to develop as separate (albeit interrelated) capabilities.

One critical concept in Vygotskian theory is the **zone of proximal development** (ZPD), which is the difference between a child's *actual developmental level,* as determined by independent problem solving, and his or her *level of potential development,* as determined through problem solving in collaboration with a more competent adult or peer (Vygotsky, 1978). The ZPD concept characterizes development dynamically by describing abilities in children that are in the process of maturing rather than by focusing solely on abilities that have already matured. Consider this example:

Lori and her 4-year-old son, Alexander, are having a conversation about rhyming words in a storybook. Without assistance from Lori, Alexander cannot produce rhymes. For instance, she asks him, "What rhymes with *cat* on this page?" to which she gets no response. However, when Lori provides Alexander with support, by telling him three words that rhyme with *cat* (*bat, fat, mat*), he can produce a rhyme (*rat*).

You might ask whether Alexander can actually recognize rhymes. On the one hand, he cannot do so independently; on the other hand, with some help from his mother, he can complete the task. From a Vygotskian perspective, examining what children can do with mediated assistance from others is necessary for identification of maturing capabilities, which provides an important window into development. Vygotsky's position is that as children learn language through social interactions, their general cognitive abilities are subsequently propelled forward.

Piaget's Cognitive Theory. Jean Piaget (1896–1980), a Swiss psychologist, is best known for his observational studies of his three children's development and his theories on **genetic epistemology,** or the study of the development of knowledge. One important element of Piaget's work is his emphasis on stages of learning and development. Piaget hypothesized a series of cognitive stages that children experience and emphasized that achievements in one stage must occur before a child can move on to the next stage.

Piaget (1923) did not believe language to be a domain-specific ability, but rather a domain-general ability that follows closely behind children's general cognitive development. His perspective on the subservience of language to cognition has been referred to as the *cognition hypothesis* because certain cognitive achievements need to be in place for language achievements to emerge (see Sinclair-de-Zwart, 1973). In essence, Piaget did not view language as a special faculty but as an ability that reflects developments in other areas of growth, such as perceptive, cognitive, and social processes. He viewed language as following the same stages he proposed for general cognitive development.

As a theorist in the nurture-inspired school of thought, Piaget viewed children as active agents in constructing their understanding of language. According to Piaget, children are egocentric and developmentally predisposed to view the world from only their perspective. For this reason, conversations between young children are essentially collective monologues, in which each child produces a monologue but cannot respond contingently or take turns with each other. The following dialogue between two preschoolers is an example of how **egocentric speech** plays out in conversations with young children:

KEVIN: Watch me score a goal!

PETE: The ground is squishy and muddy.

KEVIN: Ok, here goes. Are you watching?

PETE: My socks are getting wet!

According to Piagetian theory, children do not replace egocentric speech with true dialogue until they develop the ability to see others' perspectives. This contention supports the idea that cognitive development gives way to language achievements.

Intentionality Model of Language Acquisition. According to the intentionality model, children's abilities in language, emotional expression, cognition, social interaction, and play develop in tandem (L. Bloom, 2000; L. Bloom & Tinker, 2001a). The child is responsible for driving language learning forward. This model differs from other nurture-inspired theories in which the child's environment or peers are proposed to have the most influence in driving language development. In fact, in this model, children learn language when what they have in mind differs from what other individuals around them have in mind because they must express themselves to share this information. For example, a young child cannot assume that his or her mother will always know when he or she is thirsty and offer him or her a drink. Therefore, the child must learn how to express this intention by using language. To acquire language, then, children must be intentional, they must take strides to engage in social interaction, and they must put forth effort to construct linguistic representations for the ideas they want to express and then act to express these ideas.

Competition Model. The competition model describes specific mechanisms through which children acquire the acceptable morphological, phonological, syntactic, and lexical forms that compose their native language (MacWhinney, 1987). The competition model is nurture inspired in that language development draws heavily on the input heard. Children acquire language forms that they hear frequently and reliably early in life, and later in life they acquire forms that they hear rarely or inconsistently. In the competition model, multiple language forms compete with one another until the input strengthens the correct representation and the child no longer produces an incorrect form.

A common child language phenomenon that illustrates how the competition model works is **overgeneralization.** You have probably heard children say "I goed" instead of "I went" or "I runned" instead of "I ran." When children who are learning language make an irregular past tense verb regular by adding a /d/, /t/, or /ɪd/ sound, they are overgeneralizing the past tense rule that applies to most verbs in the English language. Eventually, though, with ongoing reliable exposures to an irregular form such as *went,* the correct past tense representation of the word is strengthened and the incorrect form (*goed*) dies out.

Usage-Based Theory. Engaging in social interactions is undoubtedly a strong impetus for attending to and learning language. Prelinguistic infants provide substantial evidence for this claim. You have probably experienced a situation similar to this scenario:

While two women were talking, the 8-month-old daughter of one of them began to interject some babbling sounds into the conversation as if to indicate that she, too, wanted to take part in the social exchange.

Usage-based theories of language acquisition, a term Tomasello (2003) coined, emphasize the social nature of language as an impetus for furthering children's language abilities, contending that children learn language because they have reason to talk (e.g., Budwig, 1995; Halliday & Hasan, 1985).

Tomasello's (2003) usage-based theory of language development is based on evidence concerning the emergence of intentionality during the first year of life. For example, in their first year, infants engage in periods of sustained joint attention with other individuals, actively direct the attention of other people to objects and events, and begin to use communication intentions to achieve various ends. Usage-based theories suggest that children's knowledge of language form and meaning emerges from their use of language, during which they induce patterns of form and meaning. A critical premise of this theory is the child's skills in "intention reading." *Intention reading,* which emerges during infancy, refers to the child's ability to recognize the intentions and mental states of other people, corresponding to the increasing capacity of the infant to engage communicatively with other persons. As a child becomes aware of others' intentions, he or she begins to actively manipulate them—for example, by drawing his or her mother's attention to an object of interest. As children repeatedly and increasingly use their awareness of social conventions to engage with other people, their more general language abilities emerge.

Nature-Inspired Theories

Fodor's Modularity Theory. Fodor's (1983) modularity theory is a popular cognitive approach that emphasizes the organization of the cognitive infrastructure of the brain as comprising a series of highly specified modules, including modules for various aspects of language processing. A modularity perspective of language views it as an innate capacity localized to domain-specific processors that are encapsulated in their functions from other processors. To say that language is *localized* means that the modules composing the language system each operate by using a dedicated neural system. The concept of encapsulization means that processors operate independently of one another and do not share information. Thus, language modules operate independently to perform dedicated functions yet can interact with one another at higher levels to produce combinations of functions. Because language modules operate independently, language development in different areas (e.g., the lexicon, syntax, morphology) is driven forward by different types of input. For example, the number and kinds of words a young child hears is an environmental influence that helps shape the lexicon, whereas innately given syntactic rules help shape the child's sentence formation abilities.

Because modularity theory stipulates that separate areas of language can develop independently of one another, it has implications for understanding language development. This phenomenon is most obvious in children who have an impairment in one or more language areas (e.g., receptive language, expressive language). In Chapter 4, we present neurological evidence concerning the modularity perspective.

Universal Grammar. Noam Chomsky (1965) popularized the term **universal grammar** (UG), which describes the system of grammatical rules and constraints that are consistent in all world languages. Chomsky postulated that language acquisition depends on an innate, species-specific module dedicated to language and not other forms of learning. Unlike Fodor, who postulated language to involve a series of modules, Chomsky theorized the existence of one language module, called the **language acquisition device.**

According to UG theory, children cannot learn language simply on the basis of experience because human language grammars are so complex and the language children hear is relatively imperfect (people sometimes garble speech and use false starts). Instead, children are born with a basic set of grammatical rules and categories that exist in all languages, and the input they receive sets parameters (options) to match those of their native language. Thus, children do not actively analyze the language they hear or make inferences or inductions about their native language.

Unlike other theories, UG theory does not view language as a developmental phenomenon. Rather, UG posits that children are born with linguistic competence and that mistakes and omissions in their speech indicate performance difficulties and not a lack of competence. The disconnect between children's performance and their grammatical competence may result from limitations in their processing capacities and other contextual factors that may mask competence (Brooks, 2004).

Bootstrapping Theories. You may have heard some people refer to *bootstrapping* their way to a particular accomplishment. This term means that the individuals accomplished a goal by personal effort or with minimal outside assistance. The bootstrap idiom is derived from the process of pulling your boots on with only the assistance of the small loop sewn to the top, back portion of a boot. **Syntactic bootstrapping** describes the process by which children use the syntactic frames surrounding unknown verbs to successfully constrain the possible interpretations of the verbs. This theory is a nature-inspired account of language development focused specifically on syntactic development. Nurture-inspired theorists suggest that children learn the meaning of an unfamiliar verb by examining extralinguistic cues, such as observing their own actions or the actions of other people nearby, to narrow the meaning of the verb. However, as Gleitman and Landau argued, the extralinguistic context will most likely not reveal a single, clear meaning (Gleitman, 1990; Landau & Gleitman, 1985). For example, the extralinguistic context surrounding the request "Are you *bringing* me the remote control?" might prompt a child to interpret the verb in the sentence to mean "hold," "carry," "walk," or "bring." Therefore, children probably use additional linguistic information—particularly the syntax of the sentence—as they learn the meanings of new verbs.

In the preceding example, information about the meaning of *bring* is available in the syntax in which *bring* appears. In this example, an indirect object (*me*) and then a direct object (*remote control*) follow the word *bring,* which suggests that *bring* is a verb of transfer (because transfer involves both the thing transferred and the person to whom it is transferred). Therefore, the meanings of *hold, carry,* and *walk* are eliminated from contention. Syntactic bootstrapping is a nature-inspired language development theory because it proposes that children arrive at the task of language learning with knowledge of syntactic categories and use this knowledge to understand the meanings of words that fill various positions in sentences.

Semantic bootstrapping is another type of bootstrapping theory. Like syntactic bootstrapping, semantic bootstrapping uses the bootstrap metaphor to illustrate how children acquire particular linguistic concepts with minimal outside assistance. However, the difference lies in what children bootstrap. With semantic bootstrapping, children deduce grammatical structures by using word

The bootstrap idiom for language development is derived from the process of pulling your boots on with only the assistance of the small loop sewn onto the top, back portion of the boot.

(*Photo Source:* Plush Studios/Getty Images Inc.—Photodisc.)

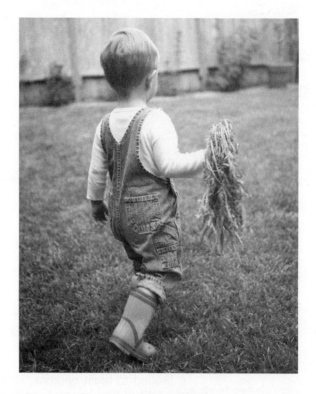

meanings they acquire from observing events around them (Pinker, 1984). After children acquire a large and diverse lexicon from their observations of objects and events in the world, they use correspondences between semantics and syntax to determine the syntactic category to which each word belongs. For example, once a child learns that *bird* describes a solid object, he or she may infer that *bird* is a count noun. Later, when the child understands the determiner *a,* he or she may infer that other words that include the determiner *a* (*a watch, a clock*) are also count nouns.

Connectionist Theories. Connectionist theories are presented in this text as nature-inspired theories, but they just as likely could be presented as nurture-inspired theories. Connectionist models of language development attempt to visually approximate the inner workings of the brain, and they model and simulate the mechanisms responsible for language growth in relationship to input. Connectionist theories are relevant to modeling an array of cognitive processes, but, in the area of language, they focus on modeling how language is organized across the brain and on describing how connections are forged among words within the lexicon, or store of words in the brain (see Chapter 3 for a discussion of the mental lexicon).

Connectionist researchers use models to represent nonlinear, dynamic, and complex development in language and other areas. One important aspect of language development that connectionist researchers have modeled is the process

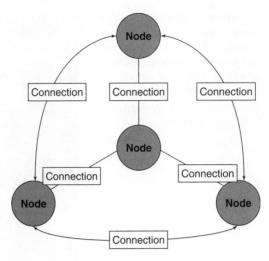

FIGURE 2.2
A connectionist network.

by which children learn both the regular (e.g., *walk–walked, cook–cooked*) and the irregular (e.g., *eat–ate, fly–flew*) forms of past tense verbs (Rumelhart & McClelland, 1986). Connectionist models are simulations of how nodes and connections are organized in larger networks (Figure 2.2). *Nodes* are simple processing units that can be likened to brain neurons. Nodes receive input from external sources through *connections*. The connections between nodes vary in strength depending on the connection weight. The network of nodes and connections adapts and transforms itself continually in response to the input it receives. For example, connections between some nodes may weaken with time from reduced input or counterevidence, and connections between other nodes may become stronger with time and contribute to a reorganization of the entire network. Elman, Bates, Johnson, Parisi, and Plunkett (1996) provide a more detailed introduction to connectionist models.

HOW DO LANGUAGE DEVELOPMENT THEORIES INFLUENCE PRACTICE?

Linkage of Theory to Practice

To this point, we have discussed some of the people who study language development and why they do so. We have described some general approaches for studying language development. We have also examined several language development theories and their premises about the predetermined abilities of infants, the mechanisms that drive language development, and the kinds of input that support language development. Next, we bridge the gaps among language development theory, science, and practice. Linking theories to practices is not a novel idea. People routinely let their ideas about particular phenomena guide their practices. You can witness this occurrence in diet trends, the medicine people take, and child-rearing practices, for example. In some cases, the connection between theory and practice is clear. For instance, Newton's first law says that an object in motion will remain in motion until acted on by an outside force. Many people, not wanting their bodies to remain in motion long enough to pass through the windshield upon impact in a car crash, faithfully wear seat belts when they travel.

However, in the case of language development, the connection between theory and practice is not always so transparent. For this reason, practitioners must make every effort to understand the theories that guide particular practices. Also important is determining whether a theory offers ample support to guide the practices in question. In the following section, we provide two examples of how language development theories influence practice in the context of second language–learning methods. Then, in the last section, we discuss practices that are informed by language theories.

Instruction in English as a Second Language: Theory and Practice

Theories of language learning influence language-teaching practices in a number of ways, although, as previously mentioned, the link between theory and practice is not always direct. Rather, the connection between theory and practice is mediated by principles of instruction, including cognitive, affective, and linguistic principles. *Cognitive principles* include ideas governing language processing and automaticity and the role of tangible and intangible rewards that the speaker gains through language use. *Affective principles* are related to the individual's confidence with language learning and his or her propensity to take risks with respect to language. *Linguistic principles* describe the role of a person's native language in simultaneously facilitating and interfering with second language acquisition. (See H. D. Brown, 2001, for a thorough discussion of language instruction principles.) When teachers of English as a second language select particular instructional practices, they consider not only language-learning theories but also relevant principles concerning all the preceding factors.

Two methods for teaching English as a second language that stem from distinct language theories are the audiolingual method and the Silent Way. Although these methods are no longer widely used, we describe them because they provide clear examples of how language development theories can be applied in practice. The *audiolingual method* was developed in response to an increasing need for translators during World War II. It emphasizes imitation, repetition, and memorization of language forms to create automatic and habitual language responses. Teachers using the audiolingual method engage students in language drills that include positive reinforcement for target verbal behavior. For example, the teacher might present lines of dialogue for students to repeat and then praise them for pronouncing the lines correctly. Teachers target more complex linguistic behavior only after students have mastered smaller, simpler chunks of language. This method has roots in behavioral psychology—more specifically in Skinner's

The audiolingual method, created during World War II, was derived from behaviorist theory and emphasizes drilling of language skills.

(*Photo Source:* Patrick White/Merrill.)

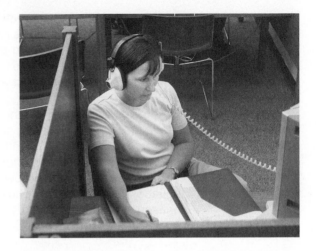

nurture-inspired theory of verbal behavior—in that it emphasizes rote, habitual responses to language forms rather than social-interactional factors or the learner's cognitive abilities.

The *Silent Way* is a language-teaching method that was popular during the cognitive revolution of the early 1970s. It emphasizes the importance of allowing students to generate hypotheses about language rules and then to apply the rules and discover errors. Using the Silent Way, teachers facilitate students' discovery of language rules, remaining mostly silent and using color-coded rods rather than words to represent vocabulary words, grammatical forms, and pronunciation rules. The Silent Way values the learner's ability to process and detect patterns in linguistic input, to generate and test hypotheses, and to correct errors by personal effort—all characteristics of nurture-inspired cognitive theories of language development.

Both the audiolingual method and the Silent Way illustrate how language development theories can be translated to educational practice. These examples also show how extremely different practices can be used in the field on the basis of a particular theory that is in vogue at the time. Sometimes, however, the connection between theory and practice is not so obvious. In Chapter 9, we discuss theories about second language development and describe additional second language teaching practices.

Practices Informed by Language Theories

Many professionals are interested in applying language development theories to practice, including clinical psychologists, speech–language pathologists, audiologists, social workers, and teachers. Parents are also interested in how theory can be linked to practice so that they can promote their children's language achievements. In this section, we consider three direct applications of language theory (and research) to practice: **prevention, intervention and remediation,** and **enrichment.**

The goal of *prevention* is to inhibit language difficulties from emerging and thus reduce the need to resolve such difficulties later in life. Preventing language difficulties is particularly important for children who are at risk for language problems because of their biological predispositions, the family's socioeconomic status, or the quality of language interactions between adults and children in the home. One popular type of prevention activity used in many preschool programs across the United States focuses on fostering phonological awareness in young children. **Phonological awareness** is the ability to focus on the sounds that make up syllables and words, and well-developed phonological awareness can help children succeed in later reading instruction. Various programs are available to promote phonological awareness in young children, which may, in turn, prevent children from experiencing later problems in reading achievement.

Intervention and remediation are programs or strategies used to help children, adolescents, and adults who exhibit difficulties with some aspect of language development. Language intervention may be appropriate for toddlers who show delays in acquiring their first words or who are slow to start combining words to make two-word utterances. For preschoolers, intervention may focus on helping children with language problems communicate more effectively with other people and improving their morphological, phonological, syntactic, and semantic development. Numerous programs and strategies are available for targeting these aspects of language development. For school-age children with language problems, intervention often focuses on helping children improve their academic language skills, such as their understanding of curricular vocabulary or their use of comprehension strategies to better understand what they read. Various interventions are also available for adults who lose their language skills because of disease or illness.

Enrichment is the process through which teachers, clinicians, and other adults provide children, adolescents, and adults with an enhanced language-learning environment that both builds on existing skills and promotes the development of new and more advanced language abilities. One example of a language enrichment program is *Learning Language and Loving It* (www.hanen.org). This program teaches preschool educators ways to promote children's language learning in the early education environment. The *Learning Language and Loving It* program, and its accompanying book by Weitzman and Greenberg (2002), takes a child-centered approach to enhancing children's early language, social, and literacy development by training educators to use specific strategies for interacting with children in responsive ways. As other examples, an enrichment program for adolescents might teach them appropriate ways to interact with peers. An enrichment program for adults who speak English with an accent (e.g., businesspersons who speak Chinese as a first language but use English for business purposes) may address improved pronunciation.

SUMMARY

In this chapter, we distinguish among theory, science, and practice and demonstrate how the three complement one another in the field of language development. A *theory* of language development is a claim or hypothesis that provides explanations for how and why children develop their capacity for language. In the field of language development, *science* describes the process of generating and testing language theories, and *practice* includes the areas of people's lives that are influenced by language development theories and science, including second language teaching methods and methods for the *prevention* of language difficulties, for *language intervention and remediation,* and for language *enrichment.*

Scientists from many disciplines (including psychology, linguistics, psycholinguistics, anthropology, speech–language pathology, education, and sociology, among others) study language development. Some scientists conduct *basic research* in language development, with the goal of generating and refining the existing knowledge base. Other scientists conduct applied research, with the goal of testing approaches and practices that pertain to real-world settings.

Scientists use various approaches to study language development. For example, to study infants' *speech perception* abilities, scientists can measure the infants' heart rate, kicking rate, and visual responses to auditory stimuli. To measure young children's *language production* abilities, scientists might use observational studies in which children's language is examined in naturalistic or semistructured contexts—or experimental studies, in which variables of interest to the researcher are manipulated. To study children's *language comprehension* abilities, scientists might measure looking time or pointing toward a stimulus.

Several nurture-inspired and nature-inspired language development theories can be examined in the context of three questions: (a) What do infants bring to the task of language learning? (b) What mechanisms drive language acquisition? (c) What types of input support the language-learning system?

Nurture-inspired, or *empiricist, theories* of language development include behaviorist theory, social-interactionist theory, cognitive theory, the intentionality model, the competition model, and usage-based theory. *Nature-inspired,* or *nativist,* theories of language development include modularity theory, universal grammar, syntactic bootstrapping, semantic bootstrapping, and connectionist theories.

Language development theories influence practices in several areas. These areas include instruction in English as a second language, prevention of language difficulties, intervention and remediation, and enrichment.

KEY TERMS

applied research, p. 43
basic research, p. 43
domain general, p. 55
egocentric speech, p. 61
enrichment, p. 68
genetic epistemology, p. 61

intervention and remediation, p. 68
language acquisition device, p. 63
language comprehension, p. 53
language production, p. 48
normative research, p. 48
operant conditioning, p. 59

For online resources related to chapter content, including audio samples, valuable Web sites, suggested readings, and self-quizzes, please go to the Companion Website at http://www.prenhall.com/pence

3

Building Blocks of Language

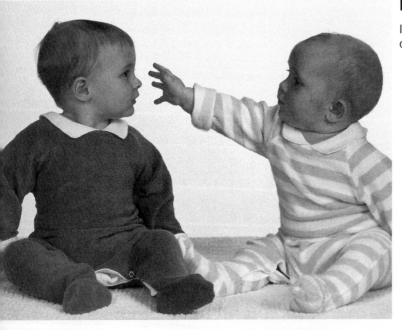

FOCUS QUESTIONS

In this chapter, we answer the following five questions:

1. What is semantic development?
2. What is morphological development?
3. What is syntactic development?
4. What is phonological development?
5. What is pragmatic development?

In Chapter 1, we discussed how language is a single dimension of human behavior that comprises three interrelated domains: content, form, and use (Lahey, 1988). Children's language development involves achieving competency in each of these domains, and, subsequently in this book, we discuss major accomplishments in each domain for infants (Chapter 5), toddlers (Chapter 6), preschoolers (Chapter 7), and school-age children (Chapter 8). In this chapter, we present these three domains in more detail, preparing you for the in-depth discussions in Chapters 5–8.

As children develop their language from infancy forward, their achievements in each language domain grow by leaps and bounds as they master and then expand on the basic building blocks of content, form, and use. Recall from Chapter 1 that the five components of the three domains are as follows: semantics, syntax, morphology, phonology, and pragmatics. Semantics and pragmatics are components of content and use, respectively, and syntax, morphology, and phonology are the components of form. In this chapter, we identify and discuss the basic building blocks for each component of the three domains. We begin by discussing the building blocks of *semantic development,* which include developing a lexicon, learning new words, and organizing the lexicon for efficient retrieval. Next, we cover the building blocks of *morphological development*—acquiring grammatical (inflectional) and derivational morphemes—and *syntactic development*—increasing utterance length, using different sentence modalities, and developing complex syntax. We then discuss the building blocks of *phonological development:* becoming sensitive to prosodic and phonotactic cues in streams of speech, developing internal representations of the phonemes of the native language, and becoming phonologically aware. Finally, we describe the *pragmatic development* building blocks: acquiring communication functions, developing conversational skills, and gaining sensitivity to extralinguistic cues. As we discuss each building block, we include a brief examination of important influences—such as gender, socioeconomic status, and language impairment—on children's achievements.

WHAT IS SEMANTIC DEVELOPMENT?

Semantic development refers to an individual's learning and storage of the meanings of words. Consider the following conversations between a mother and her 3-year-old daughter:

Friday, at home in the kitchen:

ADELAIDE: Mommy, what's this? (*points to a vent on the baseboard*)

LAURA: That's a vent. A vent lets air come into the room.

ADELAIDE: It's a vent.

Saturday, at the children's museum:

ADELAIDE: There's another went, Mommy. (*points to a speaker embedded in the wall*)

LAURA: A went? What's a went?

ADELAIDE: A went puts air into the room.

LAURA: Oh! You mean *vent*. That's a speaker; it looks like a vent, but that makes noise. People speak through it.

These two conversational snippets are useful to understanding the processes by which children learn and store new words. When encountering a new word, the child must develop an internal representation of the word that includes its phonological form (the specific sounds in it and their order), its grammatical role (e.g., verb, pronoun, noun), and its conceptual meaning. In this example, notice how readily Adelaide incorporated a new word—*vent*—into her vocabulary. These excerpts also show how knowledge of a specific word matures with time and that a child's early knowledge and use of a word may be incomplete. With additional exposure to the word in various contexts, Adelaide's initial representation will develop from a relatively immature state to a more flexible, adultlike representation.

Semantic Building Blocks

Semantic development involves three major tasks for the language learner: (a) acquiring a *mental lexicon* of about 60,000 words between infancy and adulthood, (b) learning *new words* rapidly, and (c) organizing the mental lexicon in an efficient *semantic network*.

Mental Lexicon

A person's **mental lexicon** is the volume of words he or she understands (**receptive lexicon**) and uses (**expressive lexicon**). Typically, the receptive lexicon is larger because an individual usually understands many more words than he or she actually uses. Estimates of the size of a child's lexicon show that its volume increases remarkably quickly during the first several years of life—from only several words at age 12 months to 300 words at age 24 months to 60,000 words by early adulthood (Aitchinson, 1994; Fenson, Dale, Reznick, Bates, & Thal, 1994). A typical child acquires about 860 words per year between ages 1 and 7 years, averaging about 2 new words per day during this period (Biemiller, 2005).

One long-standing perspective in the field of child language acquisition is that children undergo a **vocabulary spurt** that begins near the end of the second year and continues for several years subsequently (Choi & Gopnik, 1995). The term

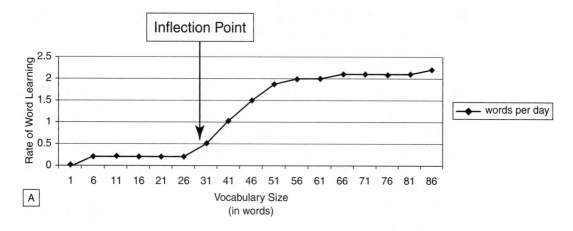

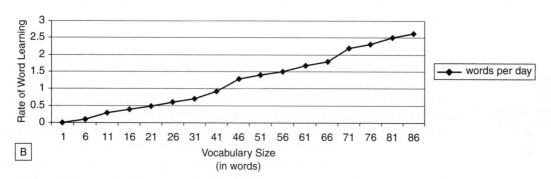

FIGURE 3.1

Lexical development featuring a vocabulary spurt (Graph A) compared with gradual linear growth (Graph B).

Source: Adapted from "Reexamining the Vocabulary Spurt," by J. Ganger and M. R. Brent, 2004, *Developmental Psychology, 40,* pp. 621–632.

spurt implies that children transition from a slow stage of development to a rapid stage of development, with an **inflection point** differentiating the stages (Ganger & Brent, 2004), as illustrated in Figure 3.1A. However, some researchers pointed out that relatively few children (25% in one study of toddlers' lexical growth) experience a vocabulary spurt (Ganger & Brent, 2004); rather, most show a continuous, linear increase in their lexical size (Figure 3.1B). These researchers argued that the concept of a vocabulary spurt is not a universal principle, but applies to only a few children. Thus, although the size of the lexicon does undergo remarkable growth, whether lexical growth is appropriately represented as a spurtlike phenomenon rather than as a more continuous, linear trajectory is unclear.

When practitioners consider the size of a child's lexicon, they consider not only its volume but also the individual lexical items it contains. A *semantic taxonomy* differentiates words on the basis of their semantic roles (Ingram, 1989). K. Nelson's (1973) semantic taxonomy differentiates children's lexical items into five categories (Ingram, 1989):

1. *Specific nominals,* which refer to a specific object (e.g., *Daddy, Fluffy*)
2. *General nominals,* which refer to all members of a category (e.g., *those, cats*)
3. *Action words,* which describe specific actions (e.g., *up*), social-action games (e.g., peekaboo), and action inhibitors (e.g., *no*)
4. *Modifiers,* which describe properties and qualities (e.g., *big, mine*)
5. *Personal–social words,* which describe affective states and relationships (e.g., *yes, bye-bye*)

Children's early lexicons, comprising the first 50 or so words, typically contain at least 1 word in each semantic category. K. Nelson's (1973) longitudinal study of 18 children's early lexical development revealed that general nominals predominated, corresponding to 51% of all words in the lexicon, and specific nominals and action words composed an additional 14% and 13%, respectively, of lexical entries. Modifiers (9% of words) and personal–social words (8% of words) composed a relatively small number of children's early lexical items. (An additional 4% of the words did not fit into any of these categories.)

New Words

DISCUSSION POINT

What are some examples of new or novel words you heard recently?

When a child encounters a word for the first time, his or her knowledge of the word is incomplete; in fact, the child's knowledge of the word is just beginning. The same is true for adults. Suppose that in a recent class lecture your professor used the word *phonotactic* and you had never heard this word before. (This term was introduced in Chapter 1.) Following your initial exposure to the word, it may seem familiar to you the next time you hear it, but you may not think you have a deepened understanding of it. In fact, you may hesitate to use the new word again, and if you do, you may use it incorrectly. This example provides a general approximation of the course of learning a new word, in which a person first achieves a general familiarity with the word—including its phonological form and its conceptual meaning—and, with time, develops a much deeper and more flexible knowledge of the word.

The process children use to learn new words is similar. Following initial exposure to a novel word, children may have a general understanding of its meaning and may even begin to express the word, albeit not always correctly (Brackenbury & Fey, 2003). Between the initial exposure to a word and the achievement of a deepened flexible understanding of the word, knowledge of a word is in a "fragile" state, meaning that errors in understanding and use of the word will likely occur (McGregor, Friedman, Reilly, & Newman, 2002). The rapidity with which a child develops a more adultlike understanding of a word is influenced by a number of factors. We consider three of them next:

1. *Concept represented by the word.* As children engage in learning a new word, some words are clearly easier to learn than others because of the concepts the words express. For instance, children learn the words *go* and *hit,* which refer to concrete actions, more easily than *think* and *know,* which represent abstract concepts (Gleitman, Cassidy, Nappa, Papafragou, & Trueswell, 2005). Words referring to abstractions are considered "hard words" (Gleitman et al., 2005) because they are relatively difficult for children to learn compared with other words. Words are "hard" when the concept to which they refer is not accessible to the child (Smiley & Huttenlocher, 1995). Words that describe beliefs and mental states—such as *think* and *know*—are often not acquired until age 3 or 4 years, whereas words such as *see* and *walk* are learned earlier (Gopnik & Meltzoff, 1997). Therefore, when an individual encounters a new word, the concept or meaning represented by the word influences the ease with which the word is learned.

2.   *Phonological form of the word.* When an individual learns a new word, he or she must acquire not only knowledge of the conceptual referent of the word, but also its phonological form (Nash & Donaldson, 2005). Two substantial differences exist among the phonological features of words. First, the relationship between the phonological form of a word and the concept to which it refers is most often arbitrary, but this is not true in all cases. Exceptions are onomatopoeic words, such as *boom* and *crash,* in which a more transparent relationship exists between the phonological form of the word and the concept it represents. Not surprisingly, many young children will use onomatopoeic words first to refer to objects (e.g., calling a cow a *moo,* or a cat a *meow*) instead of their more conventional labels. Second, some words contain sounds and sound sequences that occur relatively often in spoken language, called *common sound sequences* (e.g., the first two sounds in *sit*), whereas other words contain sounds and sound sequences that occur infrequently, called *rare sound sequences* (e.g., the first two sounds in *these;* Storkel, 2001). Children learn words containing common sound sequences more readily than words containing rare sound sequences (Storkel, 2001).

DISCUSSION POINT

What specific types of information would make a word-learning context "very" ostentive?

3.   *Contextual conditions at initial exposure.* Children's initial and subsequent exposures to a new word vary considerably according to the contextual conditions in which it is embedded. Children draw on many sources of contextual information to develop and refine their internal representations of novel words (Gleitman et al., 2005). They draw on information from the linguistic context, such as the grammar of the utterance containing a new word (e.g., "This is a vent" vs. "I dropped my ring into the vent") and the extent to which semantic features of the word are described (e.g., "A vent blows air into a room" vs. "I think the vent isn't working"). Children also draw on information from the extralinguistic context, seeking overt cues from the environment that clearly label or define the referent of a new word, such as the eye gaze and gestures of their conversational partners (Jaswal & Markman, 2001b). In **ostentive word-learning contexts,** a great deal of contextual information is provided about a novel word either linguistically or extralinguistically, whereas in **nonostentive word-learning contexts** (also called *inferential contexts*), little contextual information is provided to help a person derive the meaning of a new word (Jaswal & Markman, 2001b).

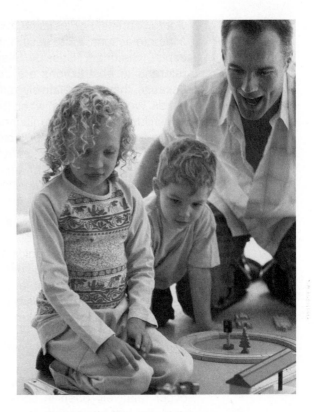

Children refine their knowledge of the meaning of a new word through repeated exposure to the word in different contexts.

(*Photo Source:* © Royalty-Free/Corbis.)

Studies of children's word learning in ostentive versus nonostentive contexts have yielded interesting findings about the remarkable ability of young children to learn new words. For example, comparisons of 3-year-olds' learning of new words show that when relatively little extralinguistic information is available, children draw on cues from the linguistic context (e.g., the phonological form or grammatical role of the word) to learn the meanings of new words, which results in similar word-learning rates in both ostentive and nonostentive contexts (Jaswal & Markman, 2001b). However, evidence also suggests that when more rather than less contextual information is provided, children's novel word learning is supported. For example, when extralinguistic cues—such as pointing—are combined with a variety of linguistic cues—such as juxtaposing a novel word against a known word: "See the bird? Look, a beak!"—children's word learning is superior to that when only one type of information is provided (Saylor & Sabbagh, 2004). In short, to develop a representation of a new word, children use various tools to draw on information from the linguistic and extralinguistic contexts in which the word is embedded.

Semantic Network

A person's mental lexicon, comprising the store of words he or she understands and uses, is not organized randomly; rather, as the human brain acquires new words, they are stored in a **semantic network** in which its entries are organized according to connective ties among them. The connections among words vary in strength from strong to weak according to the extent to which they share syntactic, phonological, or semantic features. For instance, the association between the two pronouns *him* and *her* is fairly strong because of similarities in syntactic roles; so is the association between *pin* and *pit* because of shared phonological features, and *whale* and *dolphin* because of semantic similarities. Thus, a person's mental lexicon contains a vast network of lexical entries linked by connective ties that vary in relative strength.

One important point to note is that in a semantic network, the entries themselves do not carry meaning; the links between the entries do (Harley, 2001). Theories on how an individual accesses specific entries in the semantic network emphasize a process called **spreading activation,** in which activation of specific entries spreads across the network according to the strength of connections among entries. For instance, if the word *bird* is activated, a number of additional entries in the semantic network are also activated because of semantic similarities (e.g., *wings, robin, canary;* Harley, 2001).

As a child learns new words, they are stored in his or her semantic network. Young children often make a number of naming errors (McGregor et al., 2002); such errors are particularly prominent in the second year of life (Dapretto & Bjork, 2000). For instance, a child may call a *kangaroo* a *mouse,* or a *saddle* a *chair* (McGregor et al., 2002). These types of errors provide an interesting glimpse into the organization of a child's semantic network; calling a *kangaroo* a *mouse* suggests that these two entries are stored closely and that the lexical representation of *mouse* may be stronger (i.e., more robust) than that of *kangaroo.* The strength of the word *mouse* interferes with the child's lexical access to the *kangaroo* entry, which may be relatively fragile (McGregor et al., 2002). As the child's lexical representation of *kangaroo* strengthens, naming accuracy improves and this entry becomes "less vulnerable to retrieval failure" (McGregor et al., 2002, p. 343).

Influences on Semantic Development

Several factors influence not only the rate with which children build their lexicon but also the ease with which they learn new words and their efficiency in retrieving words from the lexicon.

Gender

In the first several years of language acquisition, girls usually have larger vocabularies and learn words more easily than boys do (Bornstein, Hahn, & Haynes, 2004; J. Huttenlocher, Haight, Bryk, Seltzer, & Lyons, 1991; Reznick & Goldfield, 1992). The results of a study of 2-year-olds' expressive vocabularies showed girls know an average of 363 words versus 227 words for boys (Bornstein et al., 2004). However, these early differences often attenuate, if not disappear, by age 6–7 years (Bornstein et al., 2004). Most likely, these early differences in semantic development result from a combination of biological, psychological, and social variables (Bornstein et al., 2004). Biologically, girls' neurological development is faster than boys', including the lateralization of language to the left hemisphere

DISCUSSION POINT
What are some specific ways in which parents converse differently with boys than with girls?

(Shaywitz et al., 1995). Psychologically and socially, gender-typed interests may influence the types of interactions children experience. For instance, parent–child play with trucks, occurring more frequently for boys than for girls, may elicit fewer extended conversations compared with those elicited by parent–child play with dolls (Caldera, Huston, & O'Brien, 1989). Research results also suggest that girls in day care receive more attention from teachers than boys do (National Institute of Child Health and Human Development [NICHD] Early Child Care Research Network, 1997), which raises the possibility that early gender differences in semantic development result not only from biological differences but also from opportunities to learn language from adults.

Language Impairment

Children who exhibit a neurologically based language impairment (LI) typically have significantly smaller vocabularies than those of their peers without LI (Nash & Donaldson, 2005). Difficulties in learning new words and poorly organized semantic networks contribute to these differences in lexical size (e.g., S. Gray, 2003; Nash & Donaldson, 2005). In a study of the rate at which 4- to 5-year-old children learned new words, S. Gray (2003) determined the number of learning trials children needed to learn a new word. During each learning trial, children were exposed to a novel word during play activities in which the adult modeled the word and prompted the child to produce the word. Typically developing children required an average of 11.6 trials to produce a new word, compared with nearly 14 trials for children with LI. In addition to learning new words more slowly, many children with LI exhibit word-finding errors and slower retrieval of items from the semantic network, possibly as a result of the extended time these children require to develop a robust representation for a lexical entry (McGregor, 1997).

Language Exposure

Numerous studies have revealed a significant relationship between the number and types of words children hear in their environment and the size of their vocabulary (Hart & Risley, 1995; Hoff, 2003; J. Huttenlocher et al., 1991). Children reared in orphanages who experience relatively little language input typically show depressed vocabularies (Glennen, 2002). The same finding is true for children reared in low socioeconomic status (SES) households compared with children living in higher SES households (e.g., Hart & Risley, 1995), presumably because children in lower SES households are exposed to fewer words. Hart and Risley's (1995) seminal work in this area indicated that kindergartners' accumulated experience with words differed by more than 30 million words for children in low SES homes versus children in higher SES homes. As Neuman (2006) pointed out, one explanation for this substantial variability in children's exposure to words as a function of SES is the striking effect of poverty on parents' emotional resources, which compromises the quality and frequency of parents' conversational interactions with their children. Given that 13 million children in the United States live in poverty (DeNavas-Walt, Proctor, & Lee, 2005), this early vocabulary achievement gap is a significant educational problem in the United States. Multicultural Focus: *Language Development and Children Living in Poverty* covers this topic in more detail.

MULTICULTURAL FOCUS

Language Development and Children Living in Poverty

Often the term *multicultural* brings to mind the cultural differences that arise from religion, race, ethnicity, country of origin, and ability or disability. However, in many countries, substantial cultural differences exist between people who are economically advantaged and those who are economically disadvantaged. In the United States, children living in poverty comprise a singularly large cultural group: Twenty percent of all children younger than age 18 years (13 million) reside in households with annual incomes less than the poverty threshold ($19,157 for a family of four), and 40% live in low-income homes (twice the annual poverty threshold; DeNavas-Walt et al., 2005). Compared with White children, African American and Hispanic children are much more likely to live in poverty.

You might wonder what poverty has to do with language development, particularly the building blocks discussed in this chapter. Unfortunately, a strong negative relationship exists between poverty and language achievement. Children raised in poverty and in low-income households consistently know fewer words, produce shorter utterances, use a smaller variety of words, and have less developed phonological skills than peers raised in more advantageous circumstances do (e.g., Fazio, Naremore, & Connell, 1996; Hart & Risley, 1995; Hoff-Ginsberg, 1998; Whitehurst, 1997). Beyond language, poverty affects many other areas of child development, including cognition and learning, socioemotional functioning, and general health (Shonkoff & Phillips, 2000).

When considering how poverty most affects language, researchers point to two major influences: parental socioemotional resources and parental access to material resources. Concerning the first, poverty takes an immense toll on parents' socioemotional resources; significantly higher rates of maternal depression occur when financial resources are stressed (Mistry, Biesanz, Taylor, Burchinal, & Cox, 2004). Compared with higher income mothers, mothers living in poverty show lower levels of warmth, responsiveness, and sensitivity when interacting with their young children (Wallace, Roberts, & Lodder, 1998). High levels of maternal sensitivity and responsiveness directly support children's language development.

Poverty also undermines a family's material and financial resources. Families living in poverty do not have access to the same level of medical care as that of advantaged families, so their children often have more handicapping illnesses and injuries that may affect language development (e.g., chronic middle ear infections). Likewise, these families cannot take advantage of the "lessons, summer camps, stimulating learning materials and activities, and better quality early childhood care" available to children from advantaged backgrounds (Neuman, 2006, p. 30). Not surprisingly, literally hundreds of researchers have documented the deleterious effects of poverty on the building blocks of language and the "dramatic, linear, negative relationships between poverty and children's cognitive-developmental outcomes" (Neuman, 2006, p. 30).

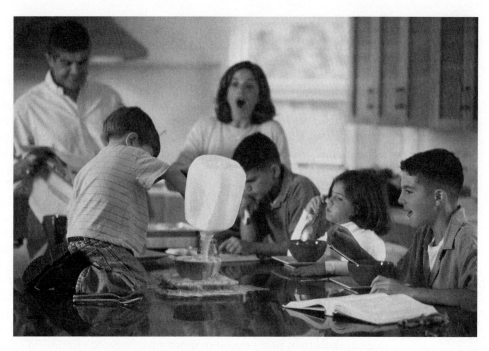

A significant relationship exists between the number and types of words children hear in their environment and the size of their vocabulary.

(*Photo Source:* © Ariel Skelley/Corbis.)

WHAT IS MORPHOLOGICAL DEVELOPMENT?

Children's *morphological development* is their internalization of the rules of language that govern word structure. *Morphemes* are the smallest meaningful units of language, and many words comprise a combination of several morphemes. Morphemes allow the grammatical inflection of words, as in adding *–ed* to *walk* to create the past tense verb *walked,* and they are used to change the syntactic class of words, as in adding *–like* to the noun *child* to create the adjective *childlike.* Morphological development thus provides children with the tools for grammatical inflection as well as a means for expanding their vocabulary from a smaller set of root words (e.g., *child*) to an exponentially larger set of derived forms (e.g., *childless, childlike, childish*).

Morphological Building Blocks

Morphological development involves acquiring two types of morphemes: **grammatical morphemes** (also called *inflectional morphemes*) and **derivational morphemes.** As discussed in Chapter 1, grammatical morphemes include the plural *-s* (*cat–cats*), the possessive *'s* (*mom–mom's*), the past tense *–ed* (*walk–walked*), and the present progressive *-ing* (*do–doing*), to name a few. Derivational morphemes are morphemes added to words to change their syntactic class and semantic meaning. For example, taking the word *like,* we can add both prefixes (*dislike, unlike*) and suffixes (*liken, likeable, likeness*) to vary its meaning and syntactic role in a sentence.

Grammatical Morphemes

Children's earliest words and sentences contain few grammatical morphemes, but only for the first year or two. At about age 2 years, children begin to use the first-appearing grammatical morpheme, the present progressive *–ing.* Whereas before then the child might ask "Where Mommy go?" he or she now asks "Where Mommy going?" In subsequent chapters, we discuss in more detail the child's timing and course of acquisition for learning the major grammatical morphemes, which include not only the present progressive *–ing,* but also the plural *-s,* the possessive *'s,* and the past tense *–ed,* as shown in Table 3.1. Note that the grammatical morphemes in Table 3.1 include not only suffixes but also several free morphemes. Suffixes (and prefixes) are called **bound morphemes** because they must be attached to other morphemes. In contrast, **free morphemes** can stand alone; they include both words with clear semantic referents (e.g., *dream, dog, walk*) and also words that serve primarily grammatical purposes (e.g., *his, the, that*). Children's early achievements in grammatical morphology include acquiring not only

TABLE 3.1

Grammatical morphemes acquired in early childhood.

Grammatical morpheme	Age (in months)	Example
Present progressive *-ing*	19–28	"Mommy eating"
Plural *-s*	27–30	"Baby shoes"
Preposition *in*	27–30	"Hat in box"
Preposition *on*	31–34	"Hat on chair"
Possessive *'s*	31–34	"Baby's ball"
Regular past tense *-ed*	43–46	"Kitty jumped"
Irregular past tense	43–46	"We ate."
Regular third person singular *-s*	43–46	"Mommy drives."
Articles *a, the, an*	43–46	"The car"
Contractible copula *be*	43–46	"She's happy."
Contractible auxiliary	47–50	"She's coming."
Uncontractible copula *be*	47–50	"We were here"
Uncontractible auxiliary	47–50	"She was coming"
Irregular third person	47–50	"She did it."

Source: From *Communication Sciences and Disorders: An Introduction* (p. 56), by L. M. Justice, 2006, Upper Saddle River, NJ: Merrill/Prentice Hall. Copyright 2006 by Pearson Education. Reprinted with permission. (Adapted from *A First Language: The Early Stages,* by R. Brown, 1973, Cambridge, MA: Harvard University Press.)

bound morphemes but also several free morphemes that serve purely grammatical purposes, including the prepositions *in* and *on* and the articles *the, a,* and *an.*

The child's acquisition of the major grammatical morphemes, which follows a fairly invariant course in both the order and the timing of acquisition, is a subtle but important achievement in early childhood. Although parents do not often applaud (or possibly even notice) when their children first begin to inflect verbs for past tense, the achievement of grammatical morphology enables the child's movement from speaking with a "telegraphic quality" (e.g., "Baby no eat") to a more adultlike quality ("The baby's not eating").

When researchers study children's achievement of grammatical morphology, they often look for **obligatory contexts** of use and determine whether the child has omitted or included the obligatory morpheme. An obligatory context occurs when a mature grammar specifies use of a grammatical marker; for instance, in the sentence *The dog's bone is lost,* the possessive *'s* is considered obligatory. Thus, if a child says "The dog bone lost," he or she is omitting the possessive *'s* morpheme in an obligatory context. When children include a grammatical morpheme in 75% or more of obligatory contexts, they are said to have mastered the morpheme.

Derivational Morphemes

DISCUSSION POINT

Using the word *school,* identify all the morphemes that can be added to it to inflect it. Classify each morpheme as grammatical or derivational.

Derivational morphemes are morphemes added to root words to create derived words. The corpus of words derived from a common root word (e.g., *friend, friendless, friendliness, befriend*) share **derivational relations.** Derived words are created by attaching morphemes, both prefixes and suffixes, to root words to yield *polysyllabic words* (words containing more than one syllable). Table 3.2 presents some common prefixes and suffixes used for derivational purposes. Because each prefix and suffix can be combined with many root words, development of derivational morphology is a powerful tool for adding precision to a person's lexical base.

Influences on Morphological Development

One of the seminal works of child language research is Roger Brown's (1973) book *Words and Things.* In this key work, Brown carefully described children's development of 14 grammatical morphemes, showing how a core of grammatical morphemes emerged in a uniform order among children. These morphemes are listed in Table 3.1. Brown's work had a tremendous influence on the field of child language research, prompting many researchers to focus their attention on describing other such universalities in child language development.

Since then, researchers have begun to appreciate the importance of studying individual differences in language acquisition and identifying specific influences that do and do not affect the normal course of language acquisition. For example, researchers have questioned whether a child's native language influences his or her development of grammatical morphology. Contrary to what you might expect, children learning languages that are richly inflected (e.g., Spanish) do not acquire novel morphemes at faster rates than those of children learning less richly inflected languages (e.g., English; see Research Paradigms: *Use of Fast Mapping to Study Morphological*

TABLE 3.2
Common derivational prefixes and suffixes.

Prefix	Examples	Suffix	Examples
un-	*unease*	*-y*	*guilty*
dis-	*disappear*	*-ly*	*happily*
re-	*rerun*	*-like*	*adultlike*
pre-	*preview*	*-tion*	*adoption*
uni-	*unitard*	*-ful*	*bountiful*
tri-	*tricycle*	*-less*	*tactless*
inter-	*intergalactic*	*-er*	*bigger*
fore-	*forecast*	*-est*	*hardest*
post-	*postcard*	*-ness*	*gentleness*
co-	*cohabitate*	*-ish*	*selfish*
im-	*immodest*	*-able*	*amicable*
anti-	*antipathy*	*-ician*	*pediatrician*
sub-	*subarctic*	*-ism*	*organism*
in-	*ineffective*	*-logy*	*anthropology*
un-	*unplug*	*-phobia*	*arachnophobia*

Source: Adapted from *Word Study for Phonics, Vocabulary, and Spelling Instruction,* by D. R. Bear, M. Invernizzi, S. Templeton, and F. Johnston, 2004, Upper Saddle River, NJ: Merrill Prentice Hall.

Development). Conversely, though, learning English as a second language does appear to affect morphological development (in English), and when children learn various English dialects, differences in morphological development are also apparent.

Second Language Acquisition

Persons learning a second language that differs considerably in its grammatical morphology from their native language may never master the grammatical morphology of the second language (Bialystok & Miller, 1999; Jia, Aaronson, & Wu, 2002). For instance, native Chinese speakers who learn English as a second language find the plural marker difficult to master because plurality is not inflected morphologically in the Chinese language (Jia, 2003). This problem is particularly true when persons learn a second language at an older age rather than at a younger age or when a specific morpheme is not inflected in a person's native language. However, even for younger children, learning the grammatical morphology of a second language can be a challenge. Jia's (2003) longitudinal study of 10 Chinese-speaking children during a 5-year period focused on the acquisition of the plural *-s,* which is not grammatically inflected in Chinese. Three of the 10 children, even after 5 years' immersion in English, never mastered the plural morpheme, and those who did so were usually younger at their initial immersion in English. The 3 children who failed to master the plural morpheme used it in fewer than 80% of obligatory contexts, typically omitting the plural marker.

RESEARCH PARADIGMS

Use of Fast Mapping to Study Morphological Development

Languages vary considerably in the extent to which words are morphologically marked (Bedore & Leonard, 2000). For instance, Spanish is a more inflectionally rich language than English. Not surprisingly, Spanish-speaking children begin to use grammatical morphemes earlier than English-speaking children do (Radford & Ploennig-Pacheco, 1995). Researchers have asked whether children learning an inflectionally rich language are better able to use morphological cues to learn new words. One research paradigm used to answer this question is **fast mapping.**

Using fast-mapping tasks, researchers examine the rate at which children learn new words. A typical scenario involves exposing children to a novel or nonsense word, often a nonsense word, and its referent. For instance, Bedore and Leonard (2000) used the nonsense word *neen* to describe a doll's twisting action at the waist. Soon after the initial exposure, experimenters study the children's learning of the word, or how the children "fast map" a new word onto its referent.

Bedore and Leonard (2000) used the fast-mapping paradigm to determine how well Spanish-speaking and English-speaking 3-year-old children used verb morphology to learn new words. In their study, they exposed children to novel words that were grammatically inflected (such as *neens*) and tested the children's understanding of the words when they were produced in an uninflected form (*neen*). If the Spanish-speaking children performed better than the English-speaking children did, this result would suggest that learning a morphologically rich language gives children a bootstrap for learning new words. However, these researchers found that Spanish-speaking and English-speaking children performed similarly in the fast-mapping task. Bedore and Leonard concluded that the Spanish-speaking children had no advantage over the English-speaking children, even though the former group used more grammatical morphemes and had more exposure to grammatical morphology at age 3 years than the latter group did. Therefore, although children who learn inflectionally rich languages produce grammatical morphemes earlier than children who learn inflectionally poor languages do, this fact does not seem to give these children an added boost in acquiring new words.

Dialect

Dialects are the variants of a single language. The dialects of a language vary in a number of important ways from the "general dialect," including their morphology. Even among speakers of a single language (e.g., English), achievement of specific morphological building blocks can vary substantially as a function of the morphological features of the dialect the speakers are acquiring. In the United States, one dialect many speakers share is African American Vernacular English (AAVE). Some morphological features of AAVE differ from

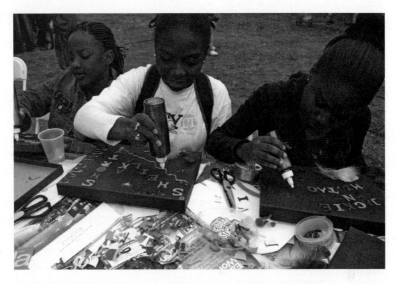

Many English dialects are spoken in the United States. One common dialect is African American Vernacular English (AAVE), which varies from other dialects in some aspects of semantics, morphology, phonology, and syntax.

(*Photo Source:* © Jeff Greenberg/PhotoEdit Inc.)

those of General American English (GAE), including the use of copulative, or *be,* auxiliary verbs; verb tense inflections; and possessive and plural inflections (Charity, Scarborough, & Griffin, 2004). For instance, a GAE speaker may say, "Tom's aunt," whereas an AAVE speaker may say, "Tom aunt," omitting the posessive marker (Reid, 2000). Some children learn only the AAVE dialect, whereas other children learn the AAVE dialect before, while, or after learning the GAE dialect. AAVE-speaking students who have more knowledge of GAE perform better in reading development, possibly because less of a mismatch occurs between the written form of language they encounter in school (which uses GAE) and the dialect they speak (Charity et al., 2004). At least in part, the mismatch between AAVE and GAE involves differences in morphology, particularly grammatical inflections.

Language Impairment

Language impairment affects morphological development, often in significant ways. In fact, one hallmark of specific language impairment (SLI), a developmental language disorder we discuss in Chapter 10, is difficulty with grammatical morphology. For instance, when typically developing children use the present progressive *-ing* with more than 80% accuracy, children with SLI use it with only 25% accuracy (Conti-Ramsden & Jones, 1997). In large part, the grammatical morphology difficulties of children with SLI involve problems with verb markings, such as the past tense inflection and the third-person singular inflection.

WHAT IS SYNTACTIC DEVELOPMENT?

Syntactic development is children's internalization of the rules of language that govern how words are organized into sentences. As Pinker (1994) stated in *The Language Instinct,*

> When a dog bites a man that is not news, but when a man bites a dog that is news. . . . The streams of words called "sentences" . . . tell you who in fact did what to whom. (p. 83)

As children develop from single-word users to conveyers of complex thoughts and ideas that involve stringing many words together, they develop a fine-tuned understanding of how to organize words into sentences that carefully specify "who did what to whom" as well as what they want ("May I please watch the Thomas video?"), remember ("Mommy, Daddy told me we couldn't go to the toy store"), and imagine ("I think if we go to the toy store I'll get to buy a new movie"). Children develop this sophisticated ability to organize words into larger propositions by gradually internalizing the grammatical system of their language. Essentially, *grammar* refers to the rules and principles that speakers of a language use to structure sentences. An example of such a rule is the use of the nominative pronoun form (e.g., *I, he, she*) rather than the objective form (e.g., *me, him, her*) when a personal pronoun follows a *be* verb; thus, "It is he" is considered "grammatically correct" instead of "It is him." These rules and principles are "in the heads" of native speakers, a "mental grammar" so to speak, allowing people to produce and comprehend grammar with remarkable rapidity and ease (Jacobs, 1995, p. 4).

Syntactic Building Blocks

The grammatical system a child acquires from birth onward is a "discrete combinatorial system" consisting of a finite number of discrete elements that allow the child to produce an infinite number of sentences (Pinker, 1994). As children internalize this combinatorial system, they exhibit three major syntactic achievements: (a) an increase in utterance length, (b) use of different sentence modalities, and (c) the development of complex syntax.

Utterance Length

A major accomplishment most children achieve with relative ease by their sixth birthday is the production of utterances that are, on average, nearly as long as those of adults. Contrast these two utterances produced by Tahim:

18 MONTHS: Daddy no.

62 MONTHS: No, put that one over there, there on the blocks I set up.

At 18 months, Tahim's utterance length averages 1.3 morphemes, whereas at 62 months his average utterance length exceeds 8 morphemes. Like Tahim, most children have an utterance length that gradually increases from ages 1 to 6 years, and these increases reflect the children's ability to chain together morphemes to produce an infinite variety of sentences.

Calculating the mean number of morphemes per utterance provides a simple proxy for estimating the syntactic complexity of children's utterances, at least in the first 5 years of development. Children with an average utterance length of two morphemes speak with a telegraphic quality in which grammatical markers (e.g., articles, conjunctions, auxiliary verbs) are omitted, as in Tahim's "Daddy no." In contrast, children with an average utterance length of four morphemes use a variety of grammatical markers to organize their sentences, including articles, conjunctions, and auxiliary verbs. In other words, when children produce longer utterances, they are not simply stringing words together haphazardly (e.g., "Daddy no go up") but are using various grammatical structures to organize sentences in precise and adultlike ways ("Daddy, I really don't think we should go up there").

Sentence Modalities

Once children begin to string together morphemes to create longer and longer utterances, they begin to produce sentences of various types, or modalities. During the early years of syntactic development, children become increasingly skilled at producing different sentence types that vary not only in their pragmatic intent, but also in their syntactic organization. In large part, the differences among sentence types reside in how words are grammatically organized at a surface level.

Declaratives. **Declarative sentences** make a statement, and simple declaratives often use these six organizational schemes (Eastwood & Mackin, 1982):

1. Subject + Verb: *I am working!*
2. Subject + Verb + Object: *She wants something.*
3. Subject + Verb + Complement: *I feel good.*
4. Subject + Verb + Adverb phrase: *I feel good today.*
5. Subject + Verb + Indirect object + Direct object: *She gave Tommy the hammer.*
6. Subject + Verb + Direct object + Indirect object: *The teacher sent me home.*

Three-year-old children have commonly mastered most of these basic declarative patterns and even use coordinating and subordinating conjunctions to link several, as in "I am working and she is too!" An important point is that during the early years of language acquisition, children are never taught explicitly *how* to produce these and other types of declarative sentences; rather, they intuit the rules from the language they experience around them and gradually become capable of producing an infinite variety of declaratives on the basis of these internalized rules.

Negatives. Any adult who has spent much time with children recognizes that many master the use of the negative sentence fairly early in development. Following are a few examples:

"No, I not going!"

"I don't want to!"

"I'm not eating that!"

"Don't do that!"

Negative sentences express negation and rely on such words as *no, not, can't, don't,* and *won't* to do so. The child's development of the art of negation involves learning where to insert these negative markers into sentences. Bellugi's (1967) extensive research on the language development of three children showed that the syntactic structure of negative sentences emerges in a predictable order. Children's first use of the negative sentence modality typically has a pattern in which the word *no* is placed at the beginning of the sentence, as in "No eat that." Soon after, the negative word moves inside the sentence next to the main verb, as in "I not eat that" and "You no do that." By age 4 years, many children use the auxiliary forms of verbs that approximate adultlike negation, as in "You can't do that" and "I don't want to go." However, other and more nuanced negative sentences may not emerge until several years later, such as passive sentences containing the modal verb *won't* ("She won't be getting a prize") and negative sentences that involve probability estimates ("I'm not sure if she'll get the prize").

Interrogatives. **Interrogative sentences** involve the act of questioning. Children become amazingly sophisticated at organizing sentences so that they can obtain information from other people:

"Why is that light green?"

"What happened?"

"Who did it?"

"Where are you going?"

"Is it snowing?"

"He's sad; isn't he?"

Although individuals can pose questions using declarative sentences by raising intonation at the end ("He's going?"), syntax provides an important vehicle for question asking that children discover early in life. Children's development of the interrogative sentence modality includes achievement of two major question types: **wh- questions** and **yes–no questions.** Many children's earliest interrogatives include the *wh-* words, such as *what, where,* and *why,* as in "What that?" "Where Daddy go?" and "Why he not here?" Children's repertoire of question words expands during the preschool years to include *who, whose, when, which,* and *how. Wh-* questions seek specific information about time, place, manner, reason, and quantity (Jacobs, 1995), whereas yes–no questions seek a yes or no response, as in "Are we going?" and "Can you see me?"

In producing interrogatives, children draw on specific syntactic rules to organize sentences for questioning purposes. To produce the *wh-* question "What may I take to school?" children must use a highly specific syntactic organization that differs significantly from the comparable declarative form ("I may take the train to school"). The interrogative sentence involves placing the *wh-* word in the initial noun phrase slot and "emptying" the object slot. Production of yes–no questions involves similar sorts of syntactic maneuvers. Consider the syntactic differences between this declarative sentence and its interrogative counterpart:

Declarative: He is going to go.

Interrogative: Is he going to go?

In forming the yes–no interrogative, children must move the auxiliary verb *is* from its place following the subject *he* and preceding its main verb *going* so that it appears before the subject (Jacobs, 1995). As simple as yes–no questions may seem, they require a sophisticated syntactic maneuver that children master at relatively young ages.

Complex Syntax: Linking Phrases and Clauses

The syntactic development of young children is often,monitored by calculating the average length of their utterances, or MLU (mean length of utterance). Though the MLU is a handy tool for estimating children's syntactic development, it does not provide much detail concerning more nuanced achievements in syntax, particularly the child's use of phrase and clause structures. A *phrase* is a cluster of words organized around a *head.* Types of phrases include noun phrases (*the tall, angry boy*), prepositional phrases (*in the bucket*), adjectival phrases (*very happy*), and verb phrases (*was saddened;* in each example, we underscored the head of the phrase). With phrasal development, sentences become increasingly elaborate, as shown in Figure 3.2. As children begin to use more elaborate phrase structures, they develop skill in **phrasal coordination,** which allows them to connect phrases, as in this sentence in which *and* links two noun phrases: *I'm putting on my coat and my hat.*

A *clause* is a syntactic structure containing a verb or a verb phrase; when we produce sentences, we often join a number of clauses by using specific rules. For instance, the sentence *I'll go and you stay* contains two independent clauses (*I'll go; you stay*) conjoined with the coordinating conjunction *and.* The sentence *That boy who hit me is in time-out* contains a dependent clause (*who hit me*) embedded within an independent clause (*That boy is in time-out*).

DISCUSSION POINT

Have you ever had to diagram a complex sentence? If so, why do so many students find this activity such a challenge when they have been able to produce complex sentences since early childhood?

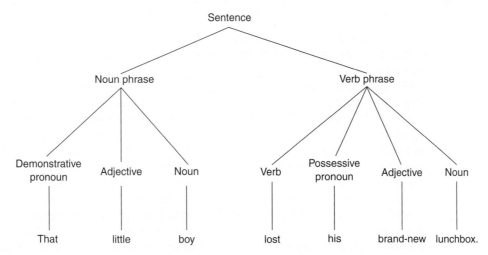

FIGURE 3.2
Example of the phrase structure of a sentence.

TABLE 3.3
Stages of grammatical development.

Stage	MLU range (midpoint)	Stage description
I	1.0–1.99 (1.75)	Single-word utterances predominate. Grammatical inflections not used.
II	2.0–2.49 (2.25)	Two- and three-word utterances predominate. Grammatical inflections emerge (e.g., present progressive marker, plural marker). Emergence of grammar as child follows basic word-order patterns (e.g., Agent + Action: "*Mommy go*"; Agent + Action + Object: "*DeeDee ate bone*").
III	2.5–2.99 (2.75)	Emergence of different sentence modalities: yes–no questions, *wh-* questions, imperatives, and negatives.
IV	3.0–3.99 (3.5)	Complex sentences emerge to feature multiclause sentences, such as object–noun phrase complements ("This is the one I made"), embedded *wh-* questions ("That's why she went outside"), and embedded relative clauses ("Clifford, who was so good, is still waiting").
V	4.0+	Emergence of coordinating conjunctions and adverbial conjuncts ("I am tired because I didn't take a nap"; "I'm helping Daddy do the dishes and make dinner").

MLU = mean length of utterance.
Source: Adapted from *A First Language: The Early Stages,* by R. Brown, 1973, Cambridge, MA: Harvard University Press.

From age 3 years onward, children begin to master the art of conjoining and embedding clauses to create sentences of not only increasing length, but also increasing syntactic complexity. Table 3.3 presents an adapted version of R. Brown's (1973) stages of grammatical development; as Table 3.3 shows, when children's utterances average 3.5 morphemes in length, the art of sentence embedding emerges. At this stage (Stage IV), children begin to use complex sentences featuring embedded subordinate clauses (*That's mine because Mommy gave it to me*), embedded *wh-* questions (*I don't know why he did it*), and relative clauses (*That boy with the crayons did it*). At this point in development, children move from using simple syntax to **complex syntax,** which refers to the use of phrase and clause structures as well as conjunctive devices for organizing internal structures of sentences. Table 3.4 presents some examples of complex syntax. Analyses of complex syntax examine children's use of different types of phrases and clauses, such as relative and infinitive clauses, as well as ways in which children embed and conjoin phrases and clauses by using coordinating and subordinating conjunctions.

TABLE 3.4
Examples of complex syntax.

Syntactic feature	Example
Double embedding	"I'm not going to think about what happened."
Infinitive clause with differing subject	"I am not sure what to think."
Object relative clause	"That's the train I lost."
Subject relative clause	"The girls who signed up didn't pay."
Wh- infinitive clause	"Tell her what you said."
Complex sentence with subordinating conjunction	"I can't go when she wants me to."
Compound sentence with coordinating conjunction	"The kids are sleeping but the teacher's about to leave."
Subject complement clause	"The kids signing up didn't know it cost money."
Perfect aspect verb	"The dog had caught it already."
Passive voice sentence	"The doll was found after we looked everywhere."
Postnoun elaboration	"Other colors like green and yellow might work too."
Multiclause sentence (+3)	"Because she didn't call first, we didn't know to wait and left without her."

Source: Adapted from "Grammar: How Can I Say That Better" by S. Eisenberg, in *Contextualized Language Intervention* (pp. 145–194), edited by T. Ukrainetz, 2006, Eau Claire, WI: Thinking Publications.

Influences on Syntactic Development

Compared with other aspects of language development, such as vocabulary, syntactic development is relatively invariant among children, proceeding in a mostly uniform pattern in both the type and the timing of developments (R. Brown, 1973; Whitehurst, 1997). This phenomenon seems particularly true during the toddler and preschool years. For instance, the results of studies suggest that the syntactic development of children reared in poverty is fairly similar to that of children raised in homes with a higher SES (Whitehurst, 1997). Comparisons of boys' and girls' syntactic achievements also show relatively few differences between the genders (Craig, Washington, & Thompson-Porter, 1998; Ely, Berko Gleason, & McCabe, 1996). These results do not mean that individual differences in children's syntactic development are nonexistent. On the contrary, even in the early years of language acquisition, differences can be seen in the length of children's sentences. Some toddlers produce utterances averaging two morphemes long, whereas other toddlers produce utterances averaging six morphemes. Individual differences among children become even more evident as children develop more complex aspects of syntax, such as clausal embedding (J. Huttenlocher, Vasilyeva, Cymerman, & Levine, 2002).

Historically, researchers emphasized the similarities in syntactic development among children. Consequently, relatively little research focused on individual differences among children and the factors that give rise to these differences.

Currently, researchers are increasingly focusing on identifying and understanding influences that affect syntactic development. We consider two of them next.

Exposure to Complex Syntax

The utterances children experience in their language-learning environments contain numerous exemplars of **simple syntax**—grammatically well-formed utterances containing simple noun phrases and verb structures (J. Huttenlocher et al., 2002). However, children vary considerably with regard to their exposure to exemplars of more complex syntax, such as embedded relative clauses, auxiliary-fronted yes–no questions, and *wh-* questions (J. Huttenlocher et al., 2002; Shatz, Hoff-Ginsberg, & MacIver, 1989). As Hoff (2004) noted, children who hear complex syntax more often in their environment produce greater amounts of complex syntax at an earlier age than do children who hear complex syntax less frequently. Hoff explained this phenomenon by using the *learning-from-input hypothesis,* which emphasizes that the grammatical properties of children's language use depend on exposure to the properties in child-directed speech. The results of two studies by J. Huttenlocher et al. (2002) substantiate this point. In these studies, researchers examined the syntactic properties of mothers' language at home and preschool teachers' language in the classroom. The researchers examined the relationship between complex syntax contained in parents' and teachers' language and children's syntactic development. The results of these studies revealed differences in maternal use of complex syntax between lower SES and middle SES parents (see Figure 3.3). The results also showed a strong linear relationship between children's exposure to complex syntax and their development of complex syntactic

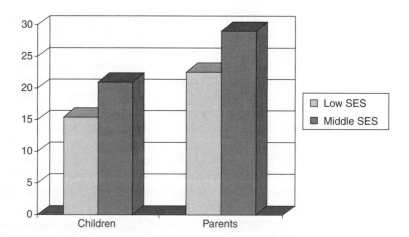

FIGURE 3.3

Percentage of mothers' and children's sentences containing complex syntax.

SES = socioeconomic status.

Source: Adapted from *Cognitive Psychology,* Vol. 45, J. Huttenlocher, M. Vasilyeva, E. Cymerman, and S. Levine, "Language Input and Child Syntax," p. 348. Copyright 2002, with permission from Elsevier.

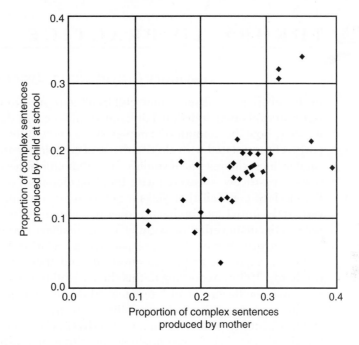

FIGURE 3.4

Relationship between mothers' and children's production of complex syntax.

Source: Reprinted from *Cognitive Psychology,* Vol. 45, J. Huttenlocher, M. Vasilyeva, E. Cymerman, and S. Levine, "Language Input and Child Syntax," p. 350, Copyright 2002, with permission from Elsevier.

forms, as depicted in Figure 3.4. Considering how such findings may translate into practice, Theory to Practice: *Auxiliary Clarification Hypothesis* provides a discussion of whether exposure to yes–no questions facilitates children's acquisition of auxiliary verbs.

Language Impairment

Although exposure is important to supporting children's developments in syntax, the environment is not all that matters. Both developmental and acquired language disorders can disrupt syntactic comprehension and production.

Developmental language disorders are present at birth. Some language disorders are specific, meaning they affect only the language faculty, a condition called *specific language impairment* (SLI). Some language disorders are secondary, resulting from other causes such as mental retardation. Both specific and secondary language impairments often affect syntactic development, sometimes profoundly. For example, children with SLI produce shorter sentences than their nonimpaired peers do (Laws & Bishop, 2003) and have particular difficulty with verbs. As a result, children with SLI may use other words to "fill in" holes in sentences created by

THEORY TO PRACTICE

Auxiliary Clarification Hypothesis

In this chapter, we discuss how children's exposure to language is an influential factor in explaining individual differences in language development. For instance, we show how the amount of complex syntax contained in mothers' utterances is positively correlated with children's use of complex syntax (see Figure 3.4). Along similar lines, the results of studies show that children's exposure to yes–no questions is positively associated with their development of auxiliary verbs (Yoder & Kaiser, 1989). Recall that yes–no questions involve movement of the auxiliary verb to the initial spot in the interrogative sentence ("*Is* he going?") from its place prior to the main verb ("He *is* going"). The auxiliary clarification hypothesis (ACH) is one theory that explains the positive correlation between the frequency of children's exposure to yes–no questions and their auxiliary verb development (Richards, 1990). According to this theory, children more readily attend to information at the beginning of utterances, therefore exposure to high frequencies of yes–no questions (which place auxiliaries at the front of the utterance) promotes children's internalization of auxiliary verbs (Fey & Frome Loeb, 2002). Extending this theory to practice, you might suppose that increasing children's exposure to yes–no questions would facilitate development of auxiliary verbs.

Fey and Frome Loeb (2002) explicitly tested this theory in a study involving 34 two- to three-year-olds that focused on the auxiliaries *is* and *will*. Children were randomly assigned to receive an 8-week enrichment program or a control program (24 sessions, each 30 min long). In each enrichment program session, children played with a research assistant who produced 30 yes–no questions ("Is Mommy flying?") by recasting children's statements ("Mommy flying"). The control program followed the same schedule and used the same play activities, but the research assistant avoided any use of yes–no questions.

On the basis of the ACH, you would expect children in the enrichment program to acquire auxiliaries at a faster rate than that of children in the control program. Instead, at the end of the 8-week program, the researchers saw no differences between the two groups. Although the ACH suggests that "high rates of these [*yes–no*] questions in children's linguistic environments should facilitate the acquisition of auxiliaries in children not already using them" (Fey & Frome Loeb, 2002), this experimental test disproved the hypothesis.

Theory often provides a framework for clinical interventions and educational practices; however, this example provides a salient illustration of the importance of explicitly testing theories by using experimental procedures. As Fey and Frome Loeb noted, "It no longer seems prudent to recommend that clinicians and caregivers increase the density of inverted *yes–no* questions. . . . [A]dult input of these forms should not be emphasized and, possibly, should be avoided in interventions" (p. 172).

verb omissions, such as "Colin lady ticket," "Lights on my camera," and "Not that the horse, where a big horse?" (Conti-Ramsden & Jones, 1997, p. 1307). Children with language impairment due to mental retardation, such as Down syndrome (DS), also show significant difficulties with syntactic development. Adolescents with DS produce sentences averaging only four morphemes long, shorter than those produced by typically developing 6-year-olds (Laws & Bishop, 2003).

Acquired language disorders occur as a result of injury or illness that damages the language centers of the brain. Stroke causing injury to Broca's area in the left hemisphere is an acquired disorder in which syntactic skills are seriously affected, leading to a condition called *agrammatic aphasia.* These individuals lose the ability to produce syntactically complex language. The results of one study of four adults with agrammatic aphasia showed their utterances to average about four morphemes in length, their complex sentences to comprise only 5% of all their sentences, and less than one third of all their sentences to be grammatically correct (Thompson, Shapiro, Kiran, & Sobecks, 2003).

WHAT IS PHONOLOGICAL DEVELOPMENT?

Phonological development involves acquiring the rules of language that govern the sound structure of syllables and words. We discuss in Chapter 1 how every language has a relatively small number of meaningful sounds, or *phonemes.* Phonemes are the individual speech sounds in a language that signal a contrast in meaning between two syllables or words. In GAE, /r/ and /l/ are two different phonemes because they create a meaning contrast in two words differing only by these two phonemes (e.g., *low* vs. *row; liver* vs. *river*). As children develop their phonological system, they develop an internal representation of each phoneme in their native language. In essence, a phonological representation is a neurological imprint of a phoneme that differentiates it from other phonemes. Thus, speakers of GAE acquire representations that signal the phonemic distinctiveness between /r/ and /l/, although speakers of other languages in which these two speech sounds are not contrastive do not.

DISCUSSION POINT

What are some additional illegal sound combinations in English?

Phonological development also involves developing sensitivity to the **phonotactic rules** of a person's native language; these rules specify "legal" (i.e., acceptable) orders of sounds in syllables and words and the places where specific phonemes can and cannot occur. Early in development, children become sensitive to both. For example, they recognize that /l/ + /h/ is an illegal combination of sounds in English, and that /t/ + /s/ is legal in the final position of a syllable (e.g., *pots*) but illegal in the initial position.

Phonological Building Blocks

Phonological development begins immediately after birth (if not prior) as the infant experiences speech beyond the womb. We next identify three key building blocks in phonological development, all of which are discussed in more detail in subsequent chapters: (a) using cues to segment streams of speech, (b) developing a phonemic inventory, and (c) becoming phonologically aware.

Cues to Segment Streams of Speech

One of the earliest phonological tasks infants face is parsing the streams of speech occurring in the world around them. Early in development, infants develop the capacity to use specific cues contained within a speech stream to parse it into smaller units (e.g., words) and to separate simultaneously occurring speech streams (e.g., the speech on the television vs. mother's speech; Hollich, Newman, & Jusczyk, 2005). One strategy infants use to parse speech streams is to draw on prosodic and phonotactic cues (Gerken & Aslin, 2005; Thiessen & Saffran, 2003).

When using **prosodic cues,** infants draw on their familiarity of word and syllable stress patterns, or the rhythm of language, to break into the speech stream. For example, infants exposed to English rapidly become sensitive to prevalent stress patterns used in English words, such as the strong–weak stress pattern in such words as *little* and *grammar* (Jusczyk, 1993; Thiessen & Saffran, 2003). During the first year of life, infants use their knowledge of predominant word-stress patterns to locate boundaries between words in running streams of speech. For example, they presume that a word boundary occurs following two syllables of a strong–weak stress pattern, given the prevalence of this word-stress pattern in English. For the infant who hears "You little boy," this cueing strategy helps him to isolate *little* and *boy* as separate words. Infants also use their knowledge of pausing to parse the speech stream, recognizing relatively early that pauses often occur at the boundaries between clauses and phrases (Gerken & Aslin, 2005). Infants' sensitivity to the way in which pausing marks linguistic boundaries within speech streams, such as clause segments, may support their syntactic development because it provides them the opportunity to analyze how smaller syntactic units combine to form larger units of speech (Gerken & Aslin, 2005).

Infants also use **phonotactic cues** to parse the speech stream. Early in development, infants become sensitive to the probability that certain sounds will occur both in general and in specific positions of syllables and words (Jusczyk, Luce, & Charles-Luce, 1994). Thus, encountering a speech stream containing the phoneme sequence of /g/ + /z/, the English-learning infant recognizes the improbability that this sequence starts a word. In contrast, this sequence is both legal and probable in the final position of a word (*dogs, eggs*), and he or she uses knowledge of these probabilities to segment a likely word boundary following the sequence. This knowledge of phonotactic probabilities and improbabilities is an important tool for the infant to use to segment novel words out of a continuous stream of speech (Thiessen & Saffran, 2003).

Phonemic Inventory

Another major building block in phonological development is the child's acquisition of internal representations of the phonemes composing his or her native language—termed **phonological knowledge**—and his or her expression of these phonemes to produce syllables and words—termed **phonological production.** Development of a full phonemic inventory occurs gradually as children make more and more fine-tuned distinctions among phonemes. When their inventory is relatively small, children use a single phoneme (e.g., /d/) to express multiple phonemes (e.g., /b/, /p/, /t/, and /d/), gradually adding more phonemes until the inventory is complete and adultlike (Ingram, 1997).

The child's phonemic inventory includes both vowels and consonants. Vowels develop prior to consonants, typically in the first year of life. Not all consonants are acquired or expressed at the same time; some emerge early in development (**early consonants**) and others emerge later (**late consonants**). The timing of development for specific phonemes is influenced by several factors, including the frequency of the occurrence of the phoneme in spoken language, the number of words a child uses that contain a given phoneme, and, to some extent, the articulatory complexity of producing the phoneme (Amayreh, 2003; Ingram, 1997). Because of these influences, the order of consonantal acquisition varies among languages; for example, English-speaking children master /z/ earlier than Arabic-speaking children do because this phoneme occurs more frequently in English words and syllables than in Arabic (Amayreh, 2003).

In general, children's phonological knowledge and production is sufficiently well developed by age 3–4 years to provide for fully intelligible speech. Although some consonantal phonemes will elude mastery for several more years, the child's inventory is large enough to allow reasonable substitutions of mastered phonemes for those yet to be mastered (e.g., /d/ for the initial sound in *that*). Figure 3.5 provides a summary of the order of mastery for the English consonantal phonemes.

Phonological Awareness

Phonological awareness is an individual's ability to attend to the phonological segments of speech through implicit or explicit analysis. For example, a child's ability to produce two words that rhyme involves phonological awareness because the child must attend to the phonological structures of words to identify two words sharing specific structural aspects (Justice & Schuele, 2004). A more challenging task that also involves phonological awareness is asking a child to identify the first sound in a word (e.g., the /b/ in *bat*) or to count the number of phonemes in a word. Again, both tasks require the child to reflect on the phonological structure of language, and the latter requires a focus on the phonemic units of words, called **phonemic awareness.**

Phonological awareness not only is an important aspect of language development but also is significant for literacy development, particularly word reading in alphabetic languages. In these languages, such as English, the written script represents phonemes by using letter-to-sound pairings for individual letters (*S* = /s/) and letter sequences (*SH* = / ʃ /; *OUGH* = /o/). Phonics instruction teaches children the relationships between letters and sounds, and children who are "phonologically aware" can better profit from phonics instruction than children who are unaware (e.g., Badian, 2000). Many children in the United States struggle to develop basic word-reading skills, and researchers contend than many of these children struggle because of a lack of phonological awareness (O'Connor & Jenkins, 1999). Systematically teaching preschoolers and kindergartners to attend to the phonological structure of language, through the use of rhyming games and other similar activities, can improve the likelihood that children will succeed during reading instruction (Byrne & Fielding-Barnsley, 1995).

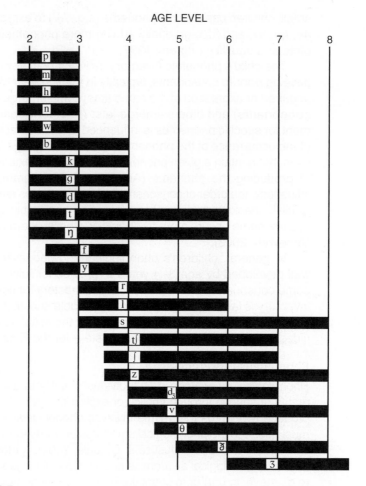

FIGURE 3.5

Order of acquisition for English consonantal phonemes.

Source: From "When Are Speech Sounds Learned?" by E. K. Sander, 1972, *Journal of Speech and Hearing Disorders, 37,* p. 62. Copyright 1972 by the American Speech–Language–Hearing Association. Reprinted with permission.

Influences on Phonological Development

Some children develop their phonological skills much more slowly than other children do, which may signal a phonological disorder if the delay is significant. Addressed in Chapter 10, such a disorder compromises the child's achievement of the building blocks discussed in the previous sections. In this section, we discuss two additional, well-established influences on phonological development.

Native Language

Infants' phonological development is influenced significantly by the phonemic composition of the language (or languages) to which the infants are exposed. Speech sounds that are phonemic in one language may not be phonemic in another.

Thus, children learning Arabic acquire representations of the phonemic inventory of Arabic and not the inventory of English (or any other language); because of this, Arabic-speaking children will not develop a phonemic representation of /p/ because it is not phonemic in their language.

Even when a given speech sound is phonemic in two languages, children may acquire it at different times, depending on the frequency with which it is used in words and its similarity to other phonemes in the language inventory. In other words, the *functional load* of a phoneme can vary among languages. *Functional load* refers essentially to the importance of a phoneme in the phonemic inventory of the language (Ingram, 1989). If we draw again on the comparison of English and Arabic, English-speaking children master /z/ by about age 4 years (Grunwell, 1997), whereas Arabic-speaking children do not master this phoneme until after age 6 years (Amayreh, 2003). In English, the phoneme /z/ has a high functional load, in part because it is used for pluralization (e.g., *vans*, *dogs*), whereas in Arabic it has a low functional load (Amayreh, 2003).

Linguistic Experience

Even among children who are learning the same language, differences can be seen in the timing of their establishment of phonological representations and in their production of different phonemes   (McCune & Vihman, 2001). Children develop phonological representations through their exposure to phonemic contrasts in their language; thus, differences in the timing of phonological development occur, at least in part, because of variability in children's phonological exposure (Nittrouer, 1996). The internal phonological representations of children reared in lower income homes are less mature and distinct than those of children of the same age reared in higher income homes, probably because of variations in the children's exposure to language (Nittrouer, 1996). The same holds true for children with a history of chronic ear infections, whose phonological representations are less mature than those of children without such a history (Nittrouer, 1996). Children with chronic ear infections experience periods in which linguistic exposure is compromised, which in turn appears to negatively affect their phonological development.

WHAT IS PRAGMATIC DEVELOPMENT?

Pragmatic development involves acquiring the rules of language that govern how language is used as a social tool. Such development involves using language for different purposes, being able to enter and hold conversations, and taking into account the circumstances and goals of the participants in a conversation.

Pragmatic Building Blocks

Three important aspects of pragmatic development are as follows: (a) using language for different communication functions, (b) developing conversational skills, and (c) gaining sensitivity to extralinguistic cues. These three areas of pragmatic development are key building blocks that emerge during early childhood and are then gradually refined during later childhood, adolescence, and adulthood.

Communication Functions

When people use language in social contexts, behind every utterance is an intention, or **communication function.** For instance, the following three utterances produced by 2-year-old Eva vary in their function:

"Give me that."

"Mommy going outside?"

"I love my doggie."

Likewise, consider these three utterances by 4-year-old Zachary:

"No, put that one up on top of the digger."

"Addie, did you bring Thomas the train to school today?"

"I actually think my mom is coming after nap."

Take a moment to study each of Eva's and Zachary's utterances and consider the intention behind it. The intentions you identify for each utterance reflect the children's mental states, beliefs, desires, and feelings (L. Bloom & Tinker, 2001b; Goldin-Meadow, 2000). These examples also reveal how children must learn to use language "differently in different situations according to the circumstances and communication goals of the participants" (L. Bloom & Tinker, 2001b, p. 14).

Early in life, children acquire a basic range of functions, and, across their life spans they become increasingly sophisticated in expressing these functions. For instance, consider the communication function of regulation, in which an individual uses communication to control other people's behavior. Consider differences in how this function might be expressed at 1, 5, 13, and 21 years. Table 3.5 defines this function and several other basic communication functions.

TABLE 3.5
Basic communication functions.

Function	Description	Example
Instrumental	Used to achieve actions or objects	"Give me that crayon over there."
Regulatory	Used to control other peoples' behavior	"Don't beat me; I want to win!"
Interactional	Used to interact with other people	"Here, I'll make room for you next to me."
Personal	Used to express a personal state	"My tummy hurts."
Heuristic	Used to gather information and explore the environment	"What's that sign say?"
Imaginative	Used to create and pretend	"You be the mommy and I'll be the baby".

Source: Adapted from *First Language Acquisition: Method, Description, and Explanation,* by D. Ingram, 1989, Cambridge, MA: Cambridge University Press.

Although many basic communication functions emerge in the first several years of life, children gain increasing competence in their ability to use these various functions successfully. Consider again, as an example, the use of regulation, in which a person uses language to direct or control other people's behaviors. Although toddlers typically use direct requests to obtain objects from other people ("Give me that"), preschoolers use direct requests with peers but indirect requests ("May I have that, please?") with adults and more dominant peers (Becker Bryant, 2005).

Developing a range of communication functions is an important aspect of language development that emerges in infancy and continues through adolescence and adulthood. As important as these functions are for children's use of language for self-expression, they may also propel other aspects of language development forward, such as vocabulary and grammar. The **intentionality hypothesis** proposes that children's development of form and content is fostered in part by their experiences with other people as they use language to engage with these people; such experiences motivate the child to "express and articulate increasingly elaborate . . . representations" (L. Bloom & Tinker, 2001b, p. 79).

Therefore, mastery of a range of communication functions is the aspect of language that allows a person to use language as an instrument for adequately conveying his or her mental state to other people and to use language as a social-interactional tool. To accurately express a communication function to another person, children draw on their language abilities in other domains, including vocabulary, morphology, syntax, and phonology (L. Bloom & Tinker, 2001b). When skills are uneven across domains, communication breakdowns may occur. For example, consider 3-year-old Hakuta, who wants his mother to read him a storybook. However, his phonological skills are underdeveloped, which renders his request completely unintelligible. Thus, expression of communication functions depends on achievements in other aspects of language.

Conversational Skills

When children express communication functions, they do so in exchanges with other people, called **conversations.** One key aspect of pragmatic development is developing understanding of a **conversational schema,** also called a *conversational framework* (Naremore, Densmore, & Harman, 1995). Schemata are the building blocks of cognition and, in essence, are internalized representations of the organizational structures of various events (Rumelhart, 1980). When children have a robust representation of a particular schema, their cognitive resources are freed from navigating the organizational structure of the event so that they can acquire new information within the event. For example, consider your first visit to the university library. The organizational schema of the library was unfamiliar; thus, during your first visit, you focused considerable cognitive effort on developing a schematic representation of the library, including how information was cataloged and where materials were located. After internalizing this schema, you could, during future visits, devote more cognitive energy to looking for and assimilating the information you were seeking (see Neuman, 2006).

Conversations have a schema as well: initiation and establishment of a topic, navigation of a series of contingent turns that maintain or shift the topic, and resolution and closure (see Figure 3.6). This macrostructural schema provides a broad

Initiation and establishment of topic	A: So, I meant to ask you, what did you think about the test? B: Boy, that was rough, wasn't it?
Navigation of a series of contingent turns that maintain or shift topic	A: Yeah, I definitely didn't study enough. I was really surprised by the essay. B: I know. I thought it was going to be on pragmatics. I didn't even study the semantic stuff. A: Well, I did, but obviously not enough. B: I went into that test with an A; it's probably shot now. A: Yeah, I feel the same way.
Resolution and closure	A: Well, we ought to go back in. B: Yeah, I definitely can't afford to miss anything. Talk to ya later. A. See ya.

FIGURE 3.6
Macrostructural schema of a conversation.

DISCUSSION POINT

Think about a conversation you had recently that did not go smoothly. What are some specific features of a less-than-optimal conversation?

organizational framework in which many additional microstructural schemata are embedded. Microstructural schemata a child must acquire include navigating topic shifts, negotiating conversational breakdowns, and knowing how much information to provide when background information is shared among listeners versus when it is not shared. An additional schema children must acquire is how to enter a conversation in which they were not previously involved. In this case, the child must identify the frame of reference for the conversation and then establish himself or herself as sharing that frame of reference (Liiva & Cleave, 2005).

Development of a conversational schematic begins soon after birth as infants engage in increasingly sustained periods of **joint attention** with their caregivers. *Joint attention* describes instances in which infants and caregivers focus attention on a mutual object; in such exchanges, the infant must coordinate his or her attention between the social partner and the object of interest (Bakeman & Adamson, 1984). Periods of joint attention, which systematically increase in duration and frequency during the first 18 months of life, provide the child with early schematic representations of conversational organization; like conversation, periods of joint attention feature a communication bid or conversational initiation, a period of sustained turn taking on a single topic, and then a resolution. Caregivers naturally assume the most control during these early *protoconversations,* often interpreting children's vocal or gestural contributions to "fill in the gaps" and using various techniques to redirect children's attention to the conversation (Tomasello, 1988).

Experiences participating in the protoconversations of infancy and toddlerhood help children develop schematic representations of mature conversations in which topics are maintained across turns by both participants. This fact is particularly true when young children participate in protoconversations embedded in highly scripted routines focused on concrete objects, such as play with a familiar toy (Tomasello, 1988). In these scripted and familiar routines, children usually take on more active conversational roles and produce longer turns than they do in less structured and unfamiliar routines.

As children increase their range of conversational partners beyond their immediate caregivers, they show gradual improvements in their ability to initiate and sustain conversations on their own. By first grade, children can successfully enter peer conversations, contributing a turn in the ongoing conversation within 1 minute of entering a conversation. Once in a conversation, first graders' verbal contributions are significant, averaging 61 utterances during only 10 minutes (Liiva & Cleave, 2005). Thus, in a relatively short period, children move from being fairly passive participants in caregiver-mediated protoconversations to active participants in extended conversations with peers.

Sensitivity to Extralinguistic Cues

When individuals use language for social-interactional purposes, they draw on a variety of extralinguistic devices to aid communication, such as posture, gesture, facial expression, eye contact, proximity, pitch, loudness, and pausing. Consequently, pragmatic development also involves developing sensitivity to these extralinguistic cues, such as how, during conversation, a person's facial expression conveys additional content beyond the words themselves.

Previously in this chapter, we discussed how children must use a variety of tactics to "break into" the streams of speech occurring around them. Attending to extralinguistic cues surrounding the speech stream is an important tool that children use early in life to make sense of the language directed at them; for instance, 6-month-olds can follow the gaze of their adult conversational partners to map adult words onto objects in the environment (Morales, Mundy, & Rojas, 1998). Infants also attend to prosodic elements of caregivers' speech to make probabilistic estimates of where word boundaries occur in the speech stream (Jusczyk et al., 1994).

Beyond infancy, children become increasingly attuned to drawing on extralinguistic information to comprehend and produce language in social-interactional contexts. They learn how to use facial expressions, gestures, stress, and loudness to convey their intentions more precisely, and they attend to these elements in conversations with other people to derive meaning beyond that contained in words alone. Interesting data concerning children's developing skills in this area of pragmatic development are provided in reports of studies in which children's register variations were examined. The term **register** refers to stylistic variations in language that occur in different situational contexts; for instance, consider how you vary your language form, content, and use when making a request of a best friend versus your college professor.

During the preschool years, children show varying registers during their dramatic play, assuming different speaking styles, for example, when playing house or school (E. Anderson, 1992). In a study of 4- to 8-year-old children, researchers observed them while they enacted a family situation, a classroom situation, and a doctor situation. The study results showed that boys and girls at all ages varied their pitch, loudness, and speaking rate as they performed different roles; for instance,

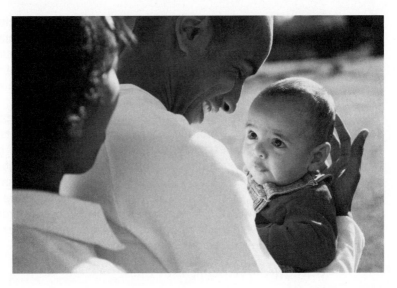

Infants use various tactics to break into the streams of speech they hear around them. For instance, early in life infants use their implicit knowledge of sound patterns in their native language to identify boundaries between words in the stream of speech.

(*Photo Source:* © A. Inden/zefa/Corbis.)

the children used higher pitches for mothers, louder voices for fathers, and the highest pitches for other children (E. Anderson, 2000). Even the youngest children in the study showed clear stylistic variations when taking on different speaker roles. Compared with the older children, the youngest relied mostly on prosodic changes for register changes, whereas the older children varied the words and syntax of utterances and were able to "stay in role" for longer periods of play. Register changes are also evident among preschoolers when the way they make requests of peers versus adults is examined. Even at age 2 years, children use a softer tone with adults than with peers (Owens, 1996). Given the importance of facial expression, posture, eye contact, and other extralinguistic cues to the success (or failure) of children's communication with other people, the fact that children acquire sensitivities to these aspects of language early in development is not surprising.

Influences on Pragmatic Development

As children become competent language users, they show differences in a range of pragmatic aspects of language. Some of these differences arise from personal disposition, particularly temperament, whereas others relate to social and cultural contexts of development. We next discuss these two influences on pragmatic development.

Temperament

Temperament is the way in which an individual approaches a situation, particularly one that is unfamiliar; put simply, *temperament* describes a person's behavioral style or personality type (Kagan & Snidman, 2004; Keogh, 2003). Some individuals are uninhibited, or bold, whereas others are inhibited, or shy. When placed in unfamiliar situations, inhibited children appear wary and fearful, have problems sustaining attention, and are verbally reticent. In contrast, uninhibited children seem eager to explore the situation, are interactive with and responsive to other people, and adjust quickly (Keogh, 2003). These individual differences in behavioral style reflect biologically based heritable variations in neurochemistry (Kagan & Snidman, 2004).

Children's temperament may be apparent in their pragmatic style. For instance, children who are shy and inhibited talk less and smile less often during communications with other people than do bold, uninhibited children (Kagan & Snidman, 2004). Within elementary classrooms, bold children interact more with teachers and peers. Such differences in temperament may give rise to individual differences in language development because bold children initiate and engage in conversations with other people more frequently than shy children do, which provides more opportunities for bold children to practice and refine their conversational abilities (Evans, 1996).

Social and Cultural Contexts of Development

Social and cultural communities have distinct rules about how language should be used during social interactions. These rules govern, for instance, how conversations are organized and how speakers address one another. When we (the authors of this book) were children, we addressed our friends' parents as "Mr. _____" and "Mrs. _____." Modern-day children often call friends' parents by their first names, which shows how this pragmatic rule has changed in one generation.

As members of specific social and cultural communities, children exhibit pragmatic development that reflects the pragmatic rules of the larger community. In one cultural community, adults may socialize children to never initiate conversations with adults, but rather to "speak when spoken to." Conversely, in another community children may be socialized to initiate conversations with adults often, and their success at doing so may be hailed as evidence of linguistic precocity. Likewise, children in one community may be socialized to limit eye contact during conversations with other people, whereas in another community children may be socialized to view maintenance of eye contact as a gesture of respect. When practitioners consider a child's achievement of specific pragmatic building blocks—including his or her development of communication functions, conversational skills, and sensitivity to extralinguistic cues—they must recognize that these skills are not developed in a vacuum. Instead, achievements in each area reflect the socialization practices children experience at home, at school, and in the community.

SUMMARY

Children's language development involves achieving competence in content (semantics), form (morphology, syntax, phonology), and use (pragmatics). In this chapter, we discuss the basic building blocks that correspond to the child's key tasks in achieving competence in these areas.

Semantic development involves three major tasks. The first is acquiring a mental lexicon of about 60,000 words between infancy and adulthood. *Mental lexicon* refers to the volume of words an individual understands and uses. The mental lexicon includes a variety of word types, which for young children includes specific nominals, general nominals, action words, modifiers, and personal–social words. The second task is acquiring words rapidly during word-learning opportunities. After children are exposed to a new word, their representation of the word emerges gradually from an immature state to an adultlike form. Some features of words influence the ease with which children learn them, including the concept represented by the word, the phonological form of the word, and contextual conditions at initial exposure. The third task is organizing the mental lexicon in an efficient semantic network so that entries can be readily retrieved. Children develop links among entries in the semantic network that reflect the strength of associations among words for syntactic, conceptual, and phonological features.

Morphological development describes internalization of the rules of language that govern word structure. Key building blocks include acquiring grammatical and derivational morphology. Grammatical morphemes are used to inflect words for grammatical purposes; they include use of past, future, and present tense markings of verbs and plural and possessive markings of nouns. Derivational morphemes are used to modify root words to change their meaning or class. Children acquire a range of grammatical and derivational morphemes during early and later childhood; such acquisition substantially increases their vocabulary size from a relatively small corpus of root words to a much larger base of derivationally related and grammatically inflected words.

Syntactic development is internalization of the rules of language that govern how words are organized into sentences. We discuss three key building blocks of syntactic development. The first is an increase in utterance length, typically estimated by calculating the mean length of utterance (MLU) in morphemes. As a child's MLU increases, the internal syntactic sophistication of sentences increases to include use of articles, conjunctions, and auxiliary verbs. The second building block is the use of different sentence modalities. During early and later childhood, children use a range of sentence types, including the declarative, negative, and interrogative. The third building block is development of complex syntax, in which children begin to use a variety of phrase types and coordinate clausal structure to produce complex and compound sentences.

Phonological development involves acquiring the rules of language that govern the sound structure of syllables and words. Infants "break into" the phonology of their language by using a range of tactics, including attending to prosodic and phonotactic cues. With ongoing exposure to the phonology of their native language, children acquire a phonemic inventory corresponding to the set of phonemes in the language. They develop a phonemic inventory of both vowels and consonants. The order of consonantal development is influenced by how frequently the phoneme occurs in the language, the number of words a child uses containing the phoneme, and the articulatory complexity of producing the phoneme. *Phonological awareness* describes a child's explicit sensitivity to or awareness of the phonological segments of spoken language.

Pragmatic development is acquisition of rules governing how language is used for social purposes. Major building blocks include developing a range of communication functions, acquiring conversational skills, and becoming sensitive to extralinguistic cues in communicative interactions. The development of communication functions involves learning how to communicate "differently in different situations according to the circumstances and communication goals of the participants" (L. Bloom & Tinker, 2001b, p. 14). Throughout childhood, children develop a range of functions and become increasingly sophisticated at using language as a social tool. Children's conversational skills emerge in early protoconversations with primary caregivers; through these interactions, children develop a conversational schema specifying the organizational structure of conversations. By late childhood, children are active conversationalists, able to enter conversations skillfully and navigate a topic across many turns. Sensitivity to extralinguistic cues—such as facial expression, posture, intonation, and loudness—also emerges early in childhood. By the end of preschool, children can readily vary their extralinguistic cues for varying communicative situations.

KEY TERMS

bound morphemes, p. 83
communication function, p. 102
complex syntax, p. 92
conversational schema, p. 103
conversations, p. 103
declarative sentences, p. 89
derivational morphemes, p. 82
derivational relations, p. 84
early consonants, p. 99
expressive lexicon, p. 74
fast mapping, p. 86
free morphemes, p. 83
grammatical morphemes, p. 82
inflection point, p. 75
intentionality hypothesis, p. 103
interrogative sentences, p. 90
joint attention, p. 104
late consonants, p. 99
mental lexicon, p. 74
negative sentences, p. 90
nonostentive word-learning
    contexts, p. 77

obligatory contexts, p. 84
ostentive word-learning
    contexts, p. 77
phonemic awareness, p. 99
phonological knowledge, p. 98
phonological production, p. 98
phonotactic cues, p. 98
phonotactic rules, p. 97
phrasal coordination, p. 91
prosodic cues, p. 98
receptive lexicon, p. 74
register, p. 105
semantic network, p. 78
simple syntax, p. 94
spreading activation, p. 79
temperament, p. 106
vocabulary spurt, p. 74
wh- questions, p. 90
yes–no questions, p. 90

For online resources related to chapter content, including audio samples, valuable Web sites, suggested readings, and self-quizzes, please go to the Companion Website at http://www.prenhall.com/pence

4

Neuroanatomy and Neurophysiology of Language

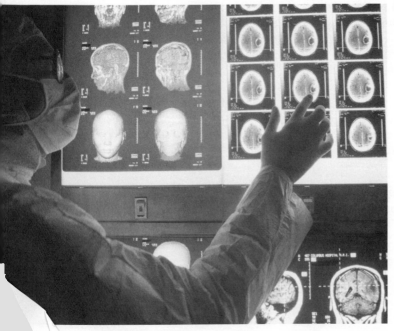

FOCUS QUESTIONS

In this chapter, we answer the following four questions:

1. What are neuroanatomy and neurophysiology?
2. What are the major structures and functions of the human brain?
3. How does the human brain process and produce language?
4. What are neurophysiological and neuroanatomical sensitive periods?

Language is a complex and distinctly human behavior that resides in the neuro-anatomical and neurophysiological architecture of the human brain. Decades of re-markable technological advances have allowed researchers to study the brain as it engages in complex linguistic activities; such studies have increased scientists' un-derstanding of and appreciation for humans' capacity for language.

Much knowledge about the neural architecture of the brain—including the neu-roanatomy and the neurophysiology of the capacity for language—stems from the focus on brain research that occurred during the 1990s. In 1990, then-President George H. Bush proclaimed the next 10 years the "Decade of the Brain" (Office of the Federal Register, 1990). Noting the powerful possibilities available through new sciences and technologies, President Bush made this official declaration:

> To enhance public awareness of the benefits to be derived from brain research, the Congress, by House Joint Resolution 174, has designated the decade beginning January 1, 1990, as the "Decade of the Brain" and has authorized and requested the President to issue a proclamation in observance of this occasion.

In his proclamation, President Bush emphasized that increased knowledge of how the brain works holds extraordinary promise for helping scientists develop im-proved treatments for various conditions. The advances in knowledge about the brain achieved during the Decade of the Brain and in subsequent years have pro-vided researchers and students of language development with unprecedented un-derstanding of how the brain processes and produces language and why, in some cases, language does not develop as expected.

For some students of language development, understanding the neuroanatomical and neurophysiological aspects of language ability may seem difficult; however, such an understanding is critical to fully appreciating and understanding the human species' biologically unique capacity for language. In this chapter, we provide a basic introduc-tion to this topic. Additional references are available on the Companion Website if you want to explore the neuroanatomy and neurophysiology of language in more depth.

WHAT ARE NEUROANATOMY AND NEUROPHYSIOLOGY?

Neuroscience is a branch of science that focuses on the anatomy and physiology of the nervous system, described, respectively, as **neuroanatomy** and **neuro-physiology.** The human nervous system includes the **central nervous system**

(comprising the brain and the spinal cord) and the **peripheral nervous system** (comprising the cranial and spinal nerves, which carry information inward to and outward from the brain and spinal cord). Neuroscientists study the anatomical structures of the nervous system (neuroanatomy) and examine the way these structures work together as a complex unit and as separate, distinct biological units (neurophysiology).

DISCUSSION POINT

What additional technological advances might improve scientists' understanding of the capacity of the brain for language?

Neuroscience is a focused branch of the more general disciplines of anatomy and physiology; anatomists and physiologists study body structures and the functions of these structures (Zemlin, 1988). Specifically, anatomists study the physical characteristics of body structures and examine how they relate to other structures to form anatomical systems. Physiologists study the way in which body structures function, both individually and in concert with other structures to form physiological systems. The fields of anatomy and physiology date back hundreds of years. Many of the terms in current use were introduced by Hippocrates, the "Father of Medicine" (c. 460 B.C.–c. 380 B.C.). In contrast, neuroscience is a relatively new science made possible by rapid and remarkable advances in imaging technologies that allow researchers to study the nervous system functions and structures. Technologies such as **magnetic resonance imaging** (MRI), positron emission tomography (PET), and computed tomography (CT) scan provide detailed images of both the anatomy and the physiology of the nervous system. Such technological tools are rapidly improving scientists' understanding of how the nervous system develops with time and how the brain acquires and processes human language. See Research Paradigms: *fMRI Studies* for information on a brain-imaging technique that allows researchers to examine brain activity when an individual is engaged in a specific processing task.

Neuroscience includes several subdisciplines, including developmental neuroscience, cognitive neuroscience, neurology, neurosurgery, neuroanatomy, neurophysiology, neuropathology, and neurolinguistics. The foci for these various subdisciplines are identified in Table 4.1. Of particular interest to the study of language acquisition is the work of **neurolinguists,** who study the structures and functions of the nervous system that relate to language. Some neurolinguists study the neuroanatomy of language to identify the nervous system structures involved with language processing. Other neurolinguists study the neurophysiology of language to identify the specific ways in which the nervous system functions, such as how language is processed in the human brain. Still other neurolinguists study the neuropathology of language to identify the ways in which diseases and injuries affect the functioning of the human nervous system; for example, some study how various brain structures reorganize and take on new language functions after injury.

Linguistics and psycholinguistics are additional disciplines that have yielded considerable advances in understanding language. *Linguistics* is a broad field concerned specifically with language as a developmental and ecological phenomenon, whereas *psycholinguistics* is a more focused field dealing with the cognitive processes involved in developing, processing, and producing human language. Psycholinguistics is the study of the psychology of language, an integration of the

RESEARCH PARADIGMS

fMRI Studies

Functional magnetic resonance imaging (fMRI) is a type of brain imaging that allows researchers and physicians to identify the brain structures involved in specific mental functions. fMRI is a noninvasive procedure that maps neural activities (i.e., functions) to specific neural regions (i.e., structures) according to changes in blood oxygen levels that correspond to changes in neural activity (Weismer, Plante, Jones, & Tomblin, 2005). fMRI uses *magnetic resonance imaging* (MRI) technology, which provides structural scans of the brain (e.g., measurements of anatomical regions of the brain). However, fMRI differs from MRI in that it maps the functioning of the brain by examining brain activity when individuals are

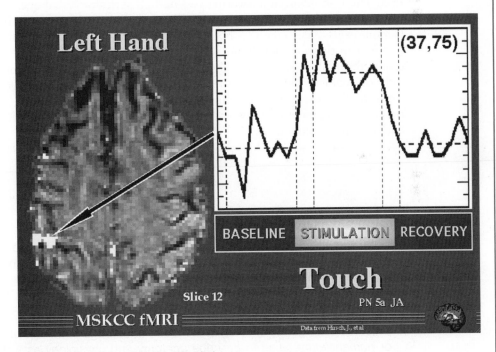

fMRI scan for left-hand tactile stimulation.
Baseline = no left-hand stimulation; Stimulation = left-hand stimulation task;
Recovery = return-to-baseline condition.

Source: From *The Future Role of functional MRI in Medical Applications,* by Functional MRI Research Center, n.d., New York: Columbia University. Copyright by Columbia University functional MRI. Reprinted with permission. http://www.fmri.org/fmri.htm

(*continued*)

engaged in a specific processing task (e.g., listening to yes–no questions). fMRI has significant benefits over other types of brain-imaging technologies, such as PET (positron emission tomography) scans because it requires no injections of radioactive materials, images can be collected relatively quickly (often with a single pass), and the resultant images are of extremely high resolution (Functional MRI Research Center, Columbia University, 2005). An example of an image obtained by using fMRI is presented in the figure accompanying this box; in this figure, areas of the brain activated by left-hand tactile stimulation are identified.

One example of the potential for fMRI to improve understanding of language functions in the brain is described in a study by Weismer and her colleagues (2005). This team of researchers used fMRI to examine verbal working memory in eight adolescents with language impairment (LI) and eight adolescents with typical language abilities (TL). These researchers collected a single functional brain scan from each adolescent while he or she completed a verbal memory task. The task involved answering yes–no to a series of verbal questions that require the use of working memory (e.g., "Do cats that are furry live in the ocean?"). Comparisons of fMRI data for both groups of adolescents showed brain activation to occur in the same left-hemisphere location. However, compared with the TL group, the adolescents with LI showed lower levels of activation (hypoactivation) in brain regions associated with attentional control and memory processing. As a result, the researchers concluded that adolescents with LI had a less functional working-memory network, which may contribute to their difficulties with language-processing tasks.

fields of psychology and linguistics. It also involves studying the language and communicative capacities of other species, such as nonhuman primates.

Terminology

Students of language development require knowledge of the specific terminology, or *nomenclature,* used to describe anatomy and physiology as well as the neuroanatomy and neurophysiology of language. As mentioned previously, much of this terminology has its roots in ancient Latin and Greek.

Nervous System Axes

The human nervous system is organized along two axes: the **horizontal axis** and the **vertical axis.** Together, these axes compose the T-shaped **neuraxis.** The horizontal axis runs from the anterior (frontal) pole of the brain to the posterior (occipital) pole. The vertical axis extends from the superior portion of the brain downward

TABLE 4.1
Areas of Study in Neuroscience

Subdiscipline	Area of study
Developmental neuroscience	Branch of neuroscience focused on identifying how the structures and functions of the nervous system develop and change with time as a function of aging and experience.
Cognitive neuroscience	Branch of neuroscience focused on identifying how the brain structures and functions support higher level cognitive functions, such as memory, reasoning, problem solving, and language processing.
Neurology	Branch of medicine focused on the nervous system. Neurologists diagnose and treat diseases that disrupt the normal functioning of the nervous system.
Neurosurgery	Branch of surgery focused on the nervous system. Neurosurgeons conduct surgery to prevent and correct diseases of the nervous system, including diseases of the brain and spinal column.
Neuroanatomy	Branch of neuroscience focused on the structures of the nervous system. Neuroanatomists study the architecture of the central and peripheral nervous systems, including the brain, to determine how their individual components work as single units and together as parts of a complex system.
Neurophysiology	Branch of neuroscience focused on the functions of the nervous system structures. Neurophysiologists study how the various units of the nervous system work as both single units and together as parts of larger systems.
Neuropathology	Branch of neuroscience and of medicine focused on identifying diseases of the nervous system, including their etiology. Clinical neuropathologists are trained medical doctors who study tissues of the nervous system to identify whether a disease is present.
Neurolinguistics	Branch of neuroscience focused specifically on human language, with a particular interest in understanding how the brain develops and processes spoken, written, and sign language.

along the entire spinal cord. Figure 4.1 depicts the horizontal and vertical axes of the neuraxis.

When experts describe specific nervous system structures, they often use the horizontal and vertical axes as reference points. They use four terms to specify locations on a specific axis: **rostral, caudal, dorsal,** and **ventral.** On the horizontal axis, *rostral* refers to the front of the brain, whereas *caudal* refers to the back of the brain. *Dorsal* refers to the top of the brain, and *ventral* refers to the bottom of the brain. On the vertical axis, *rostral* refers to the top of the spinal cord (near the brain), and *caudal* refers to the bottom of the spinal cord (near the coccyx, or tailbone). *Dorsal* refers to the back of the spinal cord (the side nearest the back), whereas *ventral* refers to the front of the spinal cord (the side nearest the belly; Bhatnagar & Andy, 1995).

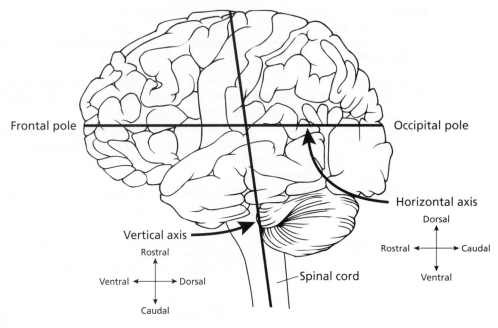

FIGURE 4.1
Vertical and horizontal axes of the neuraxis.

Directional and Positional Terms

Neuroscientists use several additional terms to discuss the directional and positional relationships among various anatomical and physiological structures. *Proximal* refers to structures relatively close to a site of reference, whereas *distal* refers to structures relatively far from a site of reference. Other terms commonly used are *anterior* (toward the front) and *posterior* (toward the back), *superior* (toward the top) and *inferior* (toward the bottom), *external* (toward the outside) and *internal* (toward the inside), and **efferent** (away from the brain) and **afferent** (toward the brain; Zemlin, 1988). The last two terms are often used to describe the pathways of information as it moves to and from the brain. Efferent pathways (also called *descending pathways*) move away from the brain, carrying motor impulses from the central nervous system to more distal body structures. Afferent pathways (also called *ascending pathways*) move toward the brain, carrying sensory information from the distal body structures to the brain.

Neuroscience Basics

The human nervous system, like that of many other species, is a complex anatomical and physiological structure that includes the brain, the spinal cord, and sets of nerves that carry information to and from the brain and spinal cord. The human nervous system mediates nearly all aspects of human behavior, with few exceptions. In this section, we provide a basic introduction to the major structures of the human

Efferent pathways carry motor impulses away from the brain, whereas afferent pathways carry sensory information toward the brain.

(*Photo Source:* Valerie Schultz/Merrill.)

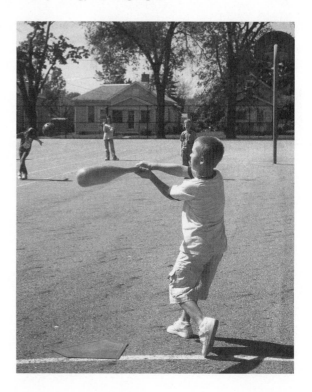

nervous system, emphasizing the aspects of the nervous system most relevant to understanding and appreciating language development.

Neurons

The billions of highly specialized cells that compose the nervous system are called **neurons.** A neuron is functionally divided into four components: cell body, axon, presynaptic terminal, and dendrites (Noback, Strominger, Demarest, & Ruggiero, 2005). The **cell body** is the center of the neuron, containing its nucleus; the nucleus contains DNA material (genes, chromosomes) and proteins. The human brain uses an estimated 30,000–40,000 genes, more than any other organ of the body (Noback et al., 2005). The **axon** and the **dendrites** are extensions from the cell body, serving as vehicles for the cell body to receive and transmit information from other neurons, as shown in Figure 4.2. The information carried by neurons is in the form of electrochemical nerve impulses; these impulses transmit information to and away from the cell body. Each neuron has a single efferent nerve extension, the axon, which carries nerve impulses away from the cell body. The axon extends from the cell body for a distance of 1 mm to 1 m, at which point it arborizes into a number of terminal branches (Noback et al., 2005). The distal end of each terminal branch is a **presynaptic terminal.** These terminals are the sites at which the axonal connection of one neuron correspond with the dendritic extension of another neuron. Dendrites are the afferent extensions of a neuron, meaning they bring nerve impulses into the cell body from the axonal projections of other neurons. A

FIGURE 4.2
The neuron.

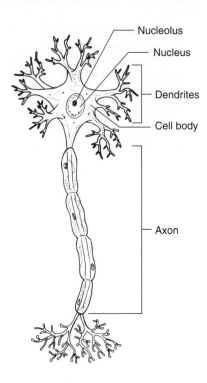

Nucleolus

Nucleus

Dendrites

Cell body

Axon

single cell body contains a number of dendritic extensions; many dendrites are studded with small protuberances (called *spines*), which increase the surface area of the afferent connections of the neuron (Noback et al., 2005).

Neurons communicate by means of electricochemical nerve impulses that travel along the dendrite of one neuron and into its cell body, then along the axon to the dendrite of another neuron. The **synapse** is the site where two neurons meet. For the two neurons to communicate, the nerve impulse must cross the synapse. **Neurotransmitters** are chemical agents that help transmit information across the **synaptic cleft,** which is the space between the axon of the transmitting neuron and the dendrite of the receiving neuron.

The tissue formed by the linkages of thousands of neurons is called *nervous tissue.* The two primary types of nervous tissue are gray matter and white matter. **Gray matter** consists of the cell bodies of neurons and the dendrites. **White matter** is the tissue that carries information among gray matter, consisting primarily of axonal fibers that carry information among gray matter tissues. Thus, gray matter is where information is generated and processed, whereas white matter serves as an information conduit.

Neurons are sheathed in a coating called **myelin.** The myelin sheath contributes to the rapid relay of nerve impulses, particularly within white matter. This sheath also helps protect the neuron. **Myelinization** refers to the growth of the myelin sheath, a slow process not complete until late childhood.

DISCUSSION POINT

To further explore the concepts of efferent and afferent pathways within the CNS, raise your right arm above your head and identify the types of information being conveyed to and away from the brain during this act.

Nervous System Divisions

As mentioned previously, the human body has two major nervous systems: the central nervous system (CNS) and the peripheral nervous system (PNS). The CNS consists of the brain and the spinal cord. The PNS comprises the nerves that emerge from the brain and the spinal cord to *innervate* the rest of the body. **Innervate** is the term in neuroscience that means "to supply nerves" to a particular region or part of the body. The 12 pairs of nerves that emerge from the brain are the **cranial nerves.** The 31 pairs of nerves that emerge from the spinal cord are called **spinal nerves.** The cranial and spinal nerves carry information back and forth among the brain, the spine, and the rest of the body. This information includes sensory information carried to the brain by afferent pathways and motor information carried away from the brain by efferent pathways. Figure 4.3 illustrates the major structures of the CNS and PNS.

Central Nervous System. The CNS consists of the brain and the spinal cord. The brain is essentially the chief operator of the entire CNS: It initiates and regulates virtually all motor, sensory, and cognitive processes (Bhatnagar & Andy, 1995). The spinal cord acts primarily as a conduit of information, carrying not only sensory information from the body to the brain through afferent pathways, but also motor commands from the brain to the rest of the body through efferent pathways.

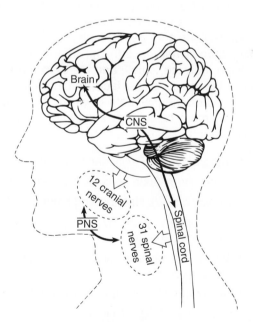

FIGURE 4.3

Major structures of the central nervous system and peripheral nervous system.

Source: From Justice, Laura M., Communication Sciences & Disorders: an Introduction, 1st Edition, © 2006. Reprinted by permission of Pearson Education, Inc., Upper Saddle River, NJ.

Given the importance of the CNS to many human functions, its design includes a series of protective shields. The first shield is bone. Both the brain and the spinal cord are protected by bone; the skull covers the brain, and the vertebral column covers the spinal cord.

The second shield is a series of layered membranes: These **meninges,** which comprise three layers, completely encase the CNS. The inside layer of membrane, called the **pia mater,** tightly wraps around the brain and spinal cord and carries the blood vessels that serve the brain. It is a thin, transparent shield that gives the brain its bright pink color. The second layer is the **arachnoid mater,** a delicate membrane separated from the pia mater by the subarachnoid space. The third and outermost layer is the **dura mater** (literally "hard mother"). The dura mater consists of thick, fibrous tissue that completely encases the brain and the spinal cord.

The third shield is a layer of fluid called **cerebrospinal fluid** (CSF). CSF circulates between the two innermost layers of the meninges: the pia mater and the arachnoid mater. CSF carries chemicals important to metabolic processes, but it is also an important buffer against jolts to the CNS.

DISCUSSION POINT
The CNS is not totally impervious to injury. What types of accidents or illnesses pose the most risk to the CNS?

Peripheral Nervous System. The peripheral nervous system, or PNS, is the system of nerves connected to the brainstem and the spinal cord. These nerves carry sensory information to the CNS and motor commands away from the CNS, thus controlling nearly all voluntary and involuntary activity of the human body.

The PNS consists of two sets of nerves: cranial nerves and spinal nerves. The 12 pairs of cranial nerves run between the brainstem and the facial and neck regions and are particularly important for speech, language, and hearing. The cranial nerves transmit information concerning four of the five senses (vision, hearing, smell, and taste) to the brain. They also carry motor impulses from the brain to the face and neck muscles, including those activating the tongue and the jaw, both of which are involved with speech. The seven cranial nerves most closely involved with speech and language production are the following:

- *Trigeminal (V):* Facial sensation; jaw movements, including chewing
- *Facial (VII):* Taste sensation; facial movements, including smiling
- *Acoustic (VIII):* Hearing and balance
- *Glossopharyngeal (IX):* Tongue sensation; palatal and pharyngeal movement, including gagging
- *Vagus (X):* Taste sensation; palatal, pharyngeal, and laryngeal movement, including voicing
- *Accessory (XI):* Palatal, pharyngeal, laryngeal, head, and shoulder movement
- *Hypoglossal (XII):* Tongue movement

The 31 pairs of spinal nerves run between the spinal cord and all peripheral areas of the human body, including the arms and the legs. These nerves mediate reflexes and volitional sensory and motor activity.

WHAT ARE THE MAJOR STRUCTURES AND FUNCTIONS OF THE HUMAN BRAIN?

The brain is the commander in chief, or mediator, of the entire human body—the "most complex organ of the human body" (Deacon, 1997, p. 147). The relatively slight volume and murky gray appearance of the brain belie its significance to the human species' capacity for thought and language. Weighing only about 2 lb (1,100–1,400 g) and comprising about 2% of the total weight of the body (Bhatnagar & Andy, 1995), the brain is extraordinarily important to the entire functioning of the human body and mind. In fact, the human brain—and its capacity for abstract thought and language—differentiates humans most significantly from other species. The growth of the human brain in both size and weight is one of the most significant evolutionary changes in the anatomy of the human species. Proportionally, the relative size of the human brain and its sheer demand for energy (consuming one fifth of the metabolic resources of the body) far exceed those of any other mammal (Lieberman, 1991).

The most important evolutionary change in the human brain, accounting for these increases in weight and mass, is the enlargement of the outer layers of the brain. These enlarged regions are called the **neocortex,** meaning "new cortex" (or, more literally, "new rind"), which has grown over the original human brain. The neocortex controls most of the functions that exemplify human thought and language, including speech, language, reasoning, planning, and problem solving (Lieberman, 1991).

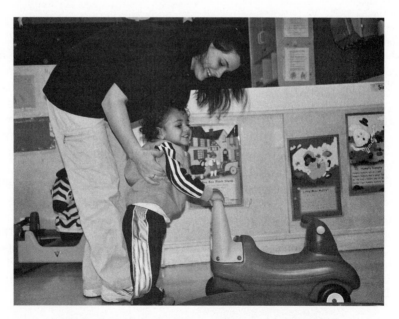

The relative size of the human brain and its sheer demand for energy—it consumes one fifth of the metabolic resources of the body—far exceed those of any other mammal.

(*Photo Source:* Lori Whitley/Merrill.)

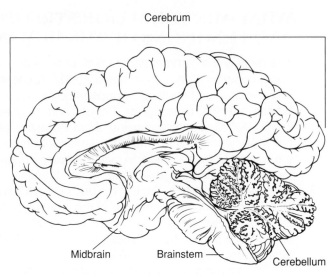

FIGURE 4.4
Cerebrum, brainstem, and cerebellum.

The brain is generally divided into three major sections: the cerebrum, the brainstem, and the cerebellum (see Figure 4.4). Next, we briefly examine these brain sections and identify the major structures and functions of each.

Cerebrum

The **cerebrum,** or cerebral cortex, is the location for the most unique human qualities; its intricate circuitry plays crucial roles in "language, conceptual thinking, creativity, planning, and the ways in which we give form and substance to our thoughts" (Noback et al., 2005, p. 439). Of the three major divisions of the brain, the cerebrum is the largest, comprising 40% of the weight of the brain and containing more than 100 billion neurons (Noback et al., 2005). The cerebrum includes both the **allocortex** and the **neocortex;** the former comprises the original and older human brain (taking up about 10% of brain matter), and the latter consists of the more newly evolved outer structures, corresponding to about 90% of brain matter.

Cerebral Hemispheres

The cerebrum consists of two mirror-image hemispheres, aptly named the **right hemisphere** and the **left hemisphere.** The two hemispheres are separated by a long cerebral crevice (or fissure) called the **longitudinal fissure.** The **corpus callosum** is a band of fibers that connects the two hemispheres, serving as a conduit for communication between them.

Cerebral Lobes

The cerebrum is organized into six lobes of four types: one frontal lobe, one occipital lobe, two temporal lobes, and two parietal lobes. Each lobe has functional specializations, as discussed in the next sections, although the neural circuitry of the

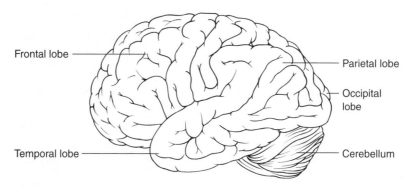

FIGURE 4.5
Lobes of the human brain.

brain features numerous and intricate associations among the lobes that result in organized and complex behavior. Figure 4.5 identifies the locations of these lobes.

DISCUSSION POINT

Provide a concrete example of a specific task that requires executive functioning.

Frontal Lobe. The **frontal lobe** is the largest lobe of the human brain; it resides in the most anterior part of the brain, behind the forehead. Two key functions of the frontal lobe are (a) activating and controlling both fine and complex motor activities, including speech output, and (b) controlling human "executive functions." **Executive functions** include solving problems, planning, creating, reasoning, making decisions, being socially aware, and rationalizing. These unique and important human qualities are *executive* functions because they govern the organized, goal-directed, and controlled execution of critical human behaviors. Executive functions provide humans with the ability to monitor and control their own purposeful behaviors, to override impulses, and to control information processing (Fernandez-Duque, Baird, & Posner, 2000). In short, executive functions are what allow you to stop your arm from reaching for a second piece of chocolate cake (if you really want to).

Several sites within the frontal lobe are important to understanding human language. The **prefrontal cortex** is the most anterior portion of the frontal lobe. It is the part of the brain that evolved most recently in the human species and is most developed relative to that of other species (E. K. Miller, 1999). The prefrontal cortex is connected with all other sensory and motor systems of the brain, which allows it to synthesize the vast stores of information needed for complex, goal-directed human behavior (E. K. Miller, 1999). This part of the brain is involved with the affective aspects of sensations, including gloom, elation, calmness, and friendliness; it thus serves as a "regulator of the depth of feeling" (Noback et al., 2005, p. 452).

Much knowledge of prefrontal cortex functions has been learned from studies of persons with damage to this area of the brain. Such persons may superficially appear normal (e.g., they can carry on a conversation; they can perform well on perceptual and memory tests) but are likely to have profound difficulties with organization, self-control, and goal-oriented tasks. They may suffer in their creativity, outlook, disposition, and drive (Noback et al., 2005).

Also located in the frontal lobe are the **primary motor cortex** and the **premotor cortex,** both important for human speech as well as other motor functions. The primary motor cortex controls the initiation of skilled, delicate voluntary movements,

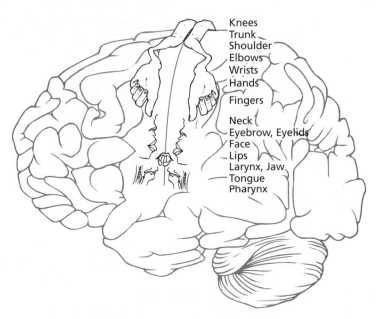

Knees
Trunk
Shoulder
Elbows
Wrists
Hands
Fingers

Neck
Eyebrow, Eyelids
Face
Lips
Larynx, Jaw
Tongue
Pharynx

FIGURE 4.6
Location of various motor functions in the left-hemisphere motor cortex of the human brain.

including not only movements of the extremities (e.g., fingers, hands, toes) but also movements used in speech. The premotor cortex is also involved with control of skilled motor functions, including control of musculature and programming patterns and sequences of movements (Noback et al., 2005). These motor areas are organized topographically, in that specific motor functions correspond to specific sites in the cortices. A *homunculus* is a map that illustrates the location of specific human functions; the motor homunculus presented in Figure 4.6 shows the location of various motor functions in the motor cortex. Because the motor functions are organized along a strip, the motor cortex is sometimes called the *motor strip*. Located on both the left and the right sides of the frontal lobe, the connections that run from the motor strip in the brain to the motor functions they control throughout the body are contralateral: The right premotor cortex controls the left side of the body, and vice versa.

The motor cortex of the left frontal lobe is also home to **Broca's area,** an especially important region of the brain for spoken communication. Broca's area, named after the French physician Paul Broca, is responsible for the fine coordination of speech output. In the mid-1800s, Paul Broca was among the first researchers to recognize the functional specializations of the brain: He identified the site of motor control of speech by autopsying a patient who lost the ability to speak following brain damage.

Occipital Lobe. The **occipital lobe** comprises the posterior portion of the brain. This lobe is functionally specialized for visual reception and processing. Located at the posterior pole of the occipital lobe is the *primary visual cortex.* This cortex receives and processes visual information received from the eyes, fusing information on depth, space, shape, movement, and color into a single visual image. Nerve fibers running from the visual cortex and associated areas project to the temporal and parietal lobes for further analysis and interpretation.

Parietal Lobes.   The two **parietal lobes** reside posterior to the frontal lobe on the left and right sides (above the ears). Key functions of the parietal lobes include perceiving and integrating sensory and perceptual information, comprehending oral and written language, and calculating mathematics.

The parietal lobes contain the locations where sensory information received from throughout the body is processed. Such processing occurs mainly in the **primary somatosensory cortex** (or, more simply, the *primary sensory cortex*) and the **sensory association cortex,** both of which reside just posterior to the primary motor cortex in the frontal lobe. The primary somatosensory cortex is sometimes called the *sensory strip.* It receives and processes sensory experiences of pain, temperature, touch, pressure, and movement from receptors throughout the body (Bhatnagar & Andy, 1995). These receptors convert sensory stimuli (e.g., heat) into neural signals and transmit this information to the sensory cortices in the parietal lobes.

The inferior part of the sensory system of the left parietal lobe is tied to language ability, particularly reading and naming abilities (Bhatnagar & Andy, 1995). This function may occur there because of the important role of the parietal lobes in integrating incoming sensory information with the executive functions of the frontal lobe. In addition, the parietal lobe is especially important to working memory, a complex system that permits individuals to "keep in mind" certain information while executing a given task (Aboitiz & Ricardo, 1997). Working memory is considered

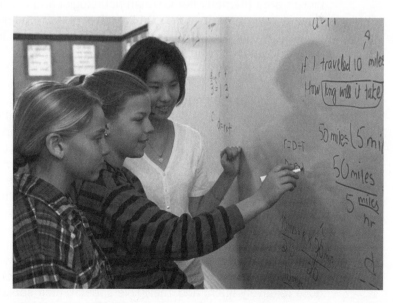

The parietal lobe is important for working memory, the complex system that allows humans to "keep in mind" information while completing a task.

(*Photo Source:* David Young-Wolff/PhotoEdit Inc.)

essential for most higher order executive functions and for acquiring and access-ing your lexicon (or known store of words). See Theory to Practice: *Differential Diagnosis of Language Disorders Using Neurophysiological Models of Language Processing* for a discussion of language disorders and working memory.

Temporal Lobes. The two **temporal lobes** also sit posterior to the frontal lobe but inferior to the parietal lobes (behind the ears). The temporal lobes are important sites for human language because they contain the functions for processing audi-tory information and language comprehension. Auditory processing, which in-volves analysis of auditory input and recognition of speech sounds, occurs in the primary auditory cortex in the superior portion of the two temporal lobes. **Heschl's gyrus,** named after Richard L. Heschl (an Austrian anatomist who identified criti-cal functions of the auditory area of the temporal lobe), is a small left temporal lobe region that appears to be specialized for processing speech, particularly its tem-poral aspects. However, evidence from brain studies shows that at least some as-pects of speech processing occur bilaterally in both the right and the left temporal lobes (Frackowiak et al., 2004). Bilateral damage to both the right and the left auditory cortices can result in *word deafness,* in which an individual has intact processing of nonword auditory stimuli but cannot understand spoken words. However, word deafness does not necessarily occur following unilateral damage (even to the left temporal lobe), thus speech processing appears to occur in both the right and the left temporal lobes (Frackowiak et al., 2004).

The left temporal lobe also contains **Wernicke's area,** sometimes called the **receptive speech area,** which is a critical site for language comprehension. Wer-nicke's area (named after German neurologist and psychiatrist Karl Wernicke), is located in the superior portion of the left temporal lobe near the intersection of the parietal, occipital, and temporal lobes. Consequently, its location is sometimes called the *parieto-occipitotemporal junction.*

Models of language circuitry identify Wernicke's area as a significant point of convergence for receiving and integrating associations from throughout the brain, including the prefrontal cortex, the sensory areas of the parietal lobes, the auditory-processing areas of the temporal lobe, and the visual-processing sys-tems of the occipital lobe. This convergence is also important for language com-prehension and production. For instance, language circuitry models detailing how a person sees an object and then names it propose that visual images are conveyed to Wernicke's area, where the name of the image is generated and then transmitted to Broca's area in the frontal lobe. There, the speech output is organized and then coordinated into motor commands for the articulators (e.g., lips, tongue; Noback et al., 2005). When Wernicke's area is damaged by stroke or other brain injury, individuals typically exhibit significant difficulty with processing and producing coherent language in both spoken and written form. This condition is called *Wernicke's aphasia.* Although persons with Wernicke's aphasia may pro-duce relatively fluent and intelligible speech, their spoken language is "obscured by the paucity of meaningful nouns and verbs, the overabundance of stock phrases and idioms, and the presence of numerous verbal errors" (Bhatnagar & Andy, 1995, p. 304).

THEORY TO PRACTICE

Differential Diagnosis of Language Disorders Using Neurophysiological Models of Language Processing

According to some theoretical models of language disorders, many children exhibit difficulties with language acquisition because of a specific weakness in verbal working memory, specifically its processing capacity. These theories hold that the ability to comprehend and produce language (particularly more complex language) requires active engagement of working memory; working memory is similar to a storage device that maintains the linguistic stimulus while it is being processed (Weismer et al., 2005). As discussed in Research Paradigms: *fMRI Studies*, data from fMRI studies support theories that implicate inefficient verbal working memory as a contributor to language impairment.

Differential diagnosis is an important aspect of psychologists' and speech–language pathologists' clinical decision making when they are identifying language impairment. *Differential diagnosis,* as the name implies, is the act of differentiating a suspected disorder from all other possible disorders. Differential diagnosis is important so that children who have language differences (e.g., who speak a nonstandard dialect) are not mistaken as having a disorder; likewise, differential diagnosis is important for setting treatment goals and approaches that effectively remediate a disorder. Nevertheless, differential diagnosis can be tricky. For instance, a child who has had limited exposure to language because of early institutionalization may appear to have grammatical development similar to that of a child with a neurologically based language impairment.

Scientific understanding of the neurophysiological correlates of language impairment can be informative to designing tasks that identify neurologically based language disorders and differentiate them from other conditions or circumstances that affect language development. For example, consider the scientific finding that deficits in verbal working memory may be a marker of neurologically based language impairment. In addition to fMRI data (Weismer et al., 2005), studies of children with language impairment have shown that verbal working-memory capacity predicts their performance on standardized language tests. Thus, measures of working memory (e.g., identifying the number of letters or digits a person can hold in working memory) have become a routine part of diagnostic procedures for identifying language impairment (e.g., Weismer & Thordardottir, 2002). By incorporating measures that examine a child's verbal working memory into language assessments, clinicians can better differentially diagnose neurologically based language impairment and develop treatment protocols that address working-memory limitations in addition to deficits in language comprehension and expression.

Brainstem

The **brainstem** sits directly on top of the spinal cord and serves as a conduit between the rest of the brain and the spinal cord. It consists of the *midbrain,* the *pons,* and the *medulla oblongata,* which together hold three primary functions (Noback et al., 2005). First, the brainstem is a key transmitter of sensory information to the brain and of motor information away from the brain. Second, the brainstem is a major relay station for the cranial nerves supplying the head and face and for controlling the visual and auditory senses. Third, the brainstem structures and functions are associated with metabolism and arousal. Three major reflex centers are located in the brainstem: the cardiac center, which controls the heart; the vasomotor center, which controls the blood vessels; and the respiratory center, which controls breathing.

Cerebellum

The **cerebellum** is an oval-shaped "little brain" that resides posterior to the brainstem. The cerebellum is primarily responsible for regulating motor and muscular activity and has little to do with the "rational" part of the brain that involves conscious planning and responses. The motor-monitoring functions of the cerebellum include coordinating motor movements, maintaining muscle tone, monitoring movement range and strength, and maintaining posture and equilibrium (Bhatnager & Andy, 1995).

HOW DOES THE HUMAN BRAIN PROCESS AND PRODUCE LANGUAGE?

Current perspectives on the anatomical and physiological organization of the brain rely on **connectionist models.** Connectionist models attempt to represent the computational architecture of the brain as it processes various types of information, particularly that which is specific to higher order human cognition (e.g., reasoning, problem solving). Although historical perspectives on the neuroanatomy and neurophysiology of the brain suggested that specific structures (e.g., Broca's area) were singularly specialized to fulfill specific functions (e.g., motor planning for speech), current scientific knowledge of how the brain works contradicts strict modularity perspectives. Rather, the results of more recent brain research challenge perspectives that isolate highly specific brain functions to specific brain structures, showing that a given brain structure (or cortical area) can vary its functions according to the other cortical areas with which it is interacting (Frackowiak et al., 2004). Likewise, more current research results suggest that most higher level cognitive functions, including that of language, involve numerous brain areas in their execution, several of which are identified in Figure 4.7.

In connectionist models, information processing within the brain (including language processing) is described as involving a network of distributed processors that interact with one another by means of excitatory and inhibitory connections (McClelland, Rumelhart, & Hinton, 1986). Connectionist models emphasize that the connectivity among units is critical to understanding how information is processed. Lieberman (1991) used the analogy of electrical power networks to discuss con-

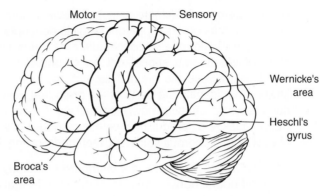

Motor — Sensory

Wernicke's area

Heschl's gyrus

Broca's area

FIGURE 4.7
Areas of the brain involved with language and other functions.

DISCUSSION POINT

Lieberman (1991) used the example of electrical power networks to discuss connectionist models. What is another example of a system that exhibits connectionist principles?

nectivity: "Through a complex interconnected network of generators and 'switching centers' the system adjusts and redirects power from other generators, and apportions output to different units" (p. 33). As Lieberman described, in electrical power networks (and other models based on connectionist principles), power is not located in a single, discrete location, but distributed through an entire network.

In contrast to the current emphasis on connectionism as a means for understanding language processes in the brain, much of the historical literature on the neuroanatomy and neurophysiology of language emphasized the correspondences between specific language functions and specific brain structures. This emphasis was the result, at least in part, of scientists' inability to closely examine the brain while it engaged in various language tasks. In the past, knowledge of brain structures and functions was based primarily on studies of what went wrong when a person's brain was damaged. Currently, because of technological advances, researchers have the tools to study exactly what happens in the brain when individuals engage in highly specific tasks, such as retrieving words corresponding to concrete or abstract labels. Although research results suggest that particular regions of the brain correspond to certain aspects of language processing or speech production, many basic language processes (e.g., word retrieval) are distributed throughout the sensory and motor cortices of the brain and are not confined to a single structure (Frackowiak et al., 2004). In the next sections, we briefly summarize the neuroanatomical and neurophysiological correlates of language processing for semantics, syntax and morphology, phonology, and pragmatics. The relevance of connectionist models to current representations of how language in each domain occurs in the human brain should be apparent.

Semantics

Semantics involves an individual's knowledge of words, or internal lexicon. A person's internal lexicon comprises thousands of words, varying in semantic features, or feature categories. For example, some words reference animate objects, whereas others reference inanimate objects. Likewise, some words reference abstract concepts, whereas others represent tangible concepts, such as size, color, and shape. Given the abundance of conceptual categories represented in a person's lexical store of words, you should not be surprised to learn that lexical knowledge is distributed across the brain. This fact has been substantiated by brain-mapping studies that identify the parts of the brain that activate when individuals engage in such tasks as retrieving newly learned words or accessing words during a decision-making task (e.g., producing a verb in response to a noun stimulus). The aggregated results from numerous studies reveal the following three findings:

1. *Semantic knowledge is a distributed modality.* Word storage involves distributed neural networks transcending the frontal and temporal lobes, with some activation in the parietal lobes. The neural networks in the various lobes seem to serve different functions in semantic processing. The frontal lobe is involved with the executive elements of word knowledge (e.g., evaluation of semantic information), and the temporal lobe is involved with the storage and organization of semantic memories and categories (Bookheimer, 2002; Frackowiak et al., 2004).

2. *Semantic knowledge is left lateralized.* Semantic processing consistently activates left-hemisphere regions, particularly left inferior portions of the frontal lobe and regions across the entire left temporal lobe. At least one region of the left temporal lobe, mapping to storage locations for semantic information, is larger than its companion site in the right hemisphere (Frackowiak et al., 2004).

3. *Some aspects of semantic knowledge involve right-hemisphere processing.* Although many aspects of semantic knowledge are left-lateralized functions, the right hemisphere also contributes to semantic processing, particularly processing figurative and abstract language. For instance, when processing an idiom (e.g., "He'll *bend over backwards* to help you"), an individual must consider the connotative meaning of the phrase rather than the strict, literal meaning (Bookheimer, 2002). Processing idioms and other types of figurative language (e.g., metaphors, proverbs) activates right-hemisphere regions, including those that anatomically correspond to the left-hemisphere Broca's and Wernicke's areas (Bookheimer, 2002). Thus, although semantic knowledge is mostly a function of the left hemisphere, when processing involves a more holistic interpretation of meaning (rather than one-to-one mappings of words to meanings), the right hemisphere becomes involved.

Although brain-imaging studies add more precision to understanding lexical organization and retrieval, current models of semantic processing are consistent with 19th-century neurological models (Frackowiak et al., 2004). Nineteenth-century models identified Wernicke's area in the left temporal lobe as a critical site for word recognition and lexical retrieval; these models further proposed that the left hemisphere was specialized for language processing. The left hemisphere and, more particularly, Wernicke's area remain an important locus for word storage, although advances also show that semantic knowledge is more widely distributed across the left hemisphere than was previously understood.

Syntax and Morphology

An individual's ability to rapidly and automatically process the rules of syntax and morphology (morphosyntax) corresponds to what experts call the *language instinct* (Pinker, 1994), or, alternatively, the *language acquisition device* (Chomsky, 1978). By many accounts, this uniquely human faculty is possible because of the genetically based adaptation of the human brain for processing the universal grammar of language. (For an alternative perspective, see Tomasello, 2003.) As some experts contend, evolutionary history has equipped humans with an innate, species-specific ability to represent the discrete rule-governed syntactic rules of a universal grammar. This remarkable neurophysiological capacity explains young children's uncanny ability to rapidly and effortlessly acquire the small, finite set of morphosyntactic rules that ultimately allow them to produce and understand an infinite variety of sentences, regardless of the specific language they develop (Glezerman & Balkoski, 1999).

The possibility of a distinct morphosyntactic brain module is supported by at least three lines of research. First, studies of language learning in nonhuman primates revealed that other species can develop a reasonably sized lexicon but that grammatical learning eludes them, a finding that supports the likelihood of a specialized neurophysiological module for morphosyntactic acquisition in the human brain (Aboitiz & Ricardo, 1997). Second, the likelihood of a specialized morphosyntactic processor is supported by study results showing specific impairments in morphosyntax as a function of focal brain damage, particularly in Broca's area (see Bookheimer, 2002). Individuals with damage to Broca's area can retain the ability to produce syntactically correct speech "automatisms" (or clichés; e.g., "Oh, my goodness!" "Good morning"), which suggests that well-rehearsed sentences and phrases are represented as whole units in the right hemisphere (Glezerman & Balkoski, 1999), whereas processing discrete morphosyntactic elements of language involves a specialized brain function in Broca's area.

DISCUSSION POINT

Provide several additional examples of sentences with legal syntactic structures that are devoid of meaning.

Third, the results of a number of studies of morphosyntactic processing showed increased activation of the language areas of the left hemisphere, notably Wernicke's area (for grammatical processing) and Broca's area (for formulating grammatically ordered speech output), as well as the parietal lobes. Likewise, the results of studies involving attempts to isolate semantic processing from syntactic processing showed distinct neuroanatomical correlates for processing complex syntax; these correlates correspond to the inferior left frontal lobe in Broca's area (Bookheimer, 2002). This region appears specialized for not only processing the morphosyntactic elements of language but also selectively attending to syntax, such as examining whether a sentence uses a "legal" syntactic structure even when the sentence is devoid of meaning (e.g., "Twas brillig, and the slithy toves . . ."; Friederici, Opitz, & von Cramon, 2000).

Nonetheless, researchers heartily disagree as to whether morphosyntactic processing should be presented as the function of a single, domain-specific module or is better represented by connectionist models that emphasize interactivity of various regions of the brain. Grammatical production and comprehension requires a person to combine fixed semantic representations into novel and complex representations of sentences; it also involves nonlinguistic symbolic and conceptual thought as well as planning and reasoning (Glezerman & Balkoski, 1999). As Aboitiz and Ricardo (1997) pointed out, although "basic components of syntactic roles are directly related to the language regions . . . the interactions between these areas and brain components involved in other cognitive tasks is probably fundamental in the development of higher-order levels of grammar" (p. 392). When individuals engage in complex linguistic tasks, left-hemisphere frontal, temporal, and parietal regions are activated, which shows an interaction of executive, semantic, and morphosyntactic processing (Bookheimer, 2002). In light of such evidence, morphosyntactic processing might best be conceived as a complex cognitive ability served by a variety of separate and specialized cortical areas transcending the right and left hemispheres. In evolutionary terms, a primitive human grammar may have once resided in a distinct language area of the brain (e.g., Broca's area). However, the higher level complex grammar in modern-day language requires integration of the traditional language areas of the brain with other cognitive systems via complex interconnections of the parietal, temporal, and frontal lobes (Abviaitiz & Ricardo, 1997).

Phonology

Processing speech sounds is qualitatively and quantitatively different from processing nonspeech sounds because speech comprises a series of overlapping, rapidly changing, and rapidly produced phonetic segments (Fitch, Miller, & Tallal, 1997). Whereas the capacity of the human brain to process sequences of nonspeech sounds is fairly limited (about 7–9 units/second), speech processing occurs at much higher rates (50–60 units/second; Lieberman, 1991; Werker & Tees, 1992). Some experts contend that the human brain has evolved a specialized processor, sometimes called the **phonetic module,** designed specifically for processing the phonetic segments of speech (Mattingly & Liberman, 1988). Experts view this specialized processor as a "biologically coherent system, specialized from top to bottom" to process the phonetic segments of speech (Liberman, 1999, p. 115).

The phonetic segments of spoken language are channeled through the human ears along the auditory pathway that culminates in the primary and secondary auditory cortices of the temporal lobe. Rapid analysis of the temporal characteristics of the speech sounds occurs in the auditory centers of the left temporal lobe, whereas the spectral characteristics of speech sounds are processed in the right temporal lobe. Therefore, both hemispheres seem to be involved in speech–sound processing, although the auditory regions of the left temporal lobe appear to be critical locations for phonetic analyses of speech sounds (Frackowiak et al., 2004).

Once speech sounds are phonetically analyzed, they must be processed as linguistic units, or phonemes. This level of processing, which occurs in Broca's area, is termed *phonological processing;* it involves analyzing phonological segments and working memory. Neuroimaging data confirm historical neuroanatomical models in which phonological processing and speech production are located at the site

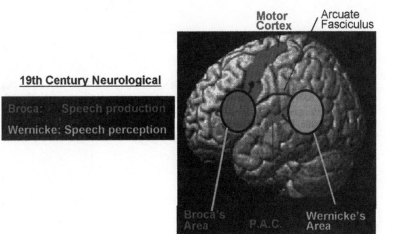

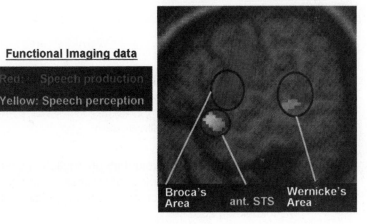

FIGURE 4.8

Historical location of Broca's area compared with that from contemporary neuroimaging data.

Source: Reprinted from *Human Brain Function* (2nd ed.), edited by R. S. J. Frackowiak, K. J. Friston, C. D. Frith, R. J. Dolan, C. J. Price, S. Zeki, J. Ashburner, and W. Penny, p. 529. Copyright 2004, with permission from Elsevier.

of Broca's area in the motor cortex of the left hemisphere (see Figure 4.8). Nevertheless, Broca's area does not work alone to process and produce speech. Heschl's gyrus, Wernicke's area, and Broca's area of the left hemisphere are connected by a series of anatomical pathways, even though they are anatomically remote, as shown in Figure 4.9 (Frackowiak et al., 2004). These interconnections support the interactions of processing mechanisms involved with auditory processing (Heschl's gyrus), language comprehension (Wernicke's area), and phonological processing (Broca's area). Recall from previous sections that Broca's area is also the site of sensorimotor encoding of phonological (speech) output, with efferent pathways to

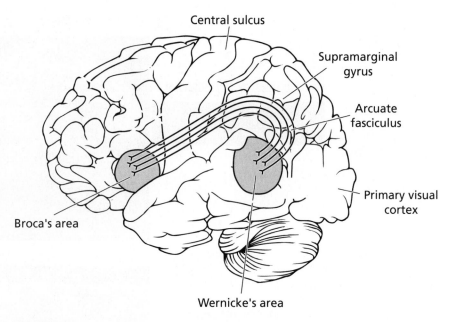

FIGURE 4.9

Anatomical connections among language areas of the brain.

Source: From *The Human Nervous System: Structure and Function* (6th ed., p. 450), by C. R. Noback, N. L. Strominger, R. J. Demarest, and D. A. Ruggiero, 2005, Totowa, NJ: Humana Press. Copyright 2005 by Humana Press, Inc. Reprinted with permission.

organize the controlled, voluntary production of speech sounds. The shared neurophysiology for both phonological processing and phonological production suggests that the motoric production of speech may play a role in phonological development (Bookheimer, 2002).

Although theoretical models of speech perception continue to emphasize the likelihood of a specialized phonetic module (likely corresponding to Broca's area), researchers have failed to identify a single structure or location in the brain specialized solely for speech processing. For instance, Broca's area activates for some nonlinguistic tasks, which suggests that its functions are not dedicated solely to phonological processing or speech production (Bookheimer, 2002). Thus, although the human brain has a specially designed phonological processor, this processor is not exclusive to this task, which casts "doubt on the concept of the language-specific [phonetic] processing module" (Bookheimer, 2002, p. 167).

Pragmatics

The pragmatics of language involves using language as a social tool. It involves understanding the rules of communication, which include following conventions related to the quantity, quality, manner, and relevance of language during communication. Although the aspects of language discussed thus far involve a significant

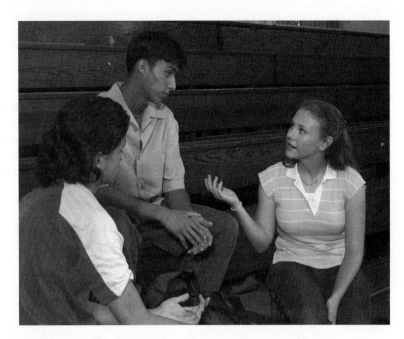

Persons with damage to the frontal lobe of the brain may use language in odd and idiosyncratic ways.

(*Photo Source:* Prentice Hall School Division.)

investment of the traditional language areas of the brain (e.g., Heschl's gyrus, Wernicke's area, and Broca's area), pragmatic ability draws primarily on frontal lobe functions. In other words, an individual who sustains damage to the language areas of the brain that results in significant impairment of semantic, phonological, and morphosyntactic abilities may have fully intact pragmatic skills. Conversely, an individual with frontal lobe damage may have intact semantic, phonological, and morphosyntactic abilities yet use language in odd and idiosyncratic ways.

As discussed previously, one major function of the frontal lobe is to control human executive functions, including solving problems, planning, creating, reasoning, making decisions, being socially aware, and rationalizing. These functions involve the organized, goal-directed, and controlled execution of critical human behaviors. Pragmatic abilities involve the organized, goal-directed, and controlled use of language as a means for communication with other people. Thus, when these more general executive functions are impaired in an individual, the social use of language is often undermined.

The results of brain-imaging studies indicate that many human executive functions involve not only the frontal lobe but also other neurophysiological functions of the brain. For example, consider the case of willful attention. *Willful attention* is what people use when they maintain attention to a given task even when competing stimuli are present (Frackowiak et al., 2004). Your attention to reading this chapter likely involves some degree of willful attention if competing thoughts (e.g., thinking about an upcoming exam) or events in the environment (e.g., friends talking, music playing) exist. Both parietal and frontal lobe regions are involved in willful attention. Together, they impose a hierarchy of control over the competing forces for attention in that the parietal lobe is involved with processing incoming stimuli, whereas the frontal lobe forces attention to the particular stimulus selected for attention (e.g., the words you are reading; Frackowiak et al., 2004). Consider an individual whose frontal lobe functions are compromised, perhaps as a result of frontal lobe injury. During communication with another person (one competing force for attention), he or she may be distracted by other competing forces for attention (e.g., noises in the environment), which thus degrades his or her ability to sustain the communication topic. Therefore, the pragmatic aspects of language are compromised.

WHAT ARE NEUROPHYSIOLOGICAL AND NEUROANATOMICAL SENSITIVE PERIODS?

Thus far in this chapter, we presented the brain as if it were a static neuroanatomical structure. This representation is far from the truth. As a human develops prenatally and postnatally, the brain undergoes significant changes. In this section, we consider the brain as a dynamic organ that changes during growth, focusing specifically on the concept of neurophysiological and neuroanatomical sensitive periods, with a particular focus on how these periods affect the capacity for language.

Sensitive Periods Defined

DISCUSSION POINT
Consider additional risks to prenatal development, such as maternal alcohol and tobacco use. For each risk you identify, consider what it might tell you about corresponding sensitive periods in prenatal development.

As applied to the development of the human brain, a **sensitive period** is a time frame of development during which a particular aspect of neuroanatomy or neurophysiology that underlies a given sensory or motoric capacity undergoes growth or change. For instance, the results of a classic study of kittens showed that deprivation of visual input during the first 6 weeks of a kitten's life resulted in permanent blindness, which indicates that this developmental time frame is a critical window of opportunity for visual development in kittens (Hubel & Wiesel, 1970). In a human analog, studies of birth defects in children born to pregnant women exposed to radiation in Nagasaki and Hiroshima in World War II showed brain damage (i.e., mental retardation, microcephaly) to be most serious when radiation occurred between 56 and 105 days postovulation (P. R. Huttenlocher, 2002). This time frame corresponds to a period of significant prenatal growth in neuron numbers in the forebrain (Schull, 1998). Thus, at least for in utero humans, the period between 56 and 105 days postovulation corresponds to a window of opportunity for supporting the child's neural development prenatally; it is also a time of significant risk.

As these examples show, sensitive periods have the following three features:

1. *Sensitive periods correspond to a time of active neuroanatomical and neurophysiological change.* Other terms used to describe this time include *critical period*, *window of opportunity*, *critical moment*, and *sensitive phase*

(Bruer, 2001). Although the term *critical period* is prevalent in the literature, it carries the connotation that changes occurring in a critical period are irreversible and permanent, which is often not the case. For instance, monkeys who experience visual deprivation during a visual critical period can regain nearly normal visual function with intense remediation (e.g., suturing closed the normal eye; Bruer, 2001). Therefore, many scientists prefer the term *sensitive period,* which carries the "window of opportunity" connotation but allows that change is possible beyond the sensitivity period (Bruer, 2001).

2. *Sensitive periods are a phase not only of opportunity but also of risk.* Some experts identify critical periods as a phase in which "normal development is most sensitive to abnormal environmental conditions" (Bruer, 2001, p. 9). Studies of sensitive periods are important not only for improving researchers' fundamental understanding of human brain development but also in identifying periods during which the brain is most vulnerable to risks. This knowledge is useful for prevention—for instance, ensuring that women prior to and in the several months following conception ingest adequate levels of folic acid to support the embryo's neural tube development. Sensitive periods therefore correspond to times in which an individual's developmental trajectory can be changed for better or for worse.

3. *Sensitive periods have a beginning and an end point, and the length of a period varies for different aspects of neuroanatomy and neurophysiology.* In the previous example, the sensitive period for neural tube development in prenatal human embryos is about 32 days; thus, this period is one of significant risk to the developing embryo if neural tube development is compromised in some way, which occurs with inadequate folic acid consumption by the mother (P. R. Huttenlocher, 2002). In contrast, the sensitive period for language acquisition is much longer, perhaps as long as 12 years for the development of grammar (Bortfeld & Whitehurst, 2001).

Neuroanatomical and Neurophysiological Concepts Related to Sensitive Periods

Synapses provide the means for neurons within the CNS to communicate, and the synaptic connections forged among neurons during development result in the complex neural circuitry that allows information processing in the human brain (P. R. Huttenlocher, 2002). Most synaptic connections do not arise randomly, nor are humans born with them already in place in the brain. Rather, **synaptogenesis** (the formation of synaptic connections) is driven by sensory and motoric experiences after birth, and synaptogenesis occurs most rapidly in the first year of life (P. R. Huttenlocher, 2002). At about the end of the first year, the infant's brain contains about twice as many synaptic connections as an adult's; from this time into adolescence, excess synapses are pruned, a process called **synaptic pruning.**

Neural plasticity is a term used to discuss the malleability of the CNS, and it relates primarily to the capacity of the sensory and motor systems to organize and reorganize themselves by generating new synaptic connections or by using existing synapses for alternative means. Consider that infants with significant left-hemisphere brain damage that destroys the language areas can achieve typical or near-typical language abilities by recruiting other neural functions to serve the purposes of language; neural plasticity accounts for this possibility (P. R. Huttenlocher, 2002). An adult who sustains a similar type of brain damage often cannot achieve normal language in his or her lifetime, which suggests that brain plasticity varies with time. Hence, plasticity relates to sensitive periods because the plasticity of the brain for reorganizing itself and for resolving injury or damage to its neurophysiology and neuroanatomy varies during development.

Plasticity is often categorized into two types: experience-expectant plasticity and experience-dependent plasticity. These two types of plasticity differentiate the effects of the environment on changes in the brain (Bruer & Greenough, 2001). **Experience-expectant plasticity** refers to changes in brain structures that occur as a result of normal experiences. As the infant develops, multitudes of synapses are present in the brain, expectantly waiting for certain normal experiences to occur for them to organize themselves into functioning circuits (P. R. Huttenlocher, 2002). This type of plasticity develops "obligatory cortical functions" (P. R. Huttenlocher, 2002, p. 176) that organize basic sensorimotor neural systems, such as vision, hearing, and language (Bruer & Greenough, 2001). Most infants develop these experience-expectant functions because the basic stimuli needed to foster their development are present in the typical environment. Once the sensitive period for a given experience-expectant brain function has passed, though, environmental experiences no longer readily modify cortical circuits, possibly because few (if any) unspecified synapses remain. Acquisition of language grammar occurs as a function of experience-expectant plasticity.

In contrast with experience-expectant plasticity, **experience-dependent plasticity** is unique to a given individual; this type of functional brain modification requires highly specific types of experiences for change. This type of plasticity is what permits humans to "learn from our personal experience and store information derived from that experience to use in later problem solving" (Bruer & Greenough, 2001, p. 212). Learning new information (whether it is novel information or information that must be relearned after brain injury) requires three mechanisms: the formation of new synaptic connections among neurons (**dendritic sprouting**), the generation of new neurons, and an increase in synaptic strength (P. R. Huttenlocher, 2002). Unlike experience-expectant plasticity, experience-dependent plasticity is a brain capacity available independent of age because, through time, the human brain retains most of its capacity to learn through experience and to adapt to change.

Some aspects of language acquisition, particularly vocabulary growth, are supported by experience-dependent plasticity. For instance, a classic work by Hart and Risley (1995) showed that the size of children's lexicon mapped to the volume and quality of words the children heard in their home environments; although the basic neural circuitry for learning new words is acquired early in development, exposure to words in the environment enriches the number of synaptic connections that support and organize the semantic store of words in the brain.

Sensitive Periods and Language Acquisition

You probably have some knowledge of how sensitive periods relate to language acquisition. For instance, if you attempted to learn a new language in high school and found doing so exceedingly difficult, you may have attributed such difficulty to your being past the "window of opportunity" for learning a new language. Moreover, you are likely aware of (or even attended) an *immersion* preschool program, in which children are exposed to two or more languages (e.g., English and Spanish) simultaneously in an effort to take advantage of sensitive periods for language acquisition.

DISCUSSION POINT
What is a *natural* experiment? How are natural experiments different from "true" experiments?

In this section, we consider the evidence on whether sensitive periods for language acquisition are a scientific reality, in that humans have a relatively brief window of time in which to acquire language, beyond which language cannot be learned. In some respects, identifying sensitive periods for language acquisition is a scientific challenge because of the ethical impossibility of actively manipulating children's language-learning environments to study the effects of language deprivation at different points to identify such periods. Nonetheless, some "natural" experiments have occurred that help scientists identify sensitive periods for language acquisition by the brain.

Linguistic Isolation

Linguistic isolation occurs when a child develops with little or no exposure to a spoken or sign language. A few cases of "feral children" (children deprived of language exposure as a result of abuse and neglect) provide support for a sensitive period for language acquisition. The most notable case is that of Genie, an adolescent in California who was discovered by social workers after having been locked in a bedroom for her entire life and presumably beaten for her attempts to vocalize or communicate. Despite substantial language therapy in subsequent years, Genie never developed age-appropriate grammatical skills. However, the extent to which concomitant cognitive disabilities combined with years of neglect may have affected Genie's capacity for language cannot be determined, thus her case provides inconclusive support for sensitive periods for language.

Evidence on sensitive periods for language acquisition is provided more conclusively in studies of children who are Deaf who are not exposed to a language, whether spoken or sign (e.g., ASL, or American Sign Language), until sometime beyond infancy and toddlerhood. Newport (1990) examined ASL fluency for three groups of individuals who were Deaf: those who learned ASL at birth, those who learned ASL between ages 4 and 6 years, and those who learned ASL after age 12 years. Newport found that age of ASL learning was associated with ASL fluency: Individuals who acquired ASL at birth exhibited nativelike language fluency, whereas those who acquired ASL later in life exhibited significant deficits in language ability, particularly in the area of grammar. Such evidence points to the period of birth through early adolescence as a sensitive period for language acquisition. Although language skills can be acquired after this period, many individuals are unlikely to acquire nativelike fluency.

Second Language Learners

One interesting approach to estimating sensitive periods for language acquisition is to compare the language abilities of groups of individuals who learned a second language at different times of life. J. S. Johnson and Newport (1989) conducted such an investigation. In their seminal study, they compared the English abilities of Asian immigrants to the United States. The immigrants had been exposed to English between age 3 and age 39 years. These researchers showed the immigrants' English abilities to be negatively associated with increased age upon learning English. However, as Hakuta (2001) pointed out, studies of second language learners have failed to reveal a specified end point for the sensitive period for language acquisition. Bialystok and Hakuta's (1994) reanalysis of Johnson and Newport's data showed gradually declining performance in language ability on the basis of age of individuals' arrival to the United States but did not identify a putative end point to the sensitive period for language learning. Other studies, including those on the language development of children who must acquire a new language (and lose their first) following a foreign-birth adoption, have also failed to identify a putative end point for the sensitive period for language acquisition. In fact, these studies have shown that "even by 7 or 8 years of age, plasticity in language areas is still sufficiently high to promote an essentially complete recovery of normal language" (Pallier et al., 2003, p. 159). Thus, although young children unequivocally exhibit a unique propensity for learning language and the capacity of the brain for rapid language acquisition slows with time, a growing number of scientists argue that "the view of a biologically constrained and specialized language acquisition device that is turned off at puberty is not correct" (Hakuta, 2001, p. 204). See Multicultural Focus: *International Adoption and Neurophysiological Sensitive Periods* for a discussion of foreign-birth adoption and sensitive periods.

Plasticity and Language

Evidence on sensitive periods for language acquisition suggests that researchers must consider both experience-expectant and experience-dependent plasticity to understand the capabilities of the brain for language during the life span. Whereas experience-expectant plasticity provides the immature brain with capacities well beyond that which is seen as people age, experience-dependent plasticity provides the human brain—even at advanced ages—with the capacity to grow and adapt to not only new experiences but also illness, disease, and injury to the brain. Although some development periods correspond to time frames in which language learning is easiest (particularly infancy through early adolescence), researchers' inability to identify a putative end point to the sensitive period for language acquisition likely reflects the experience-dependent abilities of the human brain to adapt and modify itself in response to the environment.

MULTICULTURAL FOCUS

International Adoption and Neurophysiological Sensitive Periods

One topic addressed in this chapter is sensitive periods in brain development, particularly as they apply to understanding language acquisition. We identify several approaches that researchers have used to explore sensitive periods for language acquisition, such as studies of "feral children" (e.g., Genie), children who are Deaf with delayed exposure to language (signed or spoken), and second language learners. The increase in foreign-birth adoptions in the United States—nearly 22,000 such cases occurred in 2005 (U.S. Department of State, 2005)—provides another avenue for scientists to explore the possibility of identifying sensitive periods for language acquisition.

In a foreign-birth adoption, a child is adopted from overseas, often from an institution. In the United States, most foreign-birth adoptions are from China and Eastern European countries (U.S. Department of State, 2005). In addition to the developmental challenges children experience from institutionalized care, in which they may have relatively little contact with adults and thus few experiences with healthy attachment and language–cognitive stimulation, these children often come from countries plagued by limited prenatal care and maternal exposure to infectious diseases (Glennen, 2002). Although the risks these children encounter early in life are substantial, the results of studies of outcomes for foreign adoptees suggest that many will achieve healthy developmental outcomes in cognitive and physical achievements (Glennen, 2002).

In this chapter, we discuss the concept of experience-expectant brain plasticity. In contrast with experience-dependent plasticity, experience-expectant plasticity is the developmental mechanism of the brain for achieving basic processes, including language, in relatively short time periods. Experts have failed to identify a specific end point for the sensitive period for language acquisition, which would presumably correspond to a loss of experience-expectant plasticity. Nevertheless, this sensitive period extends from at least birth to age 5 years, if not beyond, and during this period the brain exhibits an amazing capacity to make amends for early delays in language, as shown by studies of foreign-birth adoptees.

Studies of children adopted from Eastern European orphanages reveal that most of these children exhibit early and significant lags in language development, corresponding to their apparently limited exposure to language stimulation during their period of institutionalized care (Glennen & Masters, 2002). For instance, Dubrovina (as discussed in Gindis, 1999) reported that more than half of all toddlers in Eastern European orphanages were not talking by age 2 years. However, upon adoption, foreign adoptees showed rapid, substan-

(continued)

tial gains in all areas of language, including grammar and vocabulary, and the best outcomes at age 3 years occurred for children adopted earlier in life (e.g., before 12 months compared with 19–24 months; Glennen & Masters, 2002). The figure accompanying this box shows growth trajectories for expressive vocabulary from adoption to age 36–40 months for children adopted from Eastern Europe. In this figure, growth is differentiated for children adopted between birth and 12 months, 13–18 months, 19–24 months, and 25–30 months, and these statistics are compared with those for the expressive vocabulary of nonadopted children. As these data show, children show rapid vocabulary growth upon adoption; although those adopted at later ages do not exhibit the levels of expressive vocabulary seen in children adopted at earlier ages, the growth rate is similar across all groups. Data such as these, combined with the findings of studies of older children adopted from foreign locations that show normal or close-to-normal levels of language achievement by age 5 years (e.g., Roberts et al., 2005), reveal the experience-expectant plasticity of the brain for acquiring language during the sensitive period, even when it has a late start.

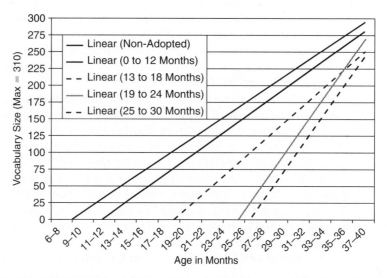

Expressive vocabulary development from time of adoption to age 36–40 months for infants and toddlers adopted from Eastern Europe.

Source: From "Typical and Atypical Language Development in Infants and Toddlers Adopted from Eastern Europe," by S. Glennen and M. G. Masters, 2002, *American Journal of Speech–Language Pathology, 11,* p. 420. Copyright 2002 by the American Speech–Language–Hearing Association. Reprinted with permission.

SUMMARY

Language, a complex and distinctly human behavior, resides in the neuroanatomical and neurophysiological architecture of the human brain. *Neuroscience* is a branch of science that focuses on the anatomy and physiology of the nervous system, described respectively as *neuroanatomy* and *neurophysiology*. The human nervous system includes the *central nervous system* (comprising the brain and the spinal cord) and the *peripheral nervous system* (comprising the cranial and spinal nerves, which carry information inward to and outward from the brain and the spinal cord). The billions of highly specialized cells that compose the nervous system are *neurons*. A neuron is functionally divided into four components: *cell body*, *axon, presynaptic terminal,* and *dendrites*. The cell body is the center of the neuron, containing its nucleus. The axon and the dendrites are extensions from the cell body. The axon transmits information away from the cell body; the *presynaptic terminals* of the axon are the sites at which the axonal connection of one neuron corresponds with another neuron. Dendrites are the afferent extensions of a neuron, bringing nerve impulses into the cell body from the axonal projections of other neurons. The *synapse* is the site where two neurons meet. For two neurons to communicate, the nerve impulse must cross the synapse.

The brain, which contains more neurons than any other organ in the human body, consists of two mirror-image hemispheres. Aptly named, the *right hemisphere* and the *left hemisphere* are separated by a long cerebral crevice (or fissure) called the *longitudinal fissure*. The *corpus callosum* is a band of fibers that connects the two hemispheres, serving as a conduit for communication between the hemispheres. The brain is further divided into six lobes: one frontal lobe, one occipital lobe, two temporal lobes, and two parietal lobes. Each lobe has functional specializations. The frontal lobe is the site of complex executive behaviors (e.g., reasoning, planning, problem solving) and contains in its left hemisphere an important site for speech production and phonological processing: Broca's area. The occipital lobe is the site of visual perception and processing. The two parietal lobes are the site for not only perceiving and integrating sensory and perceptual information but also comprehending oral and written language and calculating mathematics. The two temporal lobes contain sites critical to auditory processing as well as language comprehension; language is lateralized to the left hemisphere in Wernicke's area.

Many theorists have argued that the brain exhibits a sensitive period for language acquisition because the *experience-expectant brain plasticity* used in language development is available for a relatively short duration. In contrast, *experience-dependent plasticity* is the ability of the brain to adapt itself to new information with time. Some evidence—including that attained from studies of feral children, children who are Deaf, and second language learners—suggests that birth to early adolescence is a sensitive period for language acquisition. Nevertheless, researchers have not yet been able to identify a putative end point for this sensitive period, probably because the experience-dependent plasticity of the brain endures (more or less) throughout the lifetime. Thus, although infants, toddlers, and young children acquire language remarkably easily, the capacity to learn language (or relearn language following brain damage) is present for the entire human life span.

KEY TERMS

afferent, p. 116
allocortex, p. 122
arachnoid mater, p. 120
axon, p. 117
brainstem, p. 128
Broca's area, p. 124
caudal, p. 115
cell body, p. 117
central nervous system, p. 111
cerebellum, p. 128
cerebrospinal fluid, p. 120
cerebrum, p. 122
connectionist models, p. 128
corpus callosum, p. 122
cranial nerves, p. 119
dendrites, p. 117
dendritic sprouting, p. 138
dorsal, p. 115
dura mater, p. 120
efferent, p. 116
executive functions, p. 123
experience-dependent
 plasticity, p. 138
experience-expectant
 plasticity, p. 138
frontal lobe, p. 123
functional magnetic resonance
 imaging, p. 113
gray matter, p. 118
Heschl's gyrus, p. 126
horizontal axis, p. 114
innervate, p. 119
left hemisphere, p. 122
longitudinal fissure, p. 122
magnetic resonance imaging,
 p. 112
meninges, p. 120

myelin, p. 118
myelinization, p. 118
neocortex, p. 121
neural plasticity, p. 137
neuraxis, p. 114
neuroanatomy, p. 111
neurolinguists, p. 112
neurons, p. 117
neurophysiology, p. 111
neuroscience, p. 111
neurotransmitters, p. 118
occipital lobe, p. 124
parietal lobes, p. 125
peripheral nervous system, p. 112
phonetic module, p. 132
pia mater, p. 120
prefrontal cortex, p. 123
premotor cortex, p. 123
presynaptic terminal, p. 117
primary motor cortex, p. 123
primary somatosensory cortex,
 p. 125
receptive speech area, p. 126
right hemisphere, p. 122
rostral, p. 115
sensitive period, p. 136
sensory association cortex, p. 125
spinal nerves, p. 119
synapse, p. 118
synaptic cleft, p. 118
synaptic pruning, p. 137
synaptogenesis, p. 137
temporal lobes, p. 126
ventral, p. 115
vertical axis, p. 114
Wernicke's area, p. 126
white matter, p. 118

For online resources related to chapter content, including audio samples, valuable Web sites, suggested readings, and self-quizzes, please go to the Companion Website at http://www.prenhall.com/pence

5

Infancy

Let the Language Achievements Begin

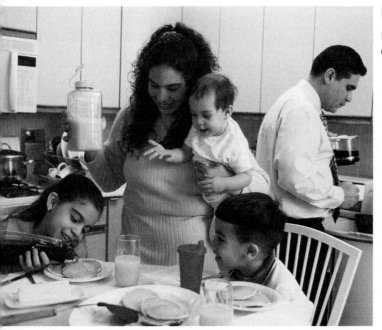

FOCUS QUESTIONS

In this chapter, we answer the following five questions:

1. What major language development milestones occur in infancy?
2. What are some of the early foundations for language development?
3. What major achievements in language content, form, and use characterize infancy?
4. What factors influence infants' individual achievements in language?
5. How do researchers and clinicians measure language development in infancy?

The first year of life is packed with spectacular prelinguistic and linguistic developments. Although infants are not yet using their language system productively, their receptive language abilities begin growing by leaps and bounds from the moment they are born. Infants need not waste any of their time maneuvering through traffic jams, preparing dinner, paying bills, walking the dog, or cutting the grass, as their parents do. As a result, they can devote all their waking hours to exploring their environment, engaging in social interactions with other people, and taking in all the sights and sounds surrounding them. In this chapter, we first provide an overview of the major language development milestones that infants achieve during their first year. Such milestones include not only using the prosodic and phonetic regularities of speech to isolate meaningful units from continuous speech but also gaining the ability to perceive speech sounds in terms of meaningful categories. We also examine infants' awareness of actions and the intentions underlying these actions, their ability to categorize items and events according to perceptual and conceptual features, and their early vocalizations. Second, we discuss some of the early foundations for language development, including infant-directed speech, joint reference and attention, the daily routines of infancy, and the responsiveness of caregivers. In the third section, we describe infants' major achievements in language content, form, and use. In the fourth part, we elucidate some reasons for the intraindividual and interindividual differences among children who are developing language. Finally, fifth, we briefly look at some of the methods researchers and clinicians use to measure language development in infancy.

WHAT MAJOR LANGUAGE-DEVELOPMENT MILESTONES OCCUR IN INFANCY?

Infant Speech Perception

Before infants are ready to speak their first word, they listen attentively to the sounds around them. As you probably know from hearing foreign languages, the speech stream is not neatly divided into words with spaces in the same way written language is. For this reason, infants learning language must be able to segment the speech they hear into meaningful phrases and words. Infants are amazingly adept at detecting speech patterns and using these patterns to their advantage as they learn to break continuous speech into smaller units. Infants' *speech perception ability*—their ability to devote attention to the **prosodic** and **phonetic regularities** of speech—develops tremendously in the first year as infants move from detecting larger patterns, such as rhythm, to detecting smaller patterns, such as combinations of specific sounds.

Attention to Prosodic Regularities

The prosodic characteristics of speech include the *frequency,* or pitch, of sounds (e.g., a low-pitched hum vs. a high-pitched squeal); the **duration,** or length, of sounds; and the *intensity,* or loudness, of sounds. Combinations of these prosodic characteristics produce distinguishable stress and intonation patterns that infants can detect. **Stress** is the prominence placed on certain syllables of multisyllabic words. For example, the first syllable of the word *over* is stressed, whereas the second syllable of the word *above* is stressed. **Intonation,** like stress, is the prominence placed on certain syllables, but it also applies to entire phrases and sentences. For instance, compare the patterns you hear in the following two sentences:

"You like sardines."

"Do you like sardines?"

Notice that the first sentence, a declarative sentence, ends in a falling intonation, whereas the second sentence, an interrogative, ends in a rising intonation.

How do infants use prosodic regularities to segment the speech stream? One way is by becoming familiar with the dominant stress patterns of their native language. Infants learning English hear many more strong–weak (*over*) stress patterns in bisyllabic words than they hear weak–strong (*above*) stress patterns. By age 9 months, infants learning English prefer to listen to words containing strong–weak stress patterns (Jusczyk, Cutler, & Redanz, 1993). A preference for the dominant stress pattern of their native language can help infants begin to isolate words in continuous speech.

Attention to Phonetic Regularities

The phonetic details of speech include *phonemes,* or speech sounds, and combinations of phonemes. According to Stager and Werker (1997), infants who are not yet learning words devote much attention to the phonetic details of speech, whereas older children concentrate their efforts on word learning at the expense of fine phonetic detail. Stager and Werker arrived at this conclusion after conducting a series of creatively designed studies. In one study, these researchers repeatedly presented an object on a television screen, accompanied by the sound "bih," to 8- and 14-month-old infants. Once the infants were accustomed to the object–sound pairing, the researchers switched the sound so that the infants saw the original object, which was paired with the sound "dih." The 14-month-olds did not seem to notice the switch in sound, but the 8-month-olds did: They watched the new pairing for a significantly longer time than they watched the original pairing. Why could the younger infants detect a change that the older infants missed? Stager and Werker hypothesized that the 14-month-olds devoted their attention to learning the object name and did not notice the fine sound difference, whereas the 8-month-olds engaged in a simple sound discrimination task and were able to notice the phonetic distinction (Figure 5.1).

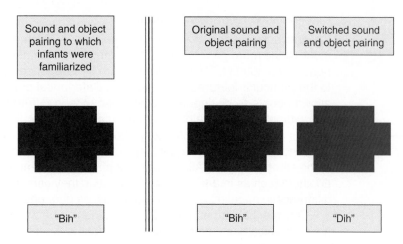

FIGURE 5.1
Stager and Werker's (1997) speech perception task.

Detection of Nonnative Phonetic Differences. Infants' ability to notice fine phonetic detail is not limited to their native language. In the first year, they can distinguish among the sounds of all world languages, an ability that adults lack. As infants develop and become attuned to the sounds they hear regularly, their ability to distinguish nonnative phonemic contrasts diminishes. The ability to discriminate nonnative contrasts appears to coincide with changes in other cognitive and perceptual abilities, such as visual categorization. Researchers suspect that discriminating nonnative contrasts may be a domain-general ability rather than an ability dedicated solely to language-learning functions because it coincides with other nonlanguage abilities (Lalonde & Werker, 1995; Werker, 1995).

Detection of Phonotactic Regularities. As infants hear their native language more and more, they also develop the ability to recognize permissible combinations of phonemes in their language, or *phonotactic regularities*. For example, infants learning English learn that the combination of sounds /ps/ (as in *maps*) must occur in a syllable-final position and never in a syllable-initial position. They also learn that the /h/ sound (as in *happy*) must begin syllables and never occur in a syllable-final position. Infants' ability to detect phonotactic regularities in their native language helps them segment words from continuous speech (Mattys & Jusczyk, 2001). For instance, in the preceding example, when infants determine that the sequence /ps/ occurs at the end of syllables and words, they can infer that the sounds that precede /ps/ are part of the same word and that the sounds following /ps/ start a new syllable or word. Infants' ability to differentiate between permissible and impermissible sound sequences in their native language is present by about age 9 months (Jusczyk, Friederici, Wessels, Svenkerud, & Jusczyk, 1993; Jusczyk & Luce, 1994).

Categorical Perception of Speech

Children's perception of speech is *categorical,* which means children categorize input. At the more general level, they categorize incoming sounds into speech and nonspeech sounds. Then, children learn to categorize speech sounds according to the particular features of the sounds. Categorical perception of speech sounds allows people to distinguish between sounds in different categories (/p/ vs. /b/), but without special training, people cannot distinguish between variations of sounds within the same category (the first and last /p/ sounds in *pup*). Variations of sounds in the same category, as in the previous example, are called *allophones* of the same phoneme. Allophones of a phoneme are measurably different from one another (such as in the amount of aspiration they contain), but they do not signal a difference in meaning between two words, as phonemes do.

One mechanism humans use to distinguish between sounds in different categories is voice onset time. **Voice onset time** is the interval between the release of a stop consonant (e.g., *p, b, t, d*) and the onset of vocal cord vibrations. The voice onset time for the sound /b/ is much shorter than that for the sound /p/. This temporal difference helps people distinguish between these two seemingly similar sounds. See Figure 5.2 for an illustration of voice onset time for the phonemes /p/ and /b/. The arrows to the left on the diagrams show the point at which the consonant is released, whereas the arrows to the right show the point at which the vocal cords

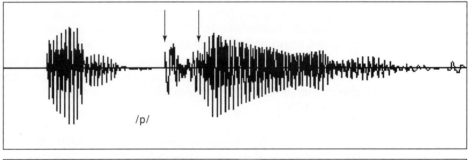

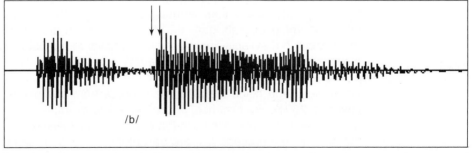

100 ms

FIGURE 5.2
Voice onset time for the consonant sounds /p/ and /b/.

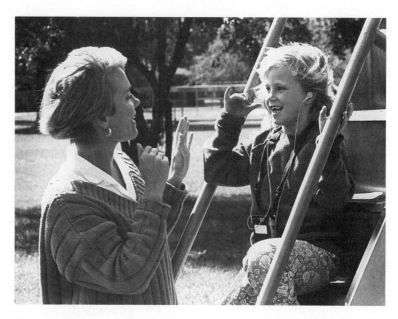

From infancy, humans can categorize speech sounds into meaningful categories. Persons who are Deaf likewise categorize hand shapes into meaningful categories.

(*Photo Source:* Barbara Schwartz/Merrill.)

DISCUSSION POINT

What regularities in language might you rely on when studying a foreign language (as an adult) to isolate meaningful units from continuous speech?

begin to vibrate. Notice the wider space between the arrows for the consonant *p*, which reflects the longer voice onset time.

As mentioned previously, infants are equipped with the ability to categorize speech sounds that are and are not a part of the repertoire of their native language. This ability also holds for hand shapes in American Sign Language (S. A. Baker, Golinkoff, & Petitto, 2006; S. A. Baker, Idsardi, Golinkoff, & Petitto, 2005). Subsequently in this chapter, we discuss the impact of category formation abilities on language development in more detail.

Awareness of Actions and Intentions

Although infants are far less mobile than their toddler counterparts, they are sensitive to actions and movement surrounding them. By age 4 months, infants can distinguish between purposeful and accidental actions, and they appear to focus on the intentions underlying actions rather than the physical details of the actions (Woodward & Hoyne, 1999).

By age 12 months, infants understand rational actions as means to a goal, even when they cannot view the entire context in which an action occurs (Csibra, Bíró, Koós, & Gergely, 2003). For example, see Figure 5.3 for an illustration of the rational and nonrational actions infants witnessed in the study conducted by Csibra et al. (2003). In this study, researchers first familiarized infants with a ball "jumping" over an occluded obstacle. When the occlusion was removed from the

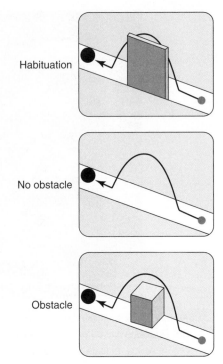

FIGURE 5.3
Rational and nonrational actions.

Source: From "One-Year-Old Infants Use Teleological Representations of Actions Productively," by G. Csibra, S. Bíró, O. Koós, and G. Gergely, 2003, *Cognitive Science, 27,* p. 125. Copyright 2003 by Lawrence Erlbaum Associates, Inc. Reprinted with permission.

DISCUSSION POINT

Consider the verbs *to chase* and *to flee.* How might an understanding of the goals underlying the actions help an infant distinguish between the two?

scene, infants were surprised to see the ball "jump" (because this action was nonrational), but they were not surprised to see the ball "jump" when the occlusion was removed and an obstacle was present (because this action was rational). Infants' awareness of movement and understanding of the goals underlying actions is an important precursor for language development because once they understand the intentions behind actions, they, too, can engage in intentional communication by pointing, gesturing, and eventually using language.

Category Formation

The ability to form categories, or to group items and events according to the perceptual and conceptual features they share, is crucial for language development. In fact, this prelinguistic ability is one of the earliest to develop and perhaps one of the most robust predictors of later cognitive and linguistic outcomes. For example, the ability of infants ages 3–9 months to form categories predicts both their general cognitive and language abilities at age 2 years (Colombo, Shaddy, Richman, Maikranz, & Blaga, 2004) and their cognitive outcomes at age 2.5 years (Laucht, Esser, & Schmidt, 1995).

Hierarchical Structure of Categories

Research results support the idea that category formation is hierarchical and includes three levels: superordinate, subordinate, and basic (Figure 5.4). The

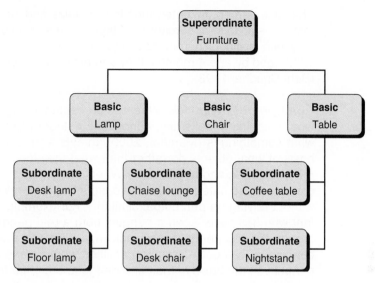

FIGURE 5.4
Hierarchical structure of categories.

superordinate level is the uppermost level in a category hierarchy. Superordinate terms describe the most general concept in a particular category and include words such as *food*, *furniture*, and *clothing*. Superordinate terms are among the later words children acquire. Children cannot successfully categorize words at the superordinate level until preschool age unless they have multiple exemplars on which to base their judgment about the appropriate superordinate category (Liu, Golinkoff, & Sak, 2001). For example, to understand that grapes are part of the category *fruit*, the child would need to see that other fruits (e.g., oranges, bananas) are part of the same category.

The *subordinate level* is the lowest level in a category hierarchy. Subordinate terms describe specific concepts in a category. For example, *garbanzo*, *pinto*, and *kidney* are subordinate terms for different types of beans.

The *basic level* lies in the center of a category hierarchy. Basic-level terms describe general concepts in a category, including words such as *apple, chair*, and *shirt*. Infants' first categories are basic-level categories, just as their first words are basic-level words (Golinkoff, Shuff-Bailey, Olguin, & Ruan, 1995; Mervis, 1987; Mervis & Crisafi, 1982).

Basic Categories at Each Hierarchical Level

In addition to using the hierarchical structure of categories to learn new concepts and words, infants use two basic categories at each level of the hierarchy: perceptual categories and conceptual categories (Mandler, 2000).

Perceptual Categories. Infants form perceptual categories on the basis of similar-appearing features, including color, shape, texture, size, and so forth.

They use perceptual categories to recognize and identify objects around them. Infants begin to form perceptual categories at a very young age: By age 3 months, they can distinguish between cats and dogs (Quinn, Eimas, & Rosenkrantz, 1993), and by age 4 months, they can distinguish between animals and furniture (Behl-Chadha, 1996).

Conceptual Categories. Whereas perceptual categorization involves knowing what something looks like, conceptual categorization requires infants to know what something is (Mandler, 2000). Infants form conceptual categories on the basis of what objects do rather than what they look like. Infants learn that balls roll, dogs bark, and airplanes fly. When infants have conceptual categories, they can use these categories to make inductive generalizations about new objects without relying on perceptual similarity. For example, suppose you show an infant who has never seen a penguin both a real penguin and a toy penguin. Although the toy penguin may look much like the real penguin, infants having conceptual category formation abilities would make inferences about the real penguin on the basis of their knowledge about other live animals. Likewise, they would understand the toy penguin in terms of other toys they already know about. They would probably not be surprised to see the real penguin move around, eat, and interact with other penguins, but they would not expect the toy penguin to do such things simply because it looks like the real penguin.

As mentioned previously, children begin to categorize language aspects at a very young age. However, because language concepts are categorized differently among the many global languages, children learning different languages perceive the world in different ways (see Multicultural Focus: *Concept Categorization Among Languages*).

MULTICULTURAL FOCUS

Concept Categorization Among Languages

All cultures do not represent concepts in the same way. As a result, languages differ in the way they label concepts with words. From a very early age, infants become aware of how their native language represents concepts. Consider the following example of how concepts are labeled differently in different languages.

The English language distinguishes between actions that characterize *containment,* or "put in," relationships and those that characterize *support,* or "put on," relationships. In contrast, the Korean language distinguishes between *tight-fit (kkita)* relationships and *loose-fit* or *contact* relationships; this distinction is not represented in English (Choi, McDonough, Bowerman, & Mandler, 1999). Children become sensitive to these language-specific spatial categories by age 18–23 months. For instance, when presented with an event in which a

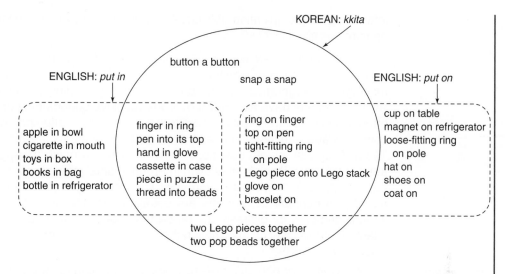

English and Korean spatial categories.

Source: Reprinted from *Cognitive Development,* Vol. 14, S. Choi, L. McDonough, M. Bowerman, and J. M. Mandler, "Early Sensitivity to Language-Specific Spatial Categories in English and Korean," p. 248, Copyright 1999, with permission from Elsevier.

book is placed *in* a tightly fitting box and an event in which rings are placed tightly *on* a pole, Korean-learning infants classify these events similarly. However, English-learning infants treat these two events differently because they perceive one event to represent a "put in" relationship and the other a "put on" relationship.

Therefore, this example suggests that language guides children from a young age as they perceive the spatial relationships around them. Bowerman and Choi (2003) call this the *language as category maker hypothesis.*

Early Vocalizations

DISCUSSION POINT

What is another example of a task that might be used to determine how infants who are learning different languages (e.g., English vs. Arabic) perceive spatial categories?

To this point, we discussed several milestones of infancy that might go unrecognized without close inspection. No one sees infants processing speech sounds or directly witnesses their category formation abilities at work. Next, however, we discuss some of the more obvious prelinguistic milestones infants achieve during the first year—namely, their early vocalizations.

Infants follow a fairly predictable pattern in their early use of *vocalizations.* Researchers who study early vocalizations often classify these sounds according to a *stage model,* which means they describe infants' vocalizations as following an observable and sequential pattern. One such stage model is the Stark Assessment of Early Vocal Development (SAEVD; Nathani, Ertmer, & Stark, 2000), which parents, researchers, and clinicians can use to classify vocalizations and assess an infant's oral communication abilities. According to the SAEVD, vocalization development has six distinct stages:

1. *Reflexive (0–8 weeks).* The first kinds of sounds infants produce are called *reflexive sounds,* which include sounds of discomfort and distress (crying, fussing) and vegetative sounds produced during feeding (burping, coughing). Although infants have no control over the reflexive sounds they produce, adults often respond as if these reflexes are true communication attempts. Parents ascribe communicative functions to even the earliest of infants' vocalizations (C. L. Miller, 1988). They ask infants questions such as "Why so much fussing?" to engage them in dialogue. Parents may even interpret infants' reflexive sounds out loud for them: "Oh, you're saying that you want Mommy to hold you, aren't you?" Compared with nonparents, parents are usually more sensitive to infants' reflexive sounds and calls for distress and report that they base their judgments about an infant's distress level on information they gain through the crying infant's face and voice (Irwin, 2003).

CD VIDEO CLIP
To watch an infant produce cooing and gooing sounds, see the CD video clip *Language 1.*

2. *Control of phonation (6–16 weeks).* In the control of phonation stage, infants begin to produce *cooing* and *gooing* sounds. Such sounds consist mainly of vowel sounds and some *nasalized* sounds (i.e., airflow is directed through the nose). When infants produce consonant sounds, they typically do so far back in the oral cavity (e.g., "goooo"). These early consonant sounds are easier for infants to produce than are sounds that require more precise manipulation of the tongue, lips, or teeth (e.g., /t/ and /f/).

3. *Expansion (4–6 months).* In the expansion stage, infants gain more control over the articulators and begin to produce series of vowel sounds as well as *vowel glides* (e.g., "eeeey"). Infants also experiment with the loudness and pitch of their voices at this time. The infant at this stage begins to yell, to growl, to squeal, and to make "raspberries" and trills. Research results also suggest that early infant vocalizations are one component of a dynamic mother–infant communication system, whereby patterns of mother–infant communication relate to infant vocalizations. Infants' rates of syllabic (speechlike) and vocalic (nonspeechlike) vocalizations are positively associated with *symmetrical communication patterns*—which involve mutual engagement on the part of mother and infant—but are negatively associated with *unilateral communication patterns*—which involve engagement on the part of the mother but not the infant (Hsu, 2001).

4. *Control of articulation (5–8 months).* During the control of articulation stage, infants continue to experiment with sounds and the loudness of their voice as they engage in squealing. Marginal babbling begins to emerge as infants gain control of their articulation. **Marginal babbling** is an early type of babbling containing short strings of consonant-like and vowel-like sounds.

5. *Canonical syllables (6–10 months).* True **babbling,** which begins between ages 6 and 10 months, is distinguished from earlier vocalizations by the child's production of syllables that contain pairs of consonants and vowels (called

C–V sequences when the consonant precedes the vowel). Babbling may be reduplicated or nonreduplicated. **Reduplicated babbling** consists of repeating consonant–vowel pairs, as in "ma ma ma," whereas **nonreduplicated babbling** (or **variegated babbling**) consists of nonrepeating consonant–vowel combinations, such as "da ma goo ga." In many cultures, infants prefer nasal sounds (/m/, /n/, and /ŋ/ as in *sing*) and stop sounds (/p/, /b/, /t/, /d/) in their variegated babbling (Locke, 1983), combining such sounds variously with vowels to produce long vocalized sequences. Infants in the canonical syllable stage also produce *whispered vocalizations, rounded vowels* (/u/ in *pool*), and *high front vowels* (/i/ as in *beet*). Often, parents view their children as beginning to talk when the children begin to babble because such syllable combinations resemble adult speech.

Hearing infants are not the only babies to babble. Infants who are Deaf, as well as infants who hear but have parents who are profoundly Deaf, babble manually—using their hands. Just as the vocalizations of infants who hear speech mimic the specific rhythmic patterns that bind syllables, so do the hand movements of babies born to parents who are Deaf. These infants' hand movements have a slower rhythm than that of ordinary gestures, and the infants produce these movements within a tightly restricted space in front of the body (Petitto, Holowka, Sergio, & Ostry, 2001).

6. *Advanced forms (10–18 months).* In the more advanced stage of early vocalizations, infants begin to produce *diphthongs,* which are combinations of two vowel sounds within the same syllable, as in the sound /ɔɪ/ in *boy* and the sound /aɪ/ in *fine.* Infants also begin to produce more complex combinations of consonants and vowels, including C–V–C ("gom"), C–C–V ("stee"), and V–C–V ("abu"). Probably the most noticeable achievement in the advanced forms stage is jargon. **Jargon** is a special type of babbling that contains the true melodic patterns of an infant's native language. When you listen to an infant who is producing jargon, you think you are hearing questions, exclamations, and commands, even in the absence of recognizable words. Although the vocalizations infants produce while they are babbling or using jargon may sound like short words or syllables, such vocalizations are not considered true words because they are not referential, nor do they convey meaning. Rather, at this stage, infants are still experimenting with the sounds of their native language.

Additional Milestones

As you can see, infants reach many important milestones during the first year on their journey through language development. As we described in the sections on speech perception, awareness of actions and intentions, category formation, and early vocalizations, these milestones involve a series of *incremental* developments in the first year, rather than all-or-nothing capabilities. See this chapter's *Developmental Timeline* for even more milestones infants reach with regard to phonology, semantics, and pragmatics.

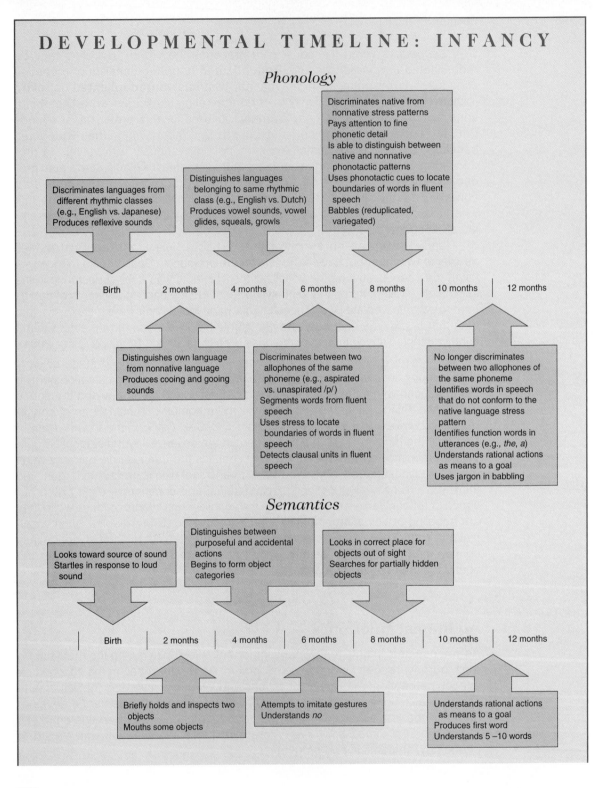

DEVELOPMENTAL TIMELINE: INFANCY

Phonology

Discriminates native from nonnative stress patterns
Pays attention to fine phonetic detail
Is able to distinguish between native and nonnative phonotactic patterns
Uses phonotactic cues to locate boundaries of words in fluent speech
Babbles (reduplicated, variegated)

Discriminates languages from different rhythmic classes (e.g., English vs. Japanese)
Produces reflexive sounds

Distinguishes languages belonging to same rhythmic class (e.g., English vs. Dutch)
Produces vowel sounds, vowel glides, squeals, growls

| Birth | 2 months | 4 months | 6 months | 8 months | 10 months | 12 months |

Distinguishes own language from nonnative language
Produces cooing and gooing sounds

Discriminates between two allophones of the same phoneme (e.g., aspirated vs. unaspirated /p/)
Segments words from fluent speech
Uses stress to locate boundaries of words in fluent speech
Detects clausal units in fluent speech

No longer discriminates between two allophones of the same phoneme
Identifies words in speech that do not conform to the native language stress pattern
Identifies function words in utterances (e.g., *the, a*)
Understands rational actions as means to a goal
Uses jargon in babbling

Semantics

Looks toward source of sound
Startles in response to loud sound

Distinguishes between purposeful and accidental actions
Begins to form object categories

Looks in correct place for objects out of sight
Searches for partially hidden objects

| Birth | 2 months | 4 months | 6 months | 8 months | 10 months | 12 months |

Briefly holds and inspects two objects
Mouths some objects

Attempts to imitate gestures
Understands *no*

Understands rational actions as means to a goal
Produces first word
Understands 5–10 words

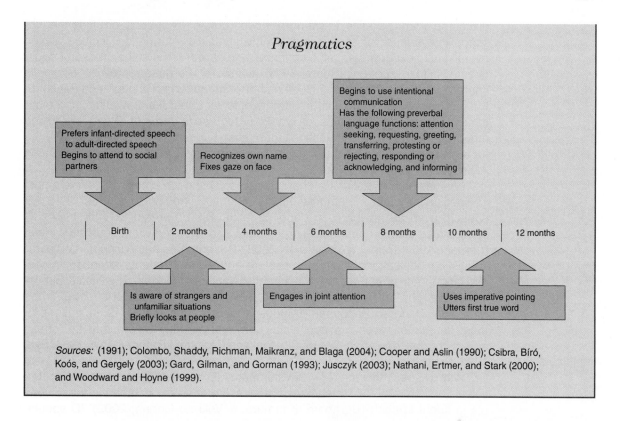

Pragmatics

Prefers infant-directed speech to adult-directed speech
Begins to attend to social partners

Recognizes own name
Fixes gaze on face

Begins to use intentional communication
Has the following preverbal language functions: attention seeking, requesting, greeting, transferring, protesting or rejecting, responding or acknowledging, and informing

| Birth | 2 months | 4 months | 6 months | 8 months | 10 months | 12 months |

Is aware of strangers and unfamiliar situations
Briefly looks at people

Engages in joint attention

Uses imperative pointing
Utters first true word

Sources: (1991); Colombo, Shaddy, Richman, Maikranz, and Blaga (2004); Cooper and Aslin (1990); Csibra, Bíró, Koós, and Gergely (2003); Gard, Gilman, and Gorman (1993); Jusczyk (2003); Nathani, Ertmer, and Stark (2000); and Woodward and Hoyne (1999).

WHAT ARE SOME OF THE EARLY FOUNDATIONS FOR LANGUAGE DEVELOPMENT?

During infancy, the quality and quantity of the input infants receive, as well as the types of social interactions in which they engage, form important early foundations for language development. Some of the foundations that pave the way for later language development are infant-directed speech, joint reference and attention, the daily routines of infancy, and caregiver responsiveness. As you read this section, think back to the language development theories you learned about in Chapter 2. Note that these early foundations for language development presuppose the importance of the environment in language development. They are also contingent on the linguistic input adults provide and the social interactions that infants engage in with other people. All these factors are central to nurture-inspired language development theories.

Infant-Directed Speech

Infant-directed (ID) speech—also called *motherese*, *baby talk*, and *child-directed speech*—is the speech adults use in communicative situations with young language learners. ID speech has several distinctive paralinguistic, syntactic, and discourse characteristics. **Paralinguistic** features of ID speech, or those that describe the manner of speech outside the linguistic information, include a high overall pitch, exaggerated pitch contours, and slower tempos than those of adult-directed (AD) speech (Snow 1972; Snow & Ferguson, 1977). *Syntactic* characteristics of ID speech include a shorter mean length of utterance (MLU), or the number of morphemes in an utterance; fewer subordinate clauses; and more content words and fewer function words. *Discourse* features of ID speech include more repetition and more questions than those used in AD speech. See Table 5.1 for a comparison of the paralinguistic, syntactic, and discourse features of ID and AD speech.

Besides having distinctive characteristics, ID speech appears to serve a host of special purposes. It attracts infants' attention, and infants prefer it to AD speech, even as newborns (Cooper & Aslin, 1990; Fernald & Kuhl, 1987). ID speech also aids in communicating emotion and speakers' communicative intent (Fernald, 1989; Trainor & Desjardins, 2002). Researchers have documented paralinguistic modifications, thought to capture and maintain infants' attention, in several languages other than American English, including German (Fernald & Simon, 1984); French, Italian, Japanese, and British English (Fernald et al., 1989); and Mandarin Chinese (Papousek, Papousek, & Symmes, 1991). Examinations of these languages reveal that adults may universally modify the prosody (i.e., stress and rhythm) of their speech to infants (but see Bernstein Ratner & Pye, 1984; Pye, 1992; Smith-Hefner, 1988).

With respect to language development, ID speech contains exaggerated vowels, which may facilitate infants' processing of words containing these vowels in fluent speech (Burnham, Kitamura, & Vollmer-Conna, 2002). ID speech also highlights content words, such as nouns and verbs, relative to function words, such as prepositions and articles (van de Weijer, 2001), and places these words on exaggerated pitch peaks at the ends of utterances, where infants are likely to remember them (Fernald & Mazzie, 1991). Moreover, ID speech exaggerates pauses, which creates a salient cue to help infants detect major syntactic units in speech (Bernstein Ratner, 1986). The rhythm of ID speech is marked by the presence of reliable acoustic correlates of both utterance and phrase boundaries in other languages as well (e.g., Japanese; Fisher & Tokura, 1996). At the very least, using ID speech to introduce new words and phrases should capture infants' attention and increase the chance that they will focus on the speech they hear.

Joint Reference and Attention

Recall from Chapter 2 the Vygotskian perspective on language development. According to Vygotsky, language development is a dynamic process that occurs within children's zone of proximal development (ZPD) as they interact socially with more advanced peers and adults. Adamson and Chance's (1998) account of infants' development of language through social interactions takes a Vygotskian approach. These researchers proposed that infancy comprises three major developmental phases with respect to joint reference and attention (Figure 5.5):

TABLE 5.1
Comparison of Infant-Directed (ID) and Adult-Directed (AD) Speech

Features	ID speech	AD speech
	Examples	Examples
Paralinguistic features		
High overall pitch	*[ID speech pitch contour graph: Frequency (Hz) 100–500 vs. Time (s) .5–2]*	*[AD speech pitch contour graph: Frequency (Hz) 100–500 vs. Time (s) .5–2]*
Exaggerated pitch contours	"You want potatoes?"	"Would you like mashed potatoes with your meal?"
Slower tempos	"I brought you a gift. Grandmom brought you a gift. Grandpop brought you a gift."	"I brought you a gift and Grandmom and Grandpop did, too."
	"See bike?"	"Do you see that bike on the sidewalk?"
Syntactic features		
Shorter mean length of utterance		
Fewer subordinate clauses		
More content words and fewer function words		
Discourse features		
More repetition	"Let's look at the book. Should we open the book? You like books?"	"I'd like to read that book."
More questions	"Is that Daddy? Is that Daddy over there?"	"Hey, there's your friend from work."

161

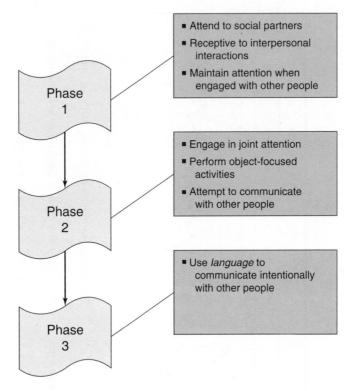

FIGURE 5.5
Adamson and Chance's (1998) three phases of language development through social interactions.

Phase 1: Attendance to social partners

Phase 2: Emergence and coordination of joint attention

Phase 3: Transition to language

In each phase, adults view infants' interactions as meaningful through the lens of their culture. Furthermore, adults support infants' expressions in each phase until infants can independently master components of the social exchange.

Phase 1: Attendance to Social Partners (Birth to Age 6 Months)

In the first phase, spanning from birth to about age 6 months, infants develop patterns of attending to social partners. In these early months of life, infants value and participate in interpersonal interactions, learning how to maintain attention and be "organized" within sustained periods of engagement. Infants are especially interested in looking at people's faces during this phase, in particular their parents' faces. Caregiver responsiveness, which we discuss later in this chapter, is an important feature of this first phase.

Phase 2: Emergence and Coordination of Joint Attention (Age 6 Months to 1 Year)

In the second phase, spanning from approximately 6 months of age through 1 year, infants begin to take more interest in looking at and manipulating the objects around them. During this phase, infants begin to move their attention between an object of interest and another person (Adamson & Chance, 1998). This activity signals the emergence of joint attention. *Joint attention* is the simultaneous engagement of two or more individuals in mental focus on a single external object of focus. For example, when a mother shakes a toy in front of her infant so that he or she will look at it, mother and infant are engaging in joint attention with respect to the toy. When parents read storybooks to their children and they look at the pictures together, they are also engaging in joint attention. This seemingly simple activity provides a critical avenue for early communication development because periods of joint attention foster important communicative exchanges, such as labeling (Ninio & Bruner, 1978). In fact, children who engage in longer periods of joint attention with their caregivers have relatively larger vocabularies at age 18 months than those of children with fewer such experiences (Tomasello & Todd, 1983).

Often, caregivers share much of the burden of sustaining the infant's participation throughout periods of joint attention. Adults may use such techniques as speaking with an animated voice or showing the infant novel objects as they engage in what is called **supported joint engagement.** The extent to which mothers use strategies to *maintain* their infant's attention is related to an infant's ability to engage in sustained attention at age 18 months (Bono & Stifter, 2003). Conversely, the extent to which mothers consistently use strategies to *redirect* their infant's attention is negatively related to an infant's ability to engage in sustained attention (Bono & Stifter, 2003).

Why is joint attention so important? In the absence of joint attention, infants may miss out on word-learning opportunities as their parents and caregivers label objects and events for them. Imagine a scenario in which a mother is pushing her infant son in a stroller. As she points upward, she utters, "Look at the birdie." Suppose the infant misses his mother's pointing gesture and hears the word *birdie* while he is carefully studying his new shoes. In this situation, the mother and her son are not jointly attending to the same entity in the world, so the baby boy will probably not learn what the word *birdie* refers to. In the worst case scenario, the boy might associate the word *birdie* with his new shoes. However, infants soon become adept at using cues—including line of regard (the direction of a person's gaze, which indicates what the person is looking at), gestures (e.g., pointing), voice direction, and body posture—to support inferences about a speaker's referential intentions, and they learn not to associate the words they hear with the objects and events on which only they are focused (Baldwin, 1991).

Before infants can use cues to infer another person's intentions, they must possess **intersubjective awareness,** or the recognition of when one person shares a mental focus on some external object or action with another person. Only after infants realize they can share a mental focus with other humans do they begin to interpret other people's referential actions as intentional and begin

CD VIDEO CLIP

To watch an infant engage in intentional communication attempts by using pointing, gestures, and advanced vocalizations, see the CD video clip *Language 2.*

DISCUSSION POINT

Why do you think declarative pointing is more challenging for infants than imperative pointing is? How could declarative pointing relate to understanding other people's intentions?

to use their own actions referentially. This skill is called *intentional communication*, or the infants' attempts to deliberately communicate with other people. Researchers who study intentional communication have devised some guidelines to determine whether infants' communicative behaviors are preintentional or intentional. Indicators of intentionality include the following: The infant alternates eye gaze between an object and a communicative partner; the infant uses ritualized gestures, such as pointing; and the infant persists toward goals by repeating or modifying his or her gestures when communicative attempts fail (Bates, Camaioni, & Volterra, 1975). Intentional communication begins to emerge around age 8–10 months.

An interesting fact is that infants are skilled in using multiple forms of pointing. They use **imperative pointing** as requests to adults to retrieve objects for them. They begin to use this type of pointing around age 10 months, for example, when they want someone to bring them a toy that is out of reach. **Declarative pointing** involves a social process between an infant and an adult. Infants use declarative pointing to call an adult's attention to objects and to comment on objects. Research results show that children produce and understand declarative pointing later than when they understand and produce imperative pointing. Furthermore, infants' production of declarative pointing, but not imperative pointing, is linked to their understanding of other people's intentions (Camaioni, Perucchini, Bellagamba, & Colonnesi, 2004).

Phase 3: Transition to Language (Age 1 Year and Beyond)

In the third phase of the development of language through social interactions, children begin to incorporate language into their communicative interactions with other

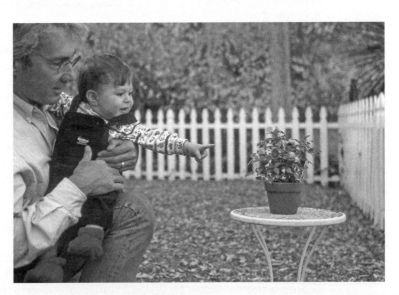

Infants' production of declarative pointing to call attention to and comment on objects is linked to their understanding of other people's intentions.

(*Photo Source:* © Michael Newman/PhotoEdit Inc.)

THEORY TO PRACTICE

Language Development and Marketing

Language development theories and the research that these theories propagate are having an increasing impact on parenting practices and even influence the products parents buy for their infants. For example, Hirsh-Pasek and Golinkoff (2003) presented compelling rationales for why "children need to play more and memorize less". Citing Albert Einstein's childhood as an example, Hirsh-Pasek and Golinkoff emphasized, "Much of his learning as a child took place through play. His parents and family paid attention to his interests and fed them with lessons and toys and books . . ." (p. 245).

Even the toy industry is changing in response to the continually increasing understanding of how language develops in infants. For example, Fisher-Price has a series of *Laugh & Learn* products that encourage language development (www.fisher-price.com/us/learning/). The Laugh & Learn Learning Phone, for instance, is designed to help infants understand cause-and-effect actions, make connections between words and images, and experience the give-and-take of a conversation.

people. Having joint attention and an understanding of intentionality well established, infants in this phase shift to being able to engage socially with other individuals and to use language to represent events and objects within these interactions. The active involvement of parents and other adults is still important during this phase. Mothers' verbal encouragement of infants' attention at age 1 year is positively related to infants' language development at that age (Karrass, Braungart-Rieker, Mullins, & Lefever, 2002).

Remarkably, research on the phases of language development has an impact on practices in many domains, including marketing, as people consider how to tailor products to best meet the needs of infants who are becoming intentional communicators. See Theory to Practice: *Language Development and Marketing* for an example of how the toy industry is taking notice of infants' developing abilities.

Daily Routines of Infancy

Infants' daily lives consist of several routines that provide a sense of comfort and predictability. As a bonus, these seemingly dull routines, such as feeding, bathing, dressing, and diaper changing, provide many opportunities for language learning. Consider a scenario in which a father is feeding his infant. During this routine, caregivers often provide a commentary for their infants similar to that of sports commentators when they talk through baseball or football games. Babies hear such things as "OK, open wide. Here comes your applesauce." "Oops, we got a little dribble there." "Wow, you ate the whole jar!" Although infants are too young even to feed themselves, they benefit from hearing the same words and phrases repeated each day as their parents feed them. Infants are adept at identifying and making sense of the patterns they hear in speech. By hearing words and phrases repeatedly, infants become attuned to where pauses occur, which helps them to segment phrases, clauses, and eventually words from the speech stream. They also learn about phonotactics, or the combinations of sounds that are acceptable in their native language. Routines allow infants not only to encounter numerous linguistic patterns but also to have many opportunities to engage in episodes of joint attention with their caregivers.

Caregiver Responsiveness

Caregiver responsiveness describes caregivers' attention and sensitivity to infants' vocalizations and communicative attempts. Caregiver responsiveness helps teach infants that other people value their behaviors and communicative attempts. Caregivers who provide consistent, contingent, and appropriate responses to their infants' communicative attempts promote their children's ability and desire to sustain long periods of joint attention and increase their children's motivation to communicate. Research results show that mothers demonstrate remarkable consistency in identifying their infants' communicative acts during the second half of the first year (Meadows, Elias, & Bain, 2000), which may in turn promote even higher levels of responsiveness.

Both the quality and the quantity of responsiveness by caregivers play a large role in early language development. More responsive maternal language input is linked—even more so than infants' own early communicative behaviors, such as vocalizations—to the time at which infants reach important language milestones, including saying their first word and producing two-word utterances (Nicely, Tamis-LeMonda, & Bornstein, 1999; Tamis-LeMonda, Bornstein, & Baumwell, 2001).

Weitzman and Greenberg (2002) described the following seven characteristics as key indicators of caregiver responsiveness. These indicators have been linked to improved rates of language development in young children (e.g., Girolametto & Weitzman, 2002):

1. *Waiting and listening.* Parents wait expectantly for initiations, use a slow pace to allow for initiations, and listen to allow the child to complete messages.

2. *Following the child's lead.* When a child initiates either verbally or nonverbally, parents follow the child's lead by responding verbally to the initiation, using animation, and avoiding vague acknowledgments.

3. *Joining in and playing.* Parents build on their child's focus of interest and play without dominating.

4. *Being face to face.* Parents adjust their physical level by sitting on the floor, leaning forward to facilitate face-to-face interaction, and bending toward the child when they are above the child's level.

5. *Using a variety of questions and labels.* Parents encourage conversation by asking a variety of *wh-* questions (e.g., "Who?" "Where?" "Why?"), by using yes–no questions only to clarify messages and obtain information, by avoiding test and rhetorical questions, and by waiting expectantly for responses.

6. *Encouraging turn taking.* Parents wait expectantly for responses, balance the number and length of adult-to-child turns, and complete their children's sentences only for children who are not yet combining words.

7. *Expanding and extending.* Parents expand and extend by repeating their children's words and correcting the grammar or by adding another idea, and use comments and questions to inform, predict, imagine, explain, and talk about feelings.

WHAT MAJOR ACHIEVEMENTS IN LANGUAGE CONTENT, FORM, AND USE CHARACTERIZE INFANCY?

Recall from Chapter 1 that language consists of three rule-governed domains that together reflect an integrated whole: content, form, and use. Language *content* is the words people use and the meanings behind them. People express content through their vocabulary system, or *lexicon,* as they retrieve and organize words to express ideas or to understand what other individuals are saying. *Form* is how people arrange words, sentences, and sounds to convey content. *Use* is language pragmatics, or how people use language in interactions with other individuals to express personal and social needs.

Language Content

Although infants reach a multitude of exciting milestones during their first year, none seems to be celebrated more than the first word. On average, infants produce their first true word at age 12 months. First words usually refer to salient people and objects in infants' everyday lives, such as *mama, dada, doggie,* and the like. Researchers consider an infant's vocalization to be a *true word* if it meets three important criteria.

First, infants must say true words with a clear intention. When a baby girl says the word *juice* while reaching for her cup of juice, she undoubtedly has the clear intention of referring to her drink. If the same baby says the word *juice* after her mother tells her "Say juice; tell me juice," researchers would consider the infant's utterance to be an imitation or a repetition rather than a true word.

Second, infants must produce true words with recognizable pronunciation that approximates the adult form. Twelve-month-olds cannot produce all sounds accurately, but their first word should sound like a close approximation of the adult form, and other people should be able to recognize it. Thus, a child's "mama" for *mommy* is a close enough approximation to be a true word. However, if a child produces *mommy* as "goo"—even consistently and while clearly referring to his or her mother—it would not meet the criteria for a true word because it does not closely approximate an adult form.

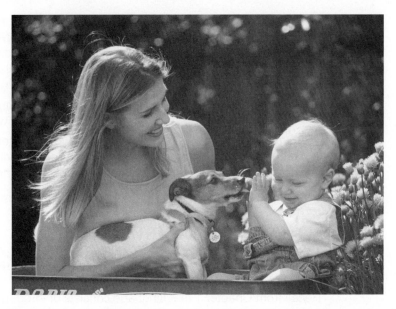

First words usually refer to salient people and objects in infants' everyday lives, such as their mother, father, pets, and so forth.

(*Photo Source:* © Michael Keller/Corbis.)

Third, a true word is a word that a child uses consistently and generalizes beyond the original context to all appropriate exemplars. In the case of the baby girl who said "Juice," she could be expected to use this word not only with her apple juice but also with orange juice, grape juice, and pictures of juice in storybooks. Because words name categories of objects, events, and activities—and not just single exemplars—infants must be able to generalize their words to several appropriate cases for their words to meet the criteria for true words.

Language Form

Infants' language form is the most simple of all. Because they do not produce their first word until about age 1 year, no real language form to speak of exists until that time. When infants do begin to use true words, they generally utter these words in isolation for several months (e.g., "Daddy") before they begin to combine words to make short phrases (e.g., "Daddy up"). However, although infants are not *producing* multiword utterances, they can typically *understand* some multiword utterances by age 1 year, particularly those they have heard many times (e.g., "Bye-bye, Mommy"; "Baby want milk?").

Language Use

Infancy is the calm before the language storm of toddlerhood, during which toddlers experiment (seemingly continuously) with all their newly acquired language skills. Although infants are not chatterboxes, they spend much of their time listening, observing, and learning how the people around them use language to communicate. Even before infants utter their first word, they are eager to communicate. Infants who are communicating intentionally (usually by age 8 months) use a variety of preverbal language functions, and include the following (Kent, 1994):

- *Attention seeking to self.* Infants may tug on an adult's clothing to gain his or her attention.
- *Attention seeking to events, objects, or other people.* Infants point to things in their environment to draw attention to them.
- *Requesting objects.* Infants use imperative pointing to indicate that they would like to have an object.
- *Requesting action.* Infants hand objects to an adult when they would like the adult to do something with the objects.
- *Requesting information.* Infants may point to an object to have an adult provide a label for it or to provide other information about the object.
- *Greeting.* Infants wave "hi" and "bye-bye" to other people.
- *Transferring.* Infants may give a toy that they were playing with to another person.
- *Protesting or rejecting.* Infants may cry to protest when someone takes away a toy that they were playing with or may push an object away to reject it.
- *Responding or acknowledging.* Infants may respond to other people and acknowledge their communicative attempts by smiling or laughing.
- *Informing.* Infants may inform other people when something is wrong—for example, by pointing to a broken wheel on a toy truck.

WHAT FACTORS INFLUENCE INFANTS' INDIVIDUAL ACHIEVEMENTS IN LANGUAGE?

Although infants develop language in a fairly predictable pattern because they meet certain milestones in the same order and at about the same age, some aspects of their language development vary. One major *intraindividual* difference in language development and three major *interindividual* differences are discussed next, along with factors that may account for such differences (Bates, Dale, & Thal, 1995).

Intraindividual Differences

If you observe an *individual* infant, you will most likely notice that he or she does not develop all aspects of language at the same rate. In this section, we discuss how an infant differs in receptive and expressive language development and three factors that may account for this difference.

As mentioned previously in this text, at all stages of life, the amount of language an individual can produce spontaneously without imitating another person's verbalizations (**expressive language**) differs from the amount of language he or she can comprehend (**receptive language**). Infancy is no exception.

For example, Figure 5.6 shows that although 1-year-olds comprehend an average of 80 words, they typically produce only about 10 words. Three factors account for why language comprehension most likely precedes language production (Golinkoff & Hirsh-Pasek, 1999). First, language comprehension requires only that people retrieve words from their lexicon, or mental dictionary, whereas language production requires people to retrieve words and apply proper pronunciation as the words are uttered. Second, with language comprehension, sentences are preorganized with lexical items, a syntactic structure, and intonation as people hear them. However, language production requires the speaker to search for words, organize them, and place stress where it is required. Third, and especially relevant to infants, language that adults use in communicative interactions with infants is usually highly contextualized, with many clues to assist comprehension. Children are generally at an advantage for comprehension because in many cases the words adults use when communicating with them have referents that are immediately available in the environment ("You want your bottle?" "Let's get your bib on"). However, in terms of production, children must construct a match between the intended referent and language to express meaning.

The theme that language comprehension precedes language production resurfaces in Chapters 6–8. In those chapters, we discuss various language developments that occur during toddlerhood, the preschool years, and the school-age years and beyond.

Interindividual Differences

If you observe a *group* of infants, you will most likely note language development differences among them. First, some children will develop language more quickly than others. Second, children will express themselves for different communicative purposes, and, third, certain children will fall at either end of the continuum for language development and be late talkers or early talkers. Following, we discuss these differences and some of the factors accounting for them.

Variation in Language Development Rate

The rate at which a group of children develop their receptive and expressive language abilities can vary considerably. One way to gauge the variability in infants' receptive and expressive vocabulary is by examining norm-referenced measures of language, such as the MacArthur–Bates Communicative Development Inventories (CDI; Fenson et al., 1993; Fenson, Pethick, et al., 2000). We describe the norming process for the CDI in Chapter 2, but what is important to note in this discussion is the variability among more than 1,800 infants' expressive and receptive vocabularies (Bates et al., 1995). In Figure 5.6, the mean developmental functions for these infants' receptive and expressive vocabularies between ages 8 and 16 months are depicted by a series of connected solid black squares. Note also in Figure 5.6 the developmental functions for children whose language development

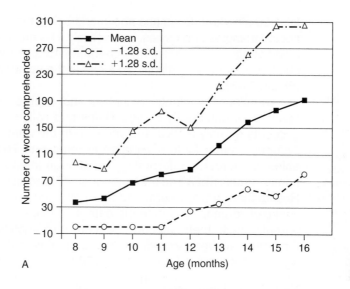

A

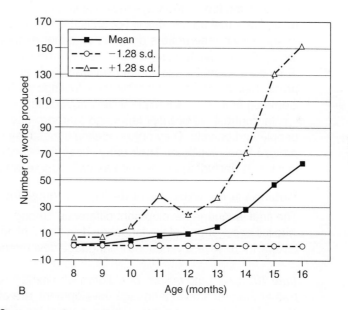

B

FIGURE 5.6
(A) Word comprehension and (B) word production on the MacArthur–Bates Communicative Development Inventory Infant Scale.

Source: From "Individual Differences and Their Implications for Theories of Language Development," by E. Bates, P. S. Dale, and D. Thal, in *Handbook of Child Language* (pp. 102–103), edited by P. Fletcher and B. MacWhinney, 1995, Oxford, England: Basil Blackwell. Copyright 1995 by Blackwell Publishing. Reprinted with permission.

DISCUSSION POINT

Besides age, SES, and the quantity of adult talk, what other factors do you think might predict some of the remaining variance *among infants* in the number of words they produce or in the number that they comprehend?

fell 1.28 standard deviations above and below the mean, represented by the connected triangles and circles, respectively. The number of words the infants understood at age 12 months ranged between 15 and 150 (Figure 5.6A), whereas the number of words the infants produced at the same age ranged between 0 and 30 (Figure 5.6B).

Variations in infants' receptive and expressive vocabularies can be accounted for only partly by age. Bates and colleagues (1995) reported that age accounts for only 22% of the variance in the number of words infants produce. Therefore, other factors explain the remaining 78% of the variance. Two variables of interest in interpreting variation in infants' vocabularies are socioeconomic status (SES) and the amount of talk parents engage in with their children. Researchers have determined that how much parents talk to their infants and young children is related to the parents' SES, but, regardless of SES, the more parents talk to their children, the more rapidly children's vocabulary grows and the better children perform on measures of verbal and cognitive competence at age 3 years (Hart & Risley, 1995, 1999).

Variation in Language-Learning Styles

Infants differ, too, in the ways they use language for communicative purposes. The main factor that affects this variation is the infants' predominant style for using language, which researchers describe as either expressive or referential (K. Nelson, 1973). *Expressive* language learners use language primarily for social exchanges. Their early vocabularies contain several words and phrases that allow them to express their needs and describe their feelings as they interact with other people. Common first words for expressive language learners include *hi* and *bye-bye.*

In contrast, *referential* language learners use language primarily to refer to people and objects. They enjoy labeling things they see, and they like when adults provide labels for them. Their early vocabularies contain a large proportion of object labels, including words such as *ball, doggie,* and *juice* (K. Nelson, 1973).

Variation at the Extremes of the Typical Range for Language Development

The final language development difference among infants involves certain children who fall at either end of the language development continuum: late talkers and early talkers. More severe variations in language development are covered in Chapter 10.

Late Talkers. Late talkers, or children who exhibit early delays in their expressive (rather than receptive) language development, are of concern to parents and clinicians. Many late talkers can achieve normal language levels by age 3 or 4 years. However, they may still exhibit delays in subtle aspects of language development and perform at significantly lower levels on measures of verbal short-term memory, sentence formulation, word retrieval, auditory processing of complex information, and elaborated verbal expression than those of their age-matched, typically developing peers at ages 6, 7, and 8 years (Rescorla, 1993b).

Early Talkers. Early talkers are children who are ahead of their peers in expressive language use. Bates and colleagues (1995) defined early talkers as children

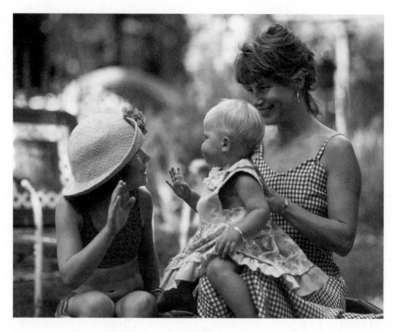

Expressive language learners use language primarily for social exchanges.
(*Photo Source:* © John Henley/Corbis.)

between ages 11 and 21 months who score in the top 10% for vocabulary production for their age on the MacArthur–Bates CDI. Although few studies on early talkers have been conducted, research results suggest that these children have an advantage over their age-matched, typically developing peers on measures of vocabulary, grammar, and verbal reasoning throughout early childhood (Robinson, Dale, & Landesman, 1990).

HOW DO RESEARCHERS AND CLINICIANS MEASURE LANGUAGE DEVELOPMENT IN INFANCY?

Many methods are available for measuring language development. In this section, we discuss ways in which researchers measure language achievements as they strive to understand the course of language development. We also describe methods clinicians use to measure language development as they seek to determine whether children are progressing typically in their receptive and expressive achievements.

Researchers

The fact that infants cannot usually tell adults what they know about language poses some interesting challenges with regard to measuring their language achievements. As a result, researchers who measure language achievements in infancy have devised an array of creative methods to shed light on infants' developing systems, including habituation–dishabituation tasks, the intermodal preferential looking paradigm, the interactive intermodal preferential looking paradigm, and naturalistic observation.

Habituation–Dishabituation Tasks

Habituation of an infant consists of presenting the same stimulus repeatedly until his or her attention to the stimulus decreases by a predetermined amount. **Dishabituation** describes the infant's renewed interest in a stimulus according to some predetermined threshold. Researchers use habituation–dishabituation tasks to determine whether infants detect differences in prelinguistic and linguistic stimuli and to determine how infants organize these stimuli categorically.

In a study by Pulverman and Golinkoff (2004), researchers were interested in determining the extent to which infants attend to potential verb referents (e.g., *bending, spinning*) as they watch motion events. These researchers habituated infants to one of nine stimulus events involving an animated starfish actor and a green ball, which serves as a point of reference (e.g., the starfish does jumping jacks over the ball). Infants were said to have *habituated* when the time of their visual fixation to the stimulus during three trials (Trials 4–6, Trials 7–9, etc.) decreased to less than 65% of their visual fixation time in the first three trials. Once the infants were habituated, researchers presented four test trials in a random order:

Test trial	Description	Example
1. Control	Same event as in habituation trials	The starfish *does jumping jacks over* the ball.
2. Path change	Same manner as in the habituation trials, but different path	The starfish does *jumping jacks under* the ball.
3. Manner change	Same path as in the habituation trials, but different manner	The starfish *spins over* the ball.
4. Path and manner change	Different path and manner than in the habituation trials	The starfish *bends alongside* the ball.

By measuring infants' dishabituation, researchers determined that young infants are sensitive to the nonlinguistic aspects of manner and path that potentially serve as verb labels in their native language. See Figure 5.7 for an illustration of the habituation–dishabituation stimuli that Pulverman and Golinkoff (2004) used in their study. Note, too, that in the study, the starfish enacted the motions in a continuous manner along the paths depicted at the bottom of the illustration.

DISCUSSION POINT
The Spanish language contains more path verbs (*exit, descend*) than manner verbs (*slither, stagger*), whereas the opposite is true for English. How might Spanish- and English-learning infants show different habituation–dishabituation patterns in a task like that presented by Pulverman and Golinkoff (2004)?

CD VIDEO CLIP
To watch an infant participating in Pulverman and Golinkoff's (2004) habituation–dishabituation study, see the CD video clip *Research 1*.

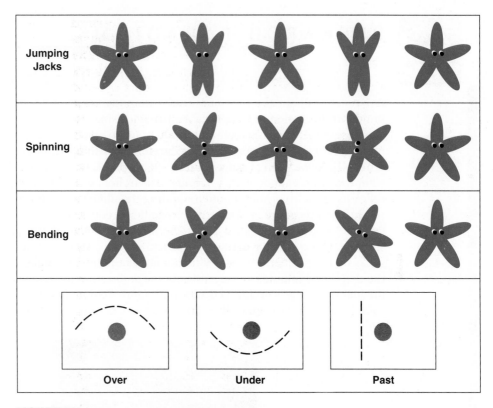

FIGURE 5.7
Sample stimuli for a habituation–dishabituation task.

Source: From *Seven-Month-Olds' Attention to Potential Verb Referents in Nonlinguistic Events,* by R. Pulverman and R. M. Golinkoff, 2004, in a paper presented at the proceedings of the 28th annual Boston University Conference on Language Development, Boston, MA. Copyright 2004 by Cascadilla Press. Reprinted with permission.

Similar to the habituation–dishabituation paradigm is the *high-amplitude nonnutritive sucking procedure,* in which a newborn's sucking rate is used as a dependent measure instead of looking time. See Research Paradigms: *The High-Amplitude Nonnutritive Sucking Procedure* for more information on this paradigm.

Intermodal Preferential Looking Paradigm

In the *intermodal preferential looking paradigm* (IPLP), an infant sits on a blindfolded parent's lap approximately 3 feet from a television screen (parents are blindfolded so that they cannot influence their infant's performance on the task; Hirsh-Pasek & Golinkoff, 1996; Spelke, 1979). The infant watches a split-screen presentation in which one stimulus is on the left side of the screen and another stimulus is on the right side. For example, the infant may see a person dancing on the left and a person jumping on the right. The audio that accompanies the presentation matches the visual information on only one side of the screen (e.g., "Find dancing!" "Where's dancing?").

RESEARCH PARADIGMS

The High-Amplitude Nonnutritive Sucking Procedure

As you read about the high-amplitude nonnutritive sucking procedure, keep in mind our discussion in Chapter 2 on behaviorism.

Researchers use the high-amplitude nonnutritive sucking procedure to determine whether infants have a priori preferences for certain sound stimuli over others. Because young infants cannot speak, point, or otherwise directly indicate what they think about speech sounds, researchers use an infant's natural sucking reflex as an indirect way of understanding the child's speech-processing abilities.

In this procedure, a nonnutritive pacifier is connected to a computer. The infant sucks on the pacifier as he or she listens to audio stimuli played on a loudspeaker. The computer delivers a particular sound stimulus each time the infant sucks on the pacifier. This stimulus reinforces the infant's sucking behavior within the first 2 or 3 minutes of the study. As the audio stimulus reinforces the behavior, the infant becomes conditioned and sucks more frequently when he or she likes the sound and sucks less often when he or she does not like or is bored with the sound.

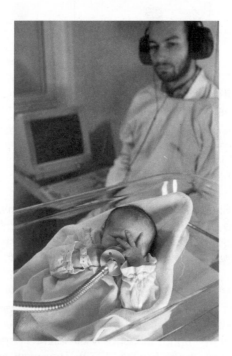

High-amplitude nonnutritive sucking procedure.

(*Photo Source:* From *Non-nutritive Sucking at Birth,* by Franck Ramus, n.d., Paris: Laboratoire de Sciences Cognitives et Psycholinguistique Ecole Normale Supérieure. Copyright F. Ramus. Reprinted with permission. http://www.lscp.net/babylab/newborns.html)

Some researchers have used this procedure to determine, for example, that 2-month-olds can distinguish between their native language and a foreign language (Mehler et al., 1988). Other researchers have determined that infants the same age can retain information about speech sounds they hear for brief intervals (Jusczyk, Jusczyk, Kennedy, Schomberg, & Koenig, 1995; Jusczyk, Kennedy, & Jusczyk, 1995; Jusczyk, Pisoni, & Mullenix, 1992) .

DISCUSSION POINT

The high-amplitude nonnutritive sucking procedure relies on behaviorist principles (which are empiricist, or nurture inspired), yet researchers argue that children demonstrate innate (or nature-inspired) language abilities during such experiments. How do you explain this relationship or discrepancy?

A hidden camera records infants' visual fixation throughout the presentation. (See Figure 5.8 for an illustration of the setup for the IPLP.) The premise behind the design is that infants will direct more visual attention to the matching side of the screen when they understand the language they hear—that is, they will find the link between the information presented in the auditory modality and that in the visual modality.

Researchers have used the IPLP to explore a variety of linguistic and prelinguistic hypotheses. For example, Kuhl and Meltzoff (1982) used the IPLP to discover that 4-month-old infants prefer to look at a face whose mouth moves in concert with

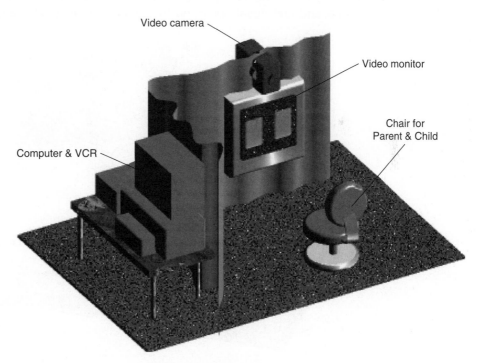

FIGURE 5.8
Intermodal preferential looking paradigm.

Source: From *Testing Language Comprehension in Infants: Introducing the Split-Screen Preferential Looking Paradigm,* by G. Hollich, C. Rocroi, K. Hirsh-Pasek, and R. Golinkoff, April 1999, in a poster session presented at the Society for Research in Child Development, Albuquerque, NM. Copyright 1999 by George Hollich. Reprinted with permission.

a speech sound than a face whose mouth produces a different speech sound. More recently, researchers have used the IPLP in studies to examine infants' understanding of action concepts and action verbs (e.g., Maguire, 2004; Naigles & Kako, 1993).

Interactive Intermodal Preferential Looking Paradigm

An interactive version of the IPLP, aptly named the *interactive intermodal preferential looking paradigm* (IIPLP), is also used (Golinkoff, Hirsh-Pasek, Cauley, & Gordon, 1987; Hirsh-Pasek & Golinkoff, 1996). In the IIPLP, an infant sits on his or her blindfolded parent's lap, facing the experimenter and the testing apparatus (again, the blindfolding is so that the parent cannot influence the child's looking). The testing apparatus is a Fagan board, to which the experimenter affixes two objects with Velcro. The experimenter can flip the board to control when and for how long the infant views the objects on the board. (See Figure 5.9 for an illustration of the IIPLP setup.) Each experiment consists of a period of object exploration, during which the infant can manipulate the objects for a specified period. After the object exploration period is a *salience trial,* which measures whether the infant has an a priori preference for one of the objects over the other object. For example, if a sparkly metallic novel object is placed on one side of the board and a relatively boring and dull novel object on the other side, infants' a priori preference for

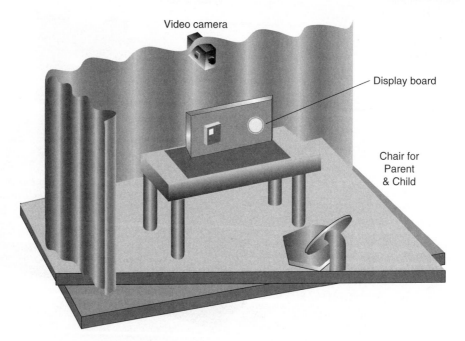

FIGURE 5.9
Interactive intermodal preferential looking paradigm.

Source: From *Testing Language Comprehension in Infants: Introducing the Split-Screen Preferential Looking Paradigm,* by G. Hollich, C. Rocroi, K. Hirsh-Pasek, and R. Golinkoff, April 1999, in poster session presented at the Society for Research in Child Development, Albuquerque, NM. Copyright 1999 by George Hollich. Reprinted with permission.

CD VIDEO CLIP

To watch an infant participate in an interactive intermodal preferential looking paradigm (IIPLP) task, see the CD video clip *Research 2*.

DISCUSSION POINT

What additional variables of interest could researchers manipulate in the IIPLP that are not possible to manipulate in the IPLP?

interesting objects may preclude them from being able to learn the name of the boring object (see Hirsh-Pasek, Golinkoff, & Hollich, 2000). Next, in the training phase, the experimenter attempts to teach the infant the name of a novel object. Finally, test trials are used to determine whether the infant has mapped the object name to the correct object. As with the IPLP, a hidden camera records infants' looking time throughout the experiment. The underlying premise of this paradigm holds that if infants understand the language they hear (e.g., "Find the glorp!" "Where's the glorp?"), they will look longer to the side of the apparatus containing the target object.

Naturalistic Observation

Naturalistic observation involves systematically observing and analyzing an infant's communicative behavior in everyday situations. Such observation usually takes place in the infant's home. Researchers may videotape, audiotape, and take notes as the infant interacts naturally with the people around him or her. The researchers may elect to gather information during specific activities, such as dinnertime or free play with a parent.

Researchers targeting specific language forms or prelinguistic behaviors may alternatively devise a semistructured or structured observation in a laboratory. During structured observations, researchers may provide the infants with specific props or ask the same questions of all infants in the study as a point of comparison.

The Child Language Data Exchange System (CHILDES) database (available at http://childes.psy.cmu.edu) is an invaluable source for researchers interested in gaining access to naturalistic and structured language samples to answer questions about language development. The CHILDES system contains transcripts of naturalistic and structured observations in several languages as well as software for coding and analyzing these transcripts.

Clinicians

As we discussed, infants in their first year absorb the language around them like sponges and begin to establish foundations for later language achievements. However, they are not true conversationalists at this age. In general, gauging whether children are lagging in their language skills is difficult before they reach toddlerhood, when their expressive language begins to emerge. However, in some instances, clinicians (including pediatricians, speech–language pathologists, and clinical psychologists) do examine infants' language skills. Such examination may be necessary for infants born with developmental disabilities (e.g., cleft palate) or infants who, for unknown reasons, seem to be lagging in meeting key milestones. Next, we discuss two informal measures of language development that clinicians use with infants: informal language screens and parent-report measures.

Informal Language Screens

Informal language screens for infants involve checklists of common early language milestones that clinicians and parents can use to check off whether or not an infant exhibits each behavior in question. The National Institute on Deafness and Other

Here is a checklist that you can follow to determine if your child's speech and language skills are developing on schedule. You should talk to your child's doctor about anything that is checked "no."

Birth to 5 months	**Yes**	**No**
Reacts to loud sounds.	○	○
Turns head toward a sound source.	○	○
Watches your face when you speak.	○	○
Vocalizes pleasure and displeasure sounds (laughs, giggles, cries, or fusses).	○	○
Makes noise when talked to.	○	○

6–11 months	**Yes**	**No**
Understands "no-no."	○	○
Babbles (says "ba-ba-ba" or "ma-ma-ma").	○	○
Tries to communicate by actions or gestures.	○	○
Tries to repeat your sounds.	○	○

FIGURE 5.10
Language screens for infants from birth to age 5 months and from age 6 months to age 11 months.

Source: From *Milestones in Your Child's Speech and Language Development,* by National Institute on Deafness and Other Communication Disorders, n.d., Bethesda, MD: Author. Copyright 2006 by National Institute on Deafness and Other Communication Disorders.
http://www.nidcd.nih.gov/health/voice/speechandlanguage.asp

Communication Disorders (www.nidcd.nih.gov) offers a series of developmental language screens that parents and clinicians can use informally. See Figure 5.10 for an example of a screen for infants from birth to age 5 months and a screen for infants ages 6–11 months.

Parent-Report Measures

Not only is having parents report directly on their infant's development a quick way to gauge the infant's progress, but researchers have proven such reporting to be a reliable and valid measure of language ability when it is compared with other direct assessments (P. Dale, 1991, 1996). Parents report on specific language behaviors, using checklists and questionnaires. Common self-report measures for infants include the Language Development Survey (LDS; Rescorla, 1993a) and the MacArthur–Bates CDI (Fenson et al., 1993; Fenson, Pethick, et al., 2000).

SUMMARY

This chapter begins with a discussion of the major language development milestones that infants achieve, including the ability to perceive speech sounds and use these sounds as a way to "break into" the continuous streams of speech they hear. Other milestones include awareness of and attention to actions that they see and the intentions underlying these actions; the ability to categorize objects, actions, and events according to perceptual and conceptual features; and production of the early vocalizations that are precursors to language.

Some early foundations for language development that follow from infants' social interactions with other people include infant-directed speech, joint reference and attention, the daily routines of infancy, and the responsiveness of caregivers. Infants' major achievements in language content, form, and use during the first year include producing their first word and using several new pragmatic functions after about age 8 months, when they are communicating intentionally.

Although infants follow a fairly predictable pattern of language development during the first year, some aspects of this development vary. An individual infant's expressive and receptive vocabularies differ in size and, among a group of infants, differences in the language development rate, language-learning style, communicative purpose, and starting time for producing speech can be seen. Various factors account for such differences.

Researchers and clinicians measure language development in infancy in a variety of ways. Four major research paradigms are habituation–dishabituation tasks, the IPLP, the IIPLP, and naturalistic observation. Two clinical methods for gathering information about infants' language progress are using informal language screens and implementing parental-report measures.

KEY TERMS

babbling, p. 156
declarative pointing, p. 164
dishabituation, p. 174
duration, p. 148
expressive language, p. 170
habituation, p. 174
imperative pointing, p. 164
intersubjective awareness, p. 163
intonation, p. 148
jargon, p. 157
marginal babbling, p. 156

nonreduplicated babbling, p. 157
paralinguistic, p. 160
phonetic regularities, p. 147
prosodic regularities, p. 147
receptive language, p. 170
reduplicated babbling, p. 157
stress, p. 148
supported joint engagement, p. 163
variegated babbling, p. 157
voice onset time, p. 150

For online resources related to chapter content, including audio samples, valuable Web sites, suggested readings, and self-quizzes, please go to the Companion Website at http://www.prenhall.com/pence

6

Toddlerhood

Exploring the World and Experimenting with Language

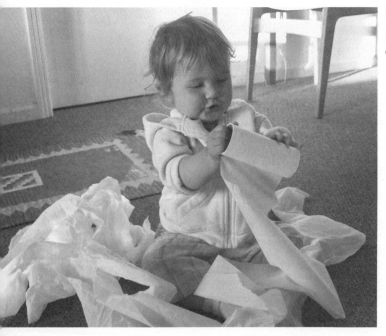

FOCUS QUESTIONS

In this chapter, we answer the following four questions:

1. What major language development milestones occur in toddlerhood?

2. What major achievements in language content, form, and use characterize toddlerhood?

3. What factors influence toddlers' individual achievements in language?

4. How do researchers and clinicians measure language development in toddlerhood?

Toddlerhood, or the period between about age 1 and age 3 years, is a time of exploration for children. Toddlers can move around by crawling or walking, and this newfound mobility heralds many new opportunities to explore the world that had not previously been available without the assistance of other people. Toddlers are inherently curious about the objects and actions around them and are likewise inquisitive about the language they hear other individuals using. During toddlerhood, children begin to consciously attempt to create matches between objects and actions in the world and the language that describes them. For example, you have probably heard toddlers ask "Wha-dat?" as they tried to link language to concepts of interest to them. In this chapter, we first provide an overview of the major language development milestones of toddlerhood, including the use of first words and gestures. Second, we explore toddlers' achievements in language content, form, and use. Such achievements involve phonological, syntactic, morphological, semantic, and pragmatic developments. We also discuss word-use errors typical of toddlers. Third, we investigate the factors that contribute to intraindividual and interindividual differences among toddlers. These factors include variation in language development rate and the effects of gender, birth order, and familial socioeconomic status on language development. Fourth, and finally, we detail the ways in which researchers and clinicians measure language development in toddlerhood. Among these measures are various production, comprehension, and judgment tasks as well as evaluation and assessment tools.

WHAT MAJOR LANGUAGE DEVELOPMENT MILESTONES OCCUR IN TODDLERHOOD?

First Words

A baby's first word marks the beginning of a transition from preverbal to verbal communication and ushers in a new and exciting period of language development. Parents may record their child's first word along with the age at which their child uttered the word and the context surrounding the word. Partly because of the excitement about this achievement, researchers know that, on average, babies produce their first word at around age 12 months.

Words are different from prelinguistic vocalizations that infants make when they babble. Although words are composed of meaningful sounds, they are also symbolic and arbitrary. They are symbolic because they represent something else in the

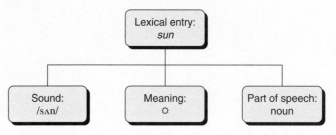

FIGURE 6.1
Lexical entry for the word *sun.*

world. They are arbitrary because the sound sequences of words do not directly stand for the concepts the words represent (one exception is onomatopoeic words, such as *whoosh* and *gurgle,* which do sound like the concepts they represent). For each word that babies learn, they create an entry in their *lexicon,* or mental dictionary. A lexical entry contains a series of symbols that compose the word, the sound of the word, the meaning of the word, and its part of speech (Pinker, 1999). Figure 6.1 illustrates how the word *sun* might appear in the lexicon.

First words usually refer to salient people and objects in babies' everyday lives, such as *mama, dada, doggie, kitty,* and the like. For a vocalization to be a *true word,* it must meet three important criteria. First, the baby must produce the word with a clear purpose. For example, when baby Zander holds up a book while saying the word *book,* he has the clear purpose of refering to the book. However, when his mom, Lori, wants to show her son's feat to a group of friends by prompting Zander, "Say book," the resulting utterance would be considered a direct imitation or repetition rather than a true word.

Second, a true word must have recognizable pronunciation similar to the adult form of the word. According to some estimates, even 18-month-old children's pronunciations are only 25% intelligible (e.g., Weiss, Gordon, & Lillywhite, 1987); however, a true word should be a close approximation of the adult form, and other people should be able to recognize it as such. Thus, a baby girl's "wawa" for *water* is close enough to the adult form of the word that it would meet one of the criteria for being a true word. In contrast, if a child produces the word *water* as "aaaah"—even consistently and while clearly using this sound to request a drink—this vocalization would not be a true word because it does not closely approximate the adult form.

The term **phonetically consistent forms** (PCFs) describes the idiosyncratic wordlike productions that children use consistently and meaningfully but that do not approximate adult forms. As the term suggests, PCFs have a consistent sound structure, but children may use them to refer to more than a single referent. For example, the baby girl who uses the PCF "aaaah" to refer to *water* might also use this sound when requesting other objects or actions, such as when requesting her mother to pick her up or someone to give her a toy. Although PCFs are not true words, they are important aspects of children's language development because, by using them, children learn the value of adopting a stable pronunciation for communicating in a particular situation (McEachern & Haynes, 2004).

CD VIDEO CLIP

To watch an 18-month-old boy engage in pretend conversation, see the CD video clip *Language* 3. As you watch, try to determine whether he uses any phonetically consistent forms (PCFs) or true words.

Third, a true word is a word that a child uses consistently and extends beyond the original context. In the case of the baby girl who said "wawa," she could be expected to use this word not only when asking for a drink of water but also when seeing her dog drinking from his water dish—and possibly even when splashing around in the bathtub.

Subsequently in this chapter, we discuss how children extend words beyond their original context. Next, however, we investigate the role of gesture use in language development. For even more milestones, see the Development Timeline: Toddlerhood.

Gestures

In Chapter 5, we discuss the emergence of gestures, such as imperative and declarative pointing, in episodes of joint attention between prelinguistic infants and other people. In this section, we examine the important role gestures continue to play in language development in the second and third year of life.

Referential Gestures

Research results indicate that gesture use precedes spoken language as children transition from the prelinguistic stage to the one-word stage of language development and then from the one-word stage to the two-word stage. As an illustration, children who are beginning to transition from the prelinguistic stage to the one-word stage use **referential gestures,** such as holding a fist to the ear to indicate *telephone* or waving the hand to indicate *bye-bye* (Caselli, 1983, as cited in Volterra, Caselli, Capirci, & Pizzuto, 2005). These gestures are different from the *deictic gestures* (e.g., pointing, showing) that characterize infancy in that they indicate a precise referent and have stable meaning across different contexts. In other words, referential gestures share some of the properties of first true words, and their use signals an impending transition from prelinguistic to linguistic communication.

Furthermore, as children are preparing to transition from the one-word stage to the two-word stage, they begin to exhibit gesture–word combinations (such as *points to chair* and says "Mommy" to request that Mommy sit on the chair) and two-gesture combinations (such as *pretend to eat–point to food* to request to be fed; Capirci, Iverson, Pizzuto, & Volterra, 1996; Caselli, Volterra, & Pizzuto, 1984, as cited in Volterra et al., 2005).

Interestingly, when children begin to use two-word utterances, they stop combining two referential gestures. The reason may be that toddlers fill in "gaps" with gestures before they develop the competence to combine words but then allow their words to dominate when they can combine them successfully. The importance of gesture use to children's developing spoken language holds not only for children who are developing typically but also for children who have developmental disabilities (Brady, Marquis, Fleming, & McLean, 2004), such as Down syndrome (Iverson, Longobardi, & Caselli, 2003).

Mirror Neurons and Gestures

Mirror neurons, a type of *visuomotor neurons* (related both to vision and to muscular movement), activate when people *perform* actions (including communicative actions)

DEVELOPMENTAL TIMELINE: TODDLERHOOD

Phonology

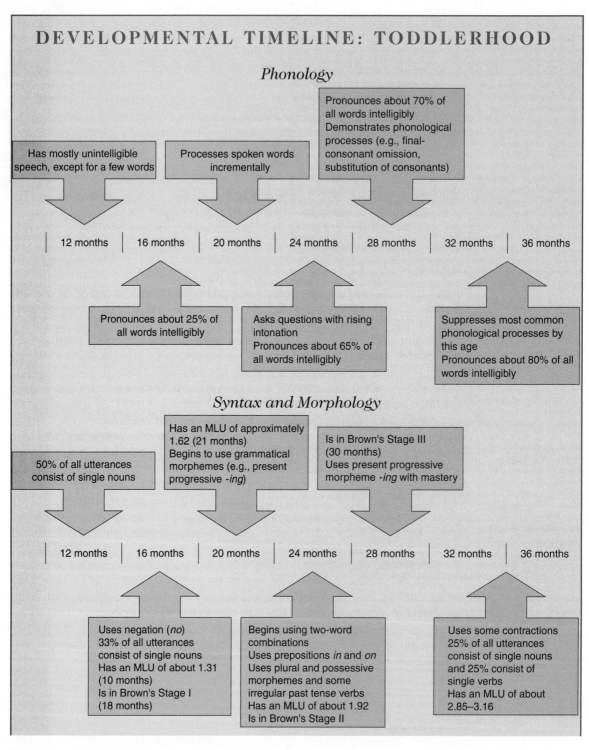

Pronounces about 70% of all words intelligibly
Demonstrates phonological processes (e.g., final-consonant omission, substitution of consonants)

Has mostly unintelligible speech, except for a few words

Processes spoken words incrementally

| 12 months | 16 months | 20 months | 24 months | 28 months | 32 months | 36 months |

Pronounces about 25% of all words intelligibly

Asks questions with rising intonation
Pronounces about 65% of all words intelligibly

Suppresses most common phonological processes by this age
Pronounces about 80% of all words intelligibly

Syntax and Morphology

Has an MLU of approximately 1.62 (21 months)
Begins to use grammatical morphemes (e.g., present progressive -ing)

Is in Brown's Stage III (30 months)
Uses present progressive morpheme -ing with mastery

50% of all utterances consist of single nouns

| 12 months | 16 months | 20 months | 24 months | 28 months | 32 months | 36 months |

Uses negation (no)
33% of all utterances consist of single nouns
Has an MLU of about 1.31 (10 months)
Is in Brown's Stage I (18 months)

Begins using two-word combinations
Uses prepositions in and on
Uses plural and possessive morphemes and some irregular past tense verbs
Has an MLU of about 1.92
Is in Brown's Stage II

Uses some contractions
25% of all utterances consist of single nouns and 25% consist of single verbs
Has an MLU of about 2.85–3.16

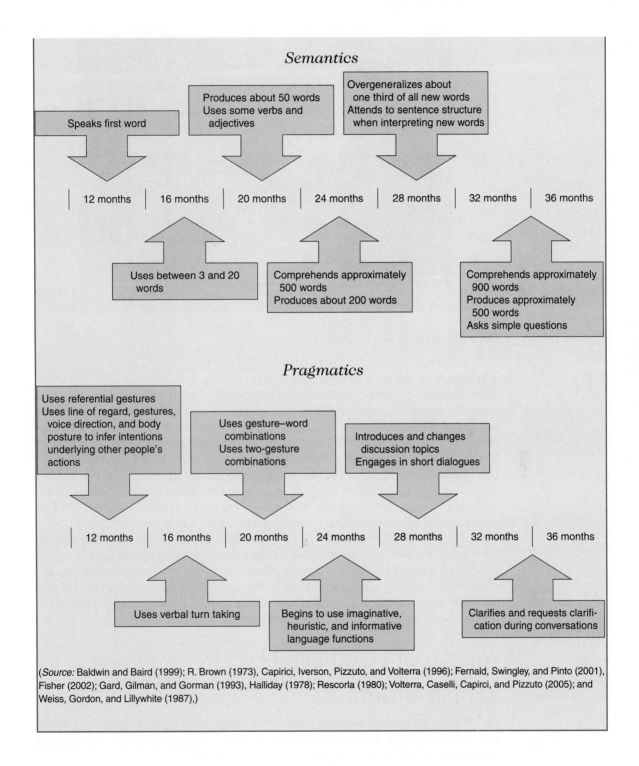

Semantics

Speaks first word

Produces about 50 words / **Uses some verbs and adjectives**

Overgeneralizes about one third of all new words / **Attends to sentence structure when interpreting new words**

| 12 months | 16 months | 20 months | 24 months | 28 months | 32 months | 36 months |

Uses between 3 and 20 words

Comprehends approximately 500 words / **Produces about 200 words**

Comprehends approximately 900 words / **Produces approximately 500 words** / **Asks simple questions**

Pragmatics

Uses referential gestures / **Uses line of regard, gestures, voice direction, and body posture to infer intentions underlying other people's actions**

Uses gesture–word combinations / **Uses two-gesture combinations**

Introduces and changes discussion topics / **Engages in short dialogues**

| 12 months | 16 months | 20 months | 24 months | 28 months | 32 months | 36 months |

Uses verbal turn taking

Begins to use imaginative, heuristic, and informative language functions

Clarifies and requests clarification during conversations

(*Source:* Baldwin and Baird (1999); R. Brown (1973), Capirici, Iverson, Pizzuto, and Volterra (1996); Fernald, Swingley, and Pinto (2001), Fisher (2002); Gard, Gilman, and Gorman (1993), Halliday (1978); Rescorla (1980); Volterra, Caselli, Capirci, and Pizzuto (2005); and Weiss, Gordon, and Lillywhite (1987),)

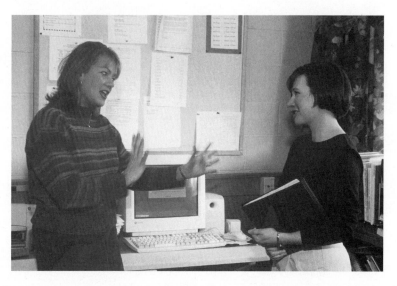

The earliest humans might have communicated with one another primarily by using hand gestures.

(*Photo Source:* Anthony Magnacca/Merrill.)

and when they *observe* other people perform actions. Evidence for a mirror neuron system in humans comes from neurophysiological and brain-imaging studies such as those discussed in Chapter 4. Some researchers have proposed that mirror neurons are responsible for the evolution of gestures and language in humans. For example, Rizzolatti and Craighero (2004) proposed that hand–arm gestures and speech share a common neural substrate. They cited evidence from transcranial magnetic stimulation (TMS) studies—which involve noninvasive electrical stimulation of the nervous system—showing that when adults read and produce spontaneous speech, the excitability of the hand motor cortex increases in the left hemisphere of the brain. Furthermore, this activation is absent in the leg motor area and in the right hemisphere of the brain. So, could humans' earliest ancestors have communicated primarily through hand gestures, and does evidence of this system remain with people today? If so, a good reason may exist for why gesture use (either alone or accompanying speech) continues throughout the preschool years, the school-age years, and adulthood as a means of communication and a way to enhance communication. Future advances in neuroscience will undoubtedly continue to shed light on this theory.

WHAT MAJOR ACHIEVEMENTS IN LANGUAGE CONTENT, FORM, AND USE CHARACTERIZE TODDLERHOOD?

Recall the three rule-governed domains that compose language: *content,* or words and their meanings; *form,* or the way in which sounds, words, and sentences are organized to convey content; and *use,* or how language is used in interactions with other people to express personal and social needs. Toddlerhood heralds important achievements in each of these three areas. In the span of just a year or two, toddlers acquire their 1st word, their 50th word, and even their 100th word. Toddlers also begin to use new speech sounds and to acquire new phonological processes as they combine these sounds in fluent speech. They move from using single-word utterances to combining words, which allows them to articulate many more communicative functions than they could in infancy.

Language Content

Toddlerhood is witness to tremendous growth in language content. During this time, toddlers progress from novice to expert word learners and make large gains in both their receptive and their expressive lexicons. In the sections that follow, we discuss the process of word learning, including strategies toddlers use to acquire words rapidly. We also discuss how toddlers learn to link meaning in the events they see with their syntactic correlates in sentences.

Receptive and Expressive Lexicons

Recall that the *receptive lexicon* is the words children comprehend, and the *expressive lexicon* is the words children produce. Although young children begin acquiring new words relatively slowly, some researchers contend that toddlers' word learning enters an explosive period between approximately 18 and 24 months of age, or around the time they can produce 50 words. This period has been aptly termed the *vocabulary spurt, word spurt,* or *naming explosion.* During this time, children may learn up to 7–9 new words per day. Parents who have begun to record their toddler's words in a diary remark that they begin to lose track of their child's new words during this period of accelerated growth. However, although children learn about 7–9 new words per day between ages 18 and 24 months, they do not always use these words the way adults do. Rather, they often overextend, underextend, and overlap words.

Overextension. **Overextension,** or *overgeneralization,* is the process by which children use words in an overly general manner. Toddlers make three major kinds of overextensions: categorical, analogical, and relational. Toddlers make *categorical overextensions* when they extend a word they know to other words in the same category. For example, if a child learns the word *dog* and then calls all four-legged animals "dog," he or she is making a categorical overextension. Another example would be if a child learned the word *milk* and called all liquids "milk."

Toddlers make *analogical overextensions* when they extend a word they know to other words that are perceptually similar. For example, a child may learn the word *ball* and then call other round objects (e.g., the moon, an orange) "ball" as well.

Toddlers make *relational overextensions* when they extend a word they know to other words that are semantically or thematically related. For instance, Zander may use the word *flower* to refer to a watering can that he sees his mother use to water flowers. He may use the same word to refer to flowerpots his mother uses to house the flowers.

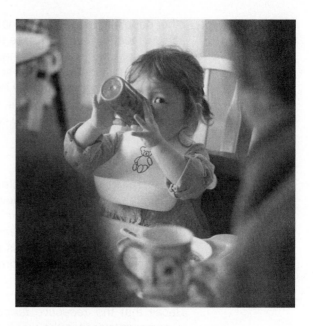

Toddlers engaging in underextension might, for example, fail to label multiple exemplars of cups as "cup."
(*Photo Source:* © Don Mason/Corbis.)

Toddlers overgeneralize about one third of all new words on the basis of categorical, analogical, and relational similarities (Rescorla, 1980). However, even more common than overextensions are underextensions.

Underextension. When toddlers learn new words, they use these words cautiously and conservatively at first. This process, whereby toddlers use words to refer to only a subset of possible referents, is called **underextension.** When a toddler girl uses the word *book* only when referring to books in her collection, or when she uses the word *bottle* to refer only to her baby bottle (and not glass bottles or plastic water bottles), she is engaging in underextension.

Overlap. When toddlers overextend a word in certain circumstances and underextend the same word in other circumstances, this process is called **overlap.** For example, when a toddler boy uses the word *candy* to refer to jelly beans *and* his grandmother's pills (overextension) but *not* to chocolate bars (underextension), he is engaging in overlap.

Reasons for Word-Use Errors. Toddlers' overextensions, underextensions, and overlaps might be viewed as types of errors in their early word use. Why do children make such errors? At least three possible explanations have been offered as to why children use words in different ways than adults (see Gershkoff-Stowe, 2001). First, children may make *category membership errors*. For instance, they may truly think that a horse and a cow are the same kind of animal and thus use the word *horse* to label a cow because they know the word *horse*.

Second, children may make *pragmatic errors*. Children make such errors when they know that two objects are conceptually different but do not yet have a name for

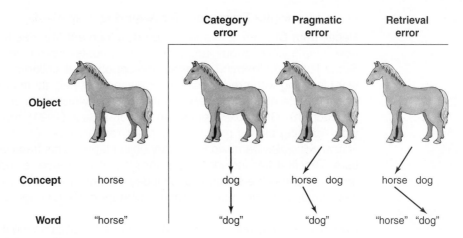

FIGURE 6.2

Types of naming errors children produce.

Source: From "The Course of Children's Naming Errors in Early Word Learning," by L. Gershkoff-Stowe, 2001, *Journal of Cognition and Development, 2,* p. 134. Copyright 2001 by Lawrence Erlbaum Associates, Inc. Reprinted with permission.

DISCUSSION POINT

What are some ways in which a parent can determine whether his or her toddler overgeneralizes and undergeneralizes new words?

one of the objects and intentionally substitute a semantically related word. For example, a young boy may know that a horse and a dog are different animals but because he does not know the word *horse,* he uses the word *dog* instead to refer to the horse.

Third, children may make a *retrieval error* when they know a certain word but for some reason cannot retrieve the word and unintentionally select a different word. For example, a child may know the word *horse* but accidentally utter the word *dog* when describing the horse. See Figure 6.2 for an example of the three types of naming errors children make. The arrows indicate the way in which information flows during production of the word.

Acquisition of New Words: The Quinean Conundrum

For a toddler to learn a new word—or create a new lexical entry—he or she must minimally do the following: segment the word from continuous speech; find objects, events, actions, and concepts in the world; and map the word in question to its corresponding object, event, action, or concept. The final task, *mapping,* is the key to learning a new word successfully and may require more than meets the eye. Imagine, as philosopher W. V. O. Quine proposed, that you encounter a native speaker of a foreign language who utters the word *gavagai* in the presence of a rabbit. Should you infer that the word *gavagai* means "rabbit," "food," "undetached rabbit part," or some other option? This dilemma—the uncertainty surrounding mapping a word to its referent in the face of seemingly endless interpretations—is called the *mapping problem, induction problem,* or *Quinean conundrum.* The mapping problem poses challenges for all people learning a new language, but especially for infants and toddlers learning their first language. Just as theories of language learning differ, so do explanations for how children overcome the Quinean conundrum as they learn new words.

Lexical Principles Framework for Acquiring New Words

Recall from Chapter 2 that language development theories have implications for how people view various language achievements. Word learning is no exception. Some language-learning theories presuppose that children arrive at the task of word learning with predispositions or biases that help them eliminate some of the nearly infinite number of referents that a novel word could describe (the Quinean conundrum). Golinkoff, Mervis, and Hirsh-Pasek (1994) organized a series of word-learning biases proposed by other researchers, into what they termed the *lexical principles framework* for early object labels. This framework consists of two tiers: The first tier includes the principles of reference, extendibility, and object scope, whereas the second tier includes the principles of conventionality, categorical scope, and novel name–nameless category (N3C) (Figure 6.3).

First Tier Principles.   The three principles that compose the first tier of the lexical principles framework do not require much linguistic sophistication. Children can use Tier 1 principles as early as when they begin to acquire words because these principles rely on cognitive-perceptual abilities (Hollich, Hirsh-Pasek, & Golinkoff, 2000). The principle of **reference** states that words symbolize objects, actions, events, and concepts. For example, the word *Daddy* stands for or symbolizes someone's father, and a child can use this word in the presence of his or her father, or the child can refer to his or her father who exists in a different place or time.

The principle of **extendibility** refers to the notion that words label categories of objects and not just the original exemplar. Therefore, the word *ball* can be used

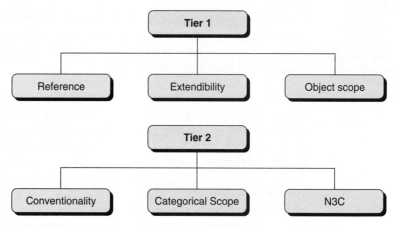

FIGURE 6.3
Lexical principles framework.

N3C = novel name–nameless category.
Source: From "An Emergentist Coalition Model for Word Learning: Mapping Words to Objects Is a Product of the Interaction of Multiple Cues," by K. Hirsh-Pasek, R. M. Golinkoff, and G. Hollich, in *Becoming a Word Learner: A Debate on Lexical Acquisition* (p. 136), edited by R. M. Golinkoff, K. Hirsh-Pasek, L. Bloom, L. B. Smith, A. L. Woodward, N. Akhtar, et al., 2000, New York: Oxford University Press. Copyright 2000 by Oxford University Press. Adapted with permission.

to describe multiple objects that fall under the basic-level category *ball*. Children commonly extend words to include objects of similar shape, size, color, smell, and material makeup; shape is the most common feature that children extend early in language development (Landau, Smith & Jones, 1998; Smith, Jones, & Landau, 1992).

The principle of **object scope** states that words map to whole objects. First, children using the principle of object scope assume that novel words label objects rather than actions. When children hear a novel label, they prefer to attach the label to an object instead of an action (e.g., Imai, Haryu, & Okada, 2002; M. Meyer et al., 2003). Second, object scope presupposes a **whole object assumption,** or the assumption that words label whole objects and not object parts (Markman, 1990, 1991). Therefore, a toddler who witnesses a bird flying in the sky as his or her mother exclaims "A bird!" will likely assume that the word *bird* refers to the bird rather than the action of flying, and, more specifically, to the whole bird rather than to the bird's wings, beak, or feet.

Second Tier Principles. The three principles that compose the second tier of the lexical principles framework are more sophisticated and become available to children as they refine their hypotheses about the nature of words. The principle of **conventionality** states that for children to communicate successfully, they must adopt the terms that people in their language community understand (see Clark, 1993). Children begin to refine their vocabulary and the Tier 1 principle of reference by using the principle of conventionality when they recognize that some of their "baby" words, such as *blankie* for *blanket,* are not conventional among other speakers in their culture.

The principle of **categorical scope** builds on the Tier 1 principle of extendibility by limiting the basis for extension to words that are taxonomically similar. Children who honor taxonomic constraints would, for example, categorize a dog and a cat similarly, instead of categorizing a dog with dog food using thematically similar properties (Markman & Hutchinson, 1984).

DISCUSSION POINT

How might toddlers, preschoolers, school-age children, and adults differ in how they try to determine the meanings of unfamiliar words?

The principle of **novel name–nameless category (N3C)** supports the Tier 1 principle of object scope by helping children select a nameless object as the recipient of a novel label. The principle of N3C rests on the principle of *mutual exclusivity*, which states that objects have only one label (Markman, 1989; Merriman & Bowman, 1989). The principle of mutual exclusivity plays out in situations in which children hear a novel label and see a series of objects in the environment for which they already possess labels. For example, suppose you present a toddler who does not know the word *thermometer* with a box containing a ball, a book, and a thermometer. If you were to subsequently request the thermometer, the toddler would likely select the thermometer because he or she knows that the ball is not called "thermometer" and that the book is not called "thermometer." The principle of N3C operates similarly to mutual exclusivity, with one exception: N3C does not presuppose that children avoid attaching more than one label to an object. See Research Paradigms: *Neuroimaging and Toddler Language Development* for a discussion on how neuroimaging studies can help researchers assess the responses of the toddler brain to known and unknown words.

RESEARCH PARADIGMS

Neuroimaging and Toddler Language Development

Neuroimaging techniques are fast becoming an important method for gaining deeper understanding about language development. Some neuroimaging techniques are even appropriate for investigating the language development of infants and toddlers. One such technique involves **event-related potentials** (ERPs). In ERP studies, participants wear a cap fitted with several electrodes that measure the electrical responses of the brain to particular linguistic stimuli. In one such study, researchers demonstrated that the electrophysiological processes of 16-month-olds differed when these toddlers heard familiar words (as assessed by parent report) and unfamiliar words (Molfese, 1990).

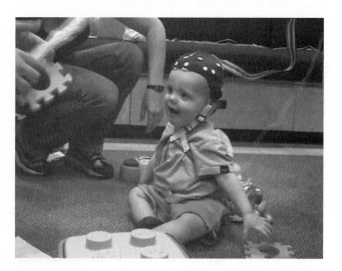

An event-related potentials (ERP) study.

(*Photo Source:* Dr. Janet F. Werker's Infant Studies Centre, Department of Psychology, University of British Columbia.)

Social-Pragmatic Framework for Acquiring New Words

Proponents of the social-pragmatic view of word learning argue that children do not require domain-specific mechanisms, including the lexical principles just mentioned, to acquire new words. Rather, these theorists propose that children can overcome the Quinean conundrum by interacting with experienced language users. According to social-pragmatic theorists, as adults interact with children, they offer many social cues to the meanings of words, which makes lexical principles unnecessary. Infants and toddlers can understand an array of sophisticated social cues at an early age. They can follow another person's gaze and pointing gestures, engage in joint attention, and imitate actions by age 9–12 months (Baldwin, 1995).

THEORY TO PRACTICE

Child Care Selection and Toddler Language Development

As we described in Chapter 2, theoretical perspectives concerning language development influence many areas of people's lives, including some of the choices parents and caregivers make. One particularly important decision surrounds selecting child care providers for developing toddlers. In 1991, the National Institute of Child Health and Human Development (NICHD) began a longitudinal study—the Study of Early Child Care (SECC). In Phase I, researchers enrolled 1,364 children from 10 locations across the United States and followed these children to gather data on their cognitive, social, emotional, and language development (among other factors), from birth through age 3 years. As a result of this intensive study, the researchers concluded that a number of important indicators were consistently associated with positive caregiving behaviors within each of the five types of nonmaternal child care they examined. These indicators included a small group size, low child–adult ratios, nonauthoritarian child-rearing beliefs, and safe, clean, and stimulating physical environments (National Institute of Child Health and Human Development Early Child Care Research Network, 1996). Furthermore, the researchers concluded that the overall quality of child care—and *language stimulation* in particular—was consistently but modestly related to toddlers' cognitive and language outcomes at ages 15, 24, and 36 months (National Institute of Child Health and Human Development Early Child Care Research Network, 2000). These research results have significant implications for the selection of quality child care, considering the impact that child care experiences can have on children's developing language competencies throughout toddlerhood.

As early as age 12 months, infants can use social cues—including line of regard (the direction of a person's gaze, which indicates what the person is looking at), gestures, voice direction, and body posture—to infer the intentions underlying other people's actions (Baldwin & Baird, 1999). Research results show that toddlers are adept at using social-pragmatic cues to word meanings, even in seemingly difficult circumstances. Such circumstances include when the referent of the word is not physically present (Akhtar & Tomasello, 1996), when an adult uses an *imperative* statement ("Put the toma down") rather than an explicit labeling statement ("That is a toma"; Callanan, Akhtar, Sussman, & Sabbagh, 2003), and when the child overhears a word by monitoring other people's conversations (Akhtar, 2005; Akhtar, Jipson, & Callanan, 2001). (See Theory to Practice: *Child Care Selection and Toddler Language Development* for a discussion on the importance of child care experiences on toddler language development.)

Fast Mapping

Have you ever used a fairly complex word in front of a toddler and later, to your amazement, heard the toddler use that word? As you undoubtedly know, toddlers' ability to pick up words after only a few incidental exposures, or even a single exposure, is remarkable. This ability is termed *fast mapping* because of the brief exposure to the novel word and its referent, for which children form a lexical representation (Carey & Bartlett, 1978).

Markson and Bloom (1997) provided evidence that although young children can fast map new words, fast mapping is not an ability specific to word learning. These researchers discovered that 3-year-olds, 4-year-olds, and adults could learn and retain a fact about an object (in this case, participants remembered who gave the object to the experimenter as a gift) as easily as they could learn and retain a new object name. Furthermore, Markson and Bloom charged that the finding that fast mapping is not restricted to word learning is consistent with other evidence for a *domain-general* word-learning mechanism. This claim spurred an interesting interchange between researchers Waxman and Booth (2000, 2001) and P. Bloom and Markson (2001) about whether word learning is a result of domain-specific or domain-general mechanisms. Waxman and Booth disagreed with P. Bloom and Markson's findings and countered that although fast mapping need not be specific to word learning, no evidence exists that word learning and fact learning rest on the same set of underlying principles. This exchange demonstrates that contention still exists among researchers with regard to the mechanisms that drive language development and whether these mechanisms are domain general or domain specific.

Thematic Roles Toddlers Acquire

A *thematic role* is the part a word plays in an event, and such roles include agent, theme, source, goal, and location (O'Grady, 1997). An **agent** is the entity that performs the action (*Nicole ate pasta*). The **theme** is the entity undergoing an action or a movement (*Tamika flew a kite*). A **source** is the starting point for movement and a **goal** is the ending point for movement (*Maurie drove from Richmond to Charlottesville*). **Location** is the place where an action occurs (*Ryan hiked through the park*).

Toddlers begin to understand thematic roles from an early age and, more important, they learn how thematic roles link to corresponding syntactic elements. For example, 2.5-year-old toddlers attend to the overall structure of sentences when interpreting new words. Moreover, they interpret novel verbs according to the number of arguments they hear (Fisher, 2002). Children who hear a novel verb in a *transitive* sentence (*Dad caught* the fish) are more likely than children who hear a novel verb in an *intransitive* sentence (*Dad swam*) to assume that the verb refers to the action of a causal agent. Having an implicit understanding of thematic roles and how thematic roles correspond to syntactic elements undoubtedly helps toddlers narrow the number of possible interpretations for the new words they hear.

Language Form

Achievements in Phonology

Recall from Chapter 5 that the human phonological system begins to solidify from early in infancy as babies take in the speech sounds they hear, learn to categorize these sounds in meaningful ways, and use their implicit knowledge of speech

CD VIDEO CLIP

To watch a toddler participate in a fast-mapping task involving novel attribute words, see the CD video clip *Research 3*.

sounds to begin to segment fluent speech into increasingly smaller units of meaning (clauses, words, morphemes). Phonological achievements in toddlerhood are much more noticeable than those that occur in infancy because people can *hear* these achievements as they are gained. Toddlers begin to acquire and refine their repertoire of speech sounds, or phonemes, and, as they do so, adults witness their **phonological processes,** or those arguably cute rule-governed errors that children make when pronouncing certain words.

Norms for Phoneme Attainment. Recall from our discussion of norms in Chapter 2 that the ages by which children can produce consonantal phonemes in English vary widely among research reports. Perhaps the most popular set of norms for phoneme attainment are Sander's (1972) customary ages of production (Figure 2.1) and ages of mastery of speech sounds (see Table 2.2, fifth column). The term **customary age of production** describes the age by which 50% of children can produce a given sound in multiple positions in words in an adultlike way. The term **age of mastery** describes the age by which most children produce a sound in an adultlike manner.

When attempting to assess toddlers' sound production abilities, practitioners must consider that phonemes are not typically produced in isolation. Neighboring sounds and combinations of sounds may affect children's production of particular sounds. Thus, to obtain an accurate picture of children's abilities, practitioners usually ask children to produce speech sounds in various positions (e.g., syllable initial, syllable final) and with a variety of neighboring sounds (e.g., followed by a vowel, after certain consonants).

Phonological Processes. As toddlers begin to gain more control over their articulators, adults witness developments in their phonology. Some people may view toddlerhood as a period during which young children talk in cute or funny ways. Cartoons even have characters, such as Tweety Bird, that emulate the phonological patterns of early childhood. However, what adults may not realize is that children who appear to make errors are in fact using systematic and rule-governed processes as they speak and are not simply making haphazard sound substitutions. The systematic and rule-governed speech patterns that characterize toddlers' speech are called phonological processes. Phonological process categories include syllable structure changes, assimilation, place-of-articulation changes, and manner-of-articulation changes. More specific types of phonological processes compose each category.

Syllable structure changes are simply changes to syllables in words. A common type of syllable structure change in child phonology is to repeat, or *reduplicate,* a stressed syllable in a word (*water* becomes "wa-wa" and *Daddy* becomes "Da-Da").

Assimilation is the process by which children change one sound in a syllable so that it takes on the features of another sound in the same syllable. For example, in *velar assimilation,* the sound /d/ in *dog* takes on the velar sound (produced at the velum near the back of the mouth) of the /g/ that follows it, and *dog* becomes "gog." Assimilation is a context-dependent change, which means children make changes to certain sounds on the basis of influential neighboring sounds. In the example in

With fronting, toddlers replace sounds produced farther back in the mouth (/k/) with sounds produced farther forward in the mouth (/t/), so that cake becomes "take."

(*Photo Source:* © Mika/zefa/Corbis.)

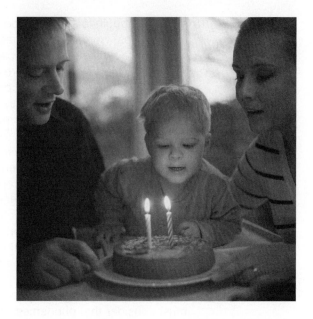

which *dog* becomes "gog," the syllable-final /g/ exerts an influence on the syllable-initial /d/, so /d/ is changed to /g/.

Children also make changes to sounds that are not context dependent, including place-of-articulation changes and manner-of-articulation changes. *Place-of-articulation changes* occur when children replace a sound produced at one location in the mouth with a sound produced at a different location in the mouth. For instance, children often replace sounds produced farther back in the mouth (e.g., /k/) with sounds produced farther forward in the mouth (e.g., /t/), so a child's pronunciation of *cake* becomes "*take*" in this process, which is called **fronting.** Place-of-articulation changes are not context dependent because children make these changes in the absence of influential neighboring sounds. In the example in which *cake* becomes "take," notice that /k/ does not change to /t/ because of the influence of any neighboring sounds that are produced closer to the front of the mouth; hence, this change is not context dependent.

Manner-of-articulation changes occur when children replace a sound produced in a particular manner with a sound produced in a different manner. A common substitution—called *stopping*—is to replace an affricate sound with a stop sound. In a *stop sound,* the airflow is temporarily stopped (e.g., the first and last sounds in the word *do͟t*). An *affricate sound* consists of a stop sound followed by a *fricative* (a sound produced by forcing air through a constricted passage; e.g., the consonant *s*). Thus, an *affricate sound* is a sound in which the airflow is temporarily stopped then forced through a constricted space in the mouth—for example, the first sound in the word *jeep* or the first and last sounds in the word *church*. Consequently, when children replace the affricate *j* in *jeep* with the stop sound *d,* they say "deep" instead of "jeep" and are making a manner-of-articulation change.

Examples of common phonological processes are provided in Table 6.1. Children typically suppress (i.e., eliminate) several of these processes by age 3 years, including final-consonant deletion, reduplication, consonant harmony, and

TABLE 6.1
Common Phonological Processes

Category	Type	Description	Example
Syllable structure changes	Weak-syllable deletion	Child deletes an unstressed syllable	*banana* = "nana"
	Final-consonant deletion	Child deletes the last consonant in a syllable	*cat* = "ca"
	Reduplication	Child repeats an entire syllable or part of a syllable	*water* = "wa-wa"
	Cluster reduction	Child reduces a cluster of consonants to include fewer consonant sounds	*splash* = "spash"
Assimilation	Consonant harmony	Child uses consonants with like features in a word	*doggie* = "doddie"
	Velar assimilation	Child produces a nonvelar consonant as a velar consonant because of a nearby velar sound	*dog* = "gog"
	Nasal assimilation	Child produces a nonnasal sound as a nasal sound because of a nearby nasal sound	*candy* = "nanny"
Place-of-articulation changes	Fronting	Child replaces a sound produced farther back in the mouth with a sound produced farther forward	*corn* = "dorn"
	Backing	Child replaces a sound produced farther forward in the mouth with a sound produced farther back	*daddy* = "gaggy"
Manner-of-articulation changes	Stopping	Child replaces a fricative or an affricate sound with a stop sound	*jeep* = "deep"
	Gliding	Child replaces a liquid sound with a glide	*love* = "wove"

DISCUSSION POINT

Do you think toddlers would notice anything strange if an adult were to use a childlike phonology? Why might they or might they not notice?

weak-syllable deletion (Stoel-Gammon & Dunn, 1985). Other phonological processes,including cluster reduction and gliding, are often not suppressed until later, although few processes persist past five years.

Phonological Perception. Although toddlers impress adults with their productive phonological achievements, such as their ability to combine sounds to produce words and phrases, they continue to make progress behind the scenes as well. Toddlers who are expanding their lexicons must possess skills to integrate incoming speech sounds with their existing linguistic and conceptual knowledge if they are to continue to acquire new words rapidly. How do toddlers process the sounds of incoming words? Experts hold one of at least two major positions with respect to how toddlers process speech.

According to the first position, toddlers use global, holistic word recognition strategies (Charles-Luce & Luce, 1990, 1996; Walley, 1993). Then, after toddlers enter the vocabulary spurt stage, a restructuring of lexical representations begins. Lexical restructuring allows more efficient storage of lexical items and recognition of words at the segmental level rather than the global level. After lexical restructuring, children can store words in their lexicons on the basis of more granular segments (e.g., combinations of particular phonemes) rather than whole units.

The second position that describes how toddlers process and recognize spoken words states that toddlers can use partial phonetic information to recognize words. For example, in one study, 18- and 21-month-olds could approximately associate the first two phonemes of a word with its corresponding picture, which indicated that toddlers process spoken words incrementally before the speaker finishes uttering the word (Fernald, Swingley, & Pinto, 2001).

One question that sometimes arises at this stage of language development is whether exposure to multiple languages confuses children who are acquiring word recognition skills. See Multicultural Focus: *Multiple Language Exposure and Toddler Language Development* for a discussion of this topic.

Achievements in Morphology

The 50-word mark for productive vocabulary, which toddlers reach between about ages 18 months and 2 years, signals some important changes, including lexical restructuring and the vocabulary spurt. The 50-word mark also usually co-occurs with the appearance of children's first grammatical morphemes. Two other morphological achievements typically occur in toddlerhood. Toddlers begin to combine words to make longer utterances, and they begin to use different types of sentence forms.

Grammatical Morphemes. A *morpheme* is a meaningful linguistic unit that cannot be divided into smaller meaningful parts. *Grammatical morphemes* are inflections added to words to indicate aspects of grammar, such as the plural -*s* (*two dogs*), the possessive '*s* (*the dog's bone*), the past tense -*ed* (*The dog barked*), and the present progressive -*ing* (*The dog is still barking*). Morphemes are added to a word to change its form, and they are an important aspect of grammatical development.

Grammatical morphemes begin to appear in children's speech between ages 18 and 24 months—at about the time when they have acquired their first 50 words.

MULTICULTURAL FOCUS

Multiple Language Exposure and Toddler Language Development

Parents sometimes express concern that exposing their children to multiple languages might have negative effects on the rate at which their children develop language, decrease the level of linguistic competency the children will be able to attain, and potentially confuse their children. Language researcher Laura Ann Pettito, M. Katerelos, et al. (2001) stated with certainty that "being exposed to two languages from birth, by itself, does not cause delay and confusion to the normal process of human language acquisition" (p. 494). These researchers studied two groups of children who were learning more than one language from birth: hearing children who were learning a sign language and a spoken language, and hearing children who were learning two spoken languages. Findings indicated that neither group was delayed in achieving early language milestones, both groups demonstrated normal vocabulary growth in both languages, and both groups demonstrated evidence of differentiating between their two languages through their sensitivity to the language that a conversational partner was using. The researchers suggested that the ability to detect temporal patterns and distributional regularities in infancy contributes to children's capacity to acquire multiple languages simultaneously.

Roger Brown (1973), a pioneer in studying early morphological development, documented the order in which and ages by which children master 14 grammatical morphemes (see Table 6.2). These grammatical morphemes develop in the same order and emerge at about the same time for English-speaking children; children do not generally master all these morphemes until about preschool age.

CD VIDEO CLIP
To watch a 2-year-old girl who is developing an understanding of grammatical morphology, including the possessive, see the CD video clip Language 4.

The first grammatical morpheme that children produce is the present progressive *-ing,* as in *Baby sleeping.* Children begin to use this morpheme around age 18 months and use it with mastery by age 28 months. Additional morphemes that appear during toddlerhood include the prepositions *in* and *on,* which children start to use at about age 2 years (*in cup, on table*). At this time, toddlers also start to use the regular plural *-s,* as in *two dogs;* the possessive *'s,* as in *kitty's bowl;* and irregular past tense verbs, as in *eat–ate* and *break–broke.*

Irregular past tense verbs do not conform to the regular verb pattern, which is to add *-ed.* Therefore, toddlers must memorize them. The English language has between 150 and 180 irregular verbs. Just as children overextend newly acquired words in categorical, analogical, and relational ways, they overgeneralize the rule for past tense verbs ("Add *-ed*") to include irregular verbs. As a result, toddlers often say things such as "I maked it" and "Mommy goed to the store." Pinker (1999) explained that children who have acquired the regular past tense rule often overgeneralize its use to irregular verbs until they have had sufficient exposure to and practice with "words" (e.g., the irregular form of a verb) and "rules" (e.g., applying the past tense ending of a regular verb, *-ed*).

TABLE 6.2
Roger Brown's (1973) Grammatical Morphemes

Grammatical morpheme	Age of appearance (months)	Example
Present progressive -ing	19–28	"Baby eating"
Plural -s	27–30	"Doggies"
Preposition in	27–30	"Toy in there"
Preposition on	31–34	"Food on table"
Possessive 's	31–34	"Mommy's book"
Regular past tense -ed	43–46	"We painted."
Irregular past tense	43–46	"I ate lunch."
Regular third person singular -s	43–46	"He runs fast."
Articles a, the, an	43–46	"I want the blocks."
Contractible copula be	43–46	"She's my friend."
Contractible auxiliary	47–50	"He's playing."
Uncontractible copula be	47–50	"He was sick."
Uncontractible auxiliary	47–50	"He was playing."
Irregular third person	47–50	"She has one."

Source: Adapted from *A First Language: The Early Stages,* by R. Brown, 1973, Cambridge, MA: Harvard University Press.

Children learn "words" and "rules" in other morphological cases as well. For example, when learning contractions, children sometimes apply a rule (e.g., "Add *n't* to change *have not* to *haven't* and add *n't* to change *has not* to *hasn't*"). Other times, children learn contractions as a unit or a "word" (e.g., *won't*), most likely because the sound of the root (*will*) is not the same in the contracted form (*won't*). So, just as children memorize irregular past tense verbs, they likewise must memorize contractions that do not conform to the typical pattern.

Combination of Words to Make Longer Utterances. In addition to inflecting words with grammatical morphemes, toddlers begin to combine words to create multiword utterances. Instead of requesting a favorite ball by saying "ball," as an infant in the one-word stage might do, toddlers might instead say "Mommy ball." This stage (sometimes called the *two-word stage*), in which toddlers begin to combine words to make utterances, marks the true beginnings of *syntax,* or the rules that govern the order of words in a child's language. Toddlers recognize the value that combining words has over using single words and can use language for many more communicative functions than they did in the one-word stage. Some simple functions that toddlers can express during the two-word stage include commenting ("Baby cry"), negating ("No juice"), requesting ("More juice"), and questioning ("What that?").

Child language researchers credit Roger Brown not only with documenting the order and ages by which children acquire grammatical morphemes, but also with creating *Brown's Stages of Language Development.* Brown's stages characterize children's language achievements according to their ability to produce utterances of varying syntactic complexity (see Table 6.3). One measure of the complexity of children's language is their mean length of utterance (MLU). MLU is the average length, in morphemes, of children's utterances. The MLU is calculated by counting the total number of morphemes used in a sample of 50–100 spontaneous utterances by a child and then dividing the total number of morphemes by the total number of utterances:

$$\text{MLU} = \frac{\text{Total number of morphemes}}{\text{Total number of utterances}}$$

Brown's rules for calculating morphemes are presented in Figure 6.4.

As children's language develops, their MLU increases systematically, as shown in Table 6.4. Researchers and clinicians alike use MLU regularly to evaluate children's language skills against the expectations, or norms, for children of the same age. As a general standard, we calculate MLU using a language sample of

TABLE 6.3
Roger Brown's (1973) Stages of Language Development

Brown's stage	Age (upper limit in months)	MLU	MLU range	Major achievements
I	18	1.31	0.99–1.64	Single-word sentences are used.
				Nouns and uninflected verbs are used ("Mommy"; "eat").
II	24	1.92	1.47–2.37	Two-element sentences are used.
				True clauses that are not evident are used ("Mommy up"; "Eat cookie").
III	30	2.54	1.97–3.11	Three-element sentences are used.
				Independent clauses emerge ("Baby want cookie").
IV	36	3.16	2.47–3.85	Four-element sentences are used.
				Independent clauses continue to emerge ("The teacher gave it to me").
V	42	3.78	2.96–4.60	Recursive elements predominate.
				Connecting devices emerge ("and"; "because").
Post-V	54	5.02	3.96–6.08	Complex syntactic patterns appear.
				Subordination and coordination continue to emerge.
				Complement clauses are used ("She's not feeling well").

MLU = mean length of utterance.
Source: Adapted from *Reference Manual for Communicative Sciences and Disorders: Speech and Language,* by R. D. Kent, 1994, Austin, TX: PRO-ED; and *The Syntax Handbook,* by L. M. Justice and H. K. Ezell, 2002, Eau Claire, WI: Thinking.

1. Start with the second page of the transcription unless that page involves a recitation of some kind. In this latter case start with the first recitation-free stretch. Count the first 100 utterances satisfying the following rules.
2. Only fully transcribed utterances are used; none with blanks. Portions of utterances, entered in parentheses to indicate doubtful transcription, are used.
3. Include all exact utterance repetitions (marked with a plus sign in records). Stuttering is marked as repeated efforts at a single word; count the word once in the most complete form produced. In the few cases where a word is produced for emphasis or the like (*no, no, no*) count each occurrence.
4. Do not count such fillers as *mm* or *oh*, but do count *no, yeah,* and *hi.*
5. All compound words (two or more free morphemes), proper names, and ritualized reduplications count as single words. Examples: *birthday, rackety-boom, choo-choo, quack-quack, right-right, pocketbook, see saw.* Justification is that no evidence that the constituent morphemes function as such for these children.
6. Count as one morpheme all irregular pasts of the verb (*got, did, went, saw*). Justification is that there is no evidence that the child relates these to present forms.
7. Count as one morpheme all diminutives (*doggie, mommie*) because these children at least do not seem to use the suffix productively. Diminutives are the standard forms used by the child.
8. Count as separate morphemes all auxiliaries (*is, have, will, can, must, would*). Also all catenatives: *gonna wanna, hafta.* These latter counted as single morphemes rather than as *going to* or *want to* because evidence is that they function so for the children. Count as separate morphemes all inflections, for example, possessive (s), plural (s), third person singular (s), regular past (d), progressive (ing).
9. The range count follows the above rules but is always calculated for the total transcription rather than for 100 utterances.

FIGURE 6.4
Roger Brown's (1973) rules for counting morphemes.

Source: From *A First Language: The Early Stages,* by R. Brown, 1973, Cambridge, MA: Harvard University Press. Copyright 1973 by Harvard University Press. Reprinted with permission.

50 utterances or more to obtain a representative sample of what the child can produce. For the sake of explanation, however, we present a short sample to demonstrate how you might calculate the MLU for a 3-year-old:

Utterance number	Utterance	Morphemes
1	"I want the ball."	4
2	"Make it go."	3
3	"No!"	1
4	"Up there."	2
5	"I want turn."	3
6	"Going over there."	4
7	"Look at that one."	4
8	"Mommy's turn."	3

TABLE 6.4
Normative References for Interpreting Mean Length of Utterance (MLU)

Age (months)	Predicted MLU	Predicted MLU ± 1 standard deviation (68% of population)
18	1.31	0.99–1.64
21	1.62	1.23–2.01
24	1.92	1.47–2.37
27	2.23	1.72–2.74
30	2.54	1.97–3.11
33	2.85	2.22–3.48
36	3.16	2.47–3.85
39	3.47	2.71–4.23
42	3.78	2.96–4.60
45	4.09	3.21–4.97
48	4.40	3.46–5.34
51	4.71	3.71–5.71
54	5.02	3.96–6.08
57	5.32	4.20–6.45
60	5.63	4.44–6.82

Source: From "The Relation Between Age and Mean Length of Utterance in Morphemes," by J. F. Miller and R. Chapman, 1981, *Journal of Speech and Hearing Research, 24,* p. 157. Copyright 1981 by American Speech–Language–Hearing Association. Adapted with permission.

In this brief sample, the child produced eight utterances and 24 morphemes, which resulted in an MLU of 3.0. The norms presented in Table 6.4 show that the predicted MLU for a child who is 3 years old is 3.16. Sixty-eight percent of children have scores within one standard deviation of 3.16, or between 2.47 and 3.85. If our sample is accurate, this child's MLU is within normal limits.

DISCUSSION POINT
Do you think speaking to toddlers at their own level—for example, by using telegraphic speech—would be beneficial? Why or why not?

Sentence Forms. When grammatical morphemes first emerge and children begin to combine words, language exhibits a telegraphic quality that results when children omit key grammatical markers. We describe toddlers' speech as telegraphic because persons sending telegrams would omit function words (e.g., *a, the*) to save money on the transmission. A toddler's "Mommy no go" and "Fishy swimming" are telegraphic reductions of "Mommy, don't go" and "The fish is swimming." Toddlers also tend to omit or misuse pronouns in their sentences ("Me do it"; "Her going"). Despite these awkward constructions, toddlers begin to use more adultlike forms for a variety of sentence types, including the yes–no question ("Are we going, Mommy?"), *wh-* questions ("What's that?"), commands ("You do it"), and negatives ("Me no want that").

Language Use

In addition to acquiring new grammatical constructions and words as they transition from the one-word stage to combining two or more words, toddlers obtain important new language, or discourse, functions and conversational skills.

CD VIDEO CLIP

To watch a 3-year-old boy use a variety of discourse functions, see the CD video clip *Language 5.* As you watch, try to identify the discourse functions.

Discourse Functions

By the time children begin to combine words, they can use a variety of language functions. These functions include instrumental, regulatory, personal-interactional, heuristic, imaginative, and informative functions (Halliday, 1978). Children can use *instrumental* functions, including requests, to satisfy their needs. They can also use *regulatory* functions, such as imperatives (commands), to control other people's behavior, and *personal-interactional* functions to share information about themselves and their feelings with other individuals. In addition, children can use *heuristic* functions by requesting information from other people to learn about the world, *imaginative* functions by telling stories to pretend, and *informative* functions to give information to other people. Children's success at using communication for a variety of purposes is one of the most important aspects of communicative development during toddlerhood.

Conversational Skills

One area in which toddlers *do not* display much skill is conversation. Conversational skill requires being able to initiate a conversational topic, sustain the topic for several turns, then appropriately take leave of the conversation. In Chapter 3, we discuss the concept of a *conversational schema,* which is a model specifying the organization of conversations. Toddlers are beginning to develop this schema, but they are relatively poor conversationalists. Anyone who has attempted to have a conversation with a young child knows it is not usually sophisticated, as in the following example:

PARENT: What did you play at Grandma's house?

TODDLER: Grandma, Uncle Tony, Pop Pop.

DISCUSSION POINT

Talking about an activity or object of interest to a toddler is one way adults might promote conversation. Can you think of other strategies adults might use to sustain conversation with a toddler?

Toddlers may demonstrate some skill in starting a conversation but cannot usually sustain it for more than one or two turns. Typically, the adult bears the burden of maintaining a particular topic. Toddlers also have difficulty keeping their audience's needs in mind: They may use pronouns without appropriately defining to whom they refer, and they may discuss topics without ensuring that the listener has a sufficient frame of reference to understand the context. You may also notice that in conversations, when you ask a toddler a specific question or give him or her an explicit opportunity to take a turn, the child will not always take the opportunity. The toddler may simply not respond or may respond *noncontingently* (off the topic). Toddlers are not yet proficient at realizing when they are not following along in a conversation and are thus not likely to seek clarification.

WHAT FACTORS INFLUENCE TODDLERS' INDIVIDUAL ACHIEVEMENTS IN LANGUAGE?

As in the case of infants, toddlers develop language in a fairly predictable pattern because they meet certain milestones in the same order and at about the same age. However, certain aspects of their language development vary. Both *intraindividual* and *interindividual* language differences among toddlers are discussed next, along with factors that may account for such differences.

Intraindividual Differences

If you observe an *individual* toddler for any length of time, you will most likely notice that his or her language development is not linear. For example, a toddler might learn several new words within a week's time, and then not learn any new words for the next few weeks. In fact, children individually experience a series of spurts and plateaus in their language abilities as they develop (Fenson, Bates, et al., 2000; Scarborough, 2002).

Likewise, as mentioned in Chapter 5, comprehension of language generally precedes production. This fact makes sense on many levels. Consider, for example, your personal abilities to comprehend and produce foreign languages. Most likely, you can understand significantly more than you can say. The idea that comprehension precedes production holds true for the sizes of toddlers' receptive and expressive lexicons as well. In fact, such disparity continues throughout the preschool and school-age years and even into adulthood.

Interindividual Differences

If you observe a *group* of toddlers, you will most likely note language development differences among them. First, boys and girls typically show differences in language acquisition and use. Second, children's birth order affects their language acquisition, and, third, the family's socioeconomic status has an impact on a child's language learning. Next, we discuss these differences and some of the factors accounting for them.

Effects of Gender

Several studies have revealed some effects of gender on language development, in terms of both the pace at which children acquire language and the communication styles they use. For example, Fenson, Bates, and colleagues (2000) found that boys both comprehend and produce fewer words than girls do. In their study, they found that girls who were 18 months old could understand an average of 65 words and produce about 27 words. However, boys of the same age understood an average of only 56 words and produced only about 18 words. Bauer, Goldfield, and Reznick (2002) also found that boys lag behind girls in lexical development. Likewise, other researchers, who conducted a study of 386 pairs of toddler twins, found that girls produce more words and more two-word combinations than boys do (Van Hulle, Goldsmith, & Lemery, 2004).

What factors underlie these gender differences? Bauer and colleagues (2002) posited that differences in boys' and girls' maturation rates, particularly with respect to neurological development, may contribute to gender differences in language acquisition. Likewise, parents may interact differently with boys and girls, and these different interaction styles may affect language development patterns. For example, parents of 3-year-old boys tend to initiate more conversation in play settings, whereas parents of 3-year-old girls typically initiate more conversation in nonplay settings. Girls may thus acquire more complex language constructions as their parents talk about objects and events outside the here and now, and boys may acquire less complex language as their parents comment on perceptually available objects and actions in the context of toy-play activities (Apel & Masterson, 2001).

Effects of Birth Order

In addition to gender, birth order may affect children's language development. First-born children are more likely to have larger vocabularies in their second year and to reach the 50-word mark sooner than their later-born counterparts do. Recall the importance of the 50-word mark: It usually signifies the beginning of the vocabulary spurt and 2-word combinations, or syntactic development.

Why might the order in which children are born relate to language development? One suggestion is that firstborn children (and only children, who are firstborn by default) receive much more one-on-one attention than do children who are not firstborn.

Effects of Socioeconomic Status

Socioeconomic status (SES), which usually includes some measure of family income, parental education, or occupational status, is associated with a variety of health, cognitive, and socioemotional outcomes in children; these effects begin before birth and continue into adulthood (Bradley & Corwyn, 2002). As is true for infants, SES is associated with toddlers' receptive and expressive language development. For example, Horton-Ikard and Ellis Weismer (2005) demonstrated that typically developing African American toddlers from low SES backgrounds perform more poorly on standardized measures of receptive and expressive language than do their counterparts from middle SES backgrounds. Analyses of spontaneous language samples show similar effects of SES. Dollaghan et al. (1999) demonstrated that even after adjustment for ethnicity in their study, toddlers from lower SES (as measured by maternal education) had shorter MLUs and used fewer words than did toddlers from higher SES backgrounds.

Why does SES make a difference? Researchers have determined that how much parents talk to their young children is related to the parents' SES, and the more parents talk to their children, the more rapidly children's vocabulary grows and the better children perform on measures of verbal and cognitive competence at age 3 years (Hart & Risley, 1995, 1999).

DISCUSSION POINT

Toddlers from low-SES backgrounds have been shown to perform more poorly on both standardized and naturalistic language measures than do their mid- and high-SES counterparts. Why is knowing this fact important?

HOW DO RESEARCHERS AND CLINICIANS MEASURE LANGUAGE DEVELOPMENT IN TODDLERHOOD?

Researchers

When studying language development in toddlerhood, researchers have a broader range of language data to consider than do researchers studying language development in infancy. The reason is that toddlers not only comprehend language but also produce it. McDaniel, McKee, and Smith (1996) classified methods for assessing children's language development (although their specific focus was on syntax) into three categories: production tasks, comprehension tasks, and judgment tasks.

Production Tasks

Production tasks allow toddlers to demonstrate their competence in various areas of language development. In these tasks, the children are asked to produce, or say, the language targets under investigation. Some production tasks are unstructured or semistructured, such as naturalistic observation, and other production tasks are structured and systematic, such as elicited imitation and elicited production tasks.

Naturalistic Observation. We introduced naturalistic observations in Chapter 5 when we described methods researchers use to study language development in infancy. Naturalistic observations of children's spontaneous productions are of great value in toddlerhood as well, when children's syntax can be analyzed for the first time. Probably the most famous naturalistic observations are Roger Brown's (1973) longitudinal observations of children with the pseudonyms Adam, Eve, and Sarah. As a result of Brown's analysis, researchers know, for example, that children's earliest utterances containing forms of the verb *to be* (*am, is, are, was, were*) include contractions (e.g., *it's*). Recall from our earlier discussion that toddlers may learn some contractions as a "word," or whole unit, rather than as two separate words to which they apply a contraction "rule."

Researchers must consider many factors when they collect, transcribe, and analyze naturalistic language samples. Such factors include the number of children to analyze, the number of recordings to collect from each child, and the variety of contexts in which to collect samples. See Demuth (1996) for some practical suggestions on how to collect spontaneous production data.

Elicited Imitation Tasks. To gauge children's underlying linguistic competence, researchers can use elicited imitation tasks, which take advantage of children's natural ability to imitate other people's movements and speech sounds. In elicited imitation tasks, the experimenter produces a target phrase and then requests that the child repeat it exactly as he or she heard it. The experimenter carefully selects sentences that vary only by the grammatical structure under investigation. Researchers have used elicited imitation tasks to explore children's competence with word order and *anaphora*, or linguistic units (such as pronouns) that refer to a previous linguistic unit. (For example, in the sentence "Doug said that *he* was happy," the word *he* refers to *Doug*.)

In elicited imitation tasks, researchers assume that for a child to successfully imitate a target, the target must be a part of the child's grammatical repertoire (Lust, Flynn, & Foley, 1996). The following two examples illustrate how an elicited imitation task might play out for one child who has acquired the rule for forming *wh*-questions in English and for a second child who has not yet acquired this rule:

ADULT 1: What is your favorite color?

CHILD 1: What is your favorite color?

ADULT 2: What is your favorite color?

CHILD 2: What your favorite color is?

In a true elicited imitation task, the experimenter would ask the child to repeat several phrases that contain the target linguistic skill under investigation and compare the child's utterances with adultlike forms.

Elicited Production Tasks. Elicited production tasks are designed to reveal aspects of children's language abilities (e.g., syntax, morphology, pragmatics) by having them produce specific sentence structures. Researchers elicit these sentence structures in the context of a game, during which the child asks questions or makes statements after receiving a prompt from the experimenter. Perhaps the most famous elicited production task is Jean Berko's (1958) **Wug Test** (Figure 6.5). Berko (now Berko Gleason) designed the Wug Test to investigate children's acquisition of English morphemes, including the plural marker. English plural nouns are marked by adding one of three *allomorphs* (variants of a morpheme with the same meaning but different sounds) of the morpheme *-s*. These allomorphs are as follows:

Allomorph of *-s*	Use	Example
/z/	Added to nouns that end in voiced consonants	pig—pig<u>s</u>
/s/	Added to nouns that end in voiceless consonants	pit—pit<u>s</u>
/ɪz/	Added to nouns that end in /s/ or /ʃ/	kiss—kiss<u>es</u> wish—*wish<u>es</u>*

Berko elicited these three allomorphs by presenting children with a pseudoword and then asking them to say what two of the same word would be called. Consider the following examples of how the Wug Test might play out with a child who is already producing the plural morpheme:

FIGURE 6.5
Wug Test.
Source: From "The Child's Learning of English Morphology," by J. Berko, 1958, *Word, 14,* p. 154. Copyright 1958 by Jean Berko. Reprinted with permission.

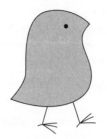

This is a wug.

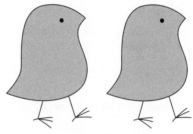

Now there is another one.
There are two of them.
There are two ___.

ADULT: This is a wug. (*points to picture of single object*)

ADULT: Now there are two of them. (*points to picture of two objects*) There are two _____.

CHILD: Wugs! [/wʌgz/]

As you can see, the adult elicits the target word with a prompt but does not provide the target for the child to repeat, as is done in elicited imitation tasks.

Comprehension Tasks

Comprehension tasks reveal toddlers' language competencies, not by asking them to produce language targets, but by having them either match or point to pictures of target words and phrases or act out phrases they hear an experimenter say.

The Picture Selection Task. In a picture selection task, the experimenter presents a language target and asks the child to choose the picture that corresponds to the target. For example, the experimenter who wants to determine whether a child understands the difference between the /l/ and /r/ sounds might ask the child to select the picture of *glass* from between a picture of *glass* and a picture of *grass.* Researchers frequently use picture selection tasks to investigate children's understanding of lexical items and syntactic constructions, including the distinction between active and passive voice. Gerken and Shady (1996) reported the results of Fraser, Bellugi, and Brown's (1963) study, which investigated 37- to 43-month-old children's understanding of several morphosyntactic contrasts and the order in which children have the most success comprehending these contrasts (see Table 6.5).

TABLE 6.5
Morphosyntactic Contrasts Tested by Using the Picture Selection Task

Contrast tested	Sample sentence pair
Affirmative vs. negative	*The girl is cooking.*
	The girl is not cooking.
Subject vs. object (active voice)	*The train bumps the car.*
	The car bumps the train.
Present progressive tense vs. future tense	*The girl is drinking.*
	The girl will drink.
Singular vs. plural possessive	*That's his wagon.*
	That's their wagon.
Present progressive tense vs. past tense	*The paint is spilling.*
	The paint spilled.
Mass noun vs. count noun	*There's some mog.*
	There's a dap.
Singular vs. plural auxiliary *be*	*The deer is running.*
	The deer are running.
Singular vs. plural inflections	*The boy draws.*
	The boys draw.
Subject vs. object (passive voice)	*The car is bumped by the train.*
	The train is bumped by the car.
Indirect vs. direct object	*The girl shows the cat the dog.*
	The girl shows the dog the cat.

Morphosyntactic contrasts are presented in order of comprehension difficulty.
Source: From "The Picture Selection Task," by L. Gerken and M. E. Shady, in *Methods for Assessing Children's Syntax* (p. 128), edited by D. McDaniel, C. McKee, and H. Smith Cairns, 1996, Cambridge: MIT Press. © 1996 Massachusetts Institute of Technology. Adapted with permission.

The Act-Out Task. In an act-out task, used to investigate the child's competence with various language constructions, an experimenter presents a child with a series of props and instructs the child to "act out" the sentences he or she hears. For instance, if you are interested in assessing a 3-year-old's ability to comprehend agent and recipient relations, you might say something such as "The dog tickled the cat," then ask the child to act out that particular sequence with a toy dog and cat.

Judgment Tasks

In judgment tasks, children are asked to decide whether certain language constructions are appropriate so that their level of grammatical competence can be assessed. Researchers can infer that children possess adultlike levels of grammatical competence when they judge adultlike constructions to be "correct" and nonadultlike sentences to be "incorrect." Two types of judgment tasks that researchers routinely use are truth value judgment tasks and grammaticality judgment tasks.

DISCUSSION POINT

What are some pros and cons of using truth value judgment tasks with toddlers?

Truth Value Judgment Tasks. In truth value judgment tasks, children are asked to judge certain language constructions to be correct or incorrect. These tasks take two forms: yes–no tasks and reward–punishment tasks. In a yes–no task, an experimenter presents a scenario and asks the child a question. For example, an experimenter who wants to gauge a child's comprehension of quantifiers might present a picture and ask "Is every mother holding a baby?" or "Is a mother holding every baby?" and note the child's response. In a reward–punishment task, an experimenter introduces a puppet and explains to a child that he or she should reward the puppet with a cookie (or some other treat) when the puppet says something "right" and should punish the puppet by withholding a treat when the puppet says something "wrong." The experimenter uses sentences containing the target linguistic construction, but such sentences are declarative rather than yes–no questions. For example, a puppet might say "Every mother is holding a baby" and if what the puppet said was correct, the child would reward the puppet with a cookie.

Grammaticality Judgment Tasks. Grammaticality judgment tasks are generally suited for preschoolers, older children, and adults, so we discuss them in Chapter 7.

Clinicians

Several tools are available to clinicians as they work with toddlers. Even though toddlers are prone to acting according to their own agendas, measuring the language development of toddlers is arguably easier than measuring that of infants. The reason is that toddlers can follow simple instructions during an assessment and are generally eager to play along when the clinician structures the assessment to resemble a game rather than a test.

Evaluation and Assessment Tools

The Individuals with Disabilities Education Act of 2004 (IDEA; 2004) differentiates between two methods of measuring language development: evaluation and assessment. **Evaluation** refers to a method used to determine a child's initial and continuing eligibility for services under IDEA and includes a determination of the child's status across developmental areas. Evaluations are generally structured and standardized and are limited in duration rather than ongoing. **Assessment** describes ongoing procedures used to identify a child's needs, family concerns, and resources. Assessments are generally less formal than evaluations and involve a variety of methods, including standardized tests and observations. Assessments also generally encourage more parental and caregiver participation than do evaluations.

The 10 most common *evaluation* tools speech–language pathologists use to evaluate children's language skills are presented in Table 6.6, and the top 10 *assessment* tools are presented in Table 6.7 (Crais, 1995). Many of the evaluation tools reported in Table 6.6 and the assessment tools reported in Table 6.7 have been revised since 1995. Although these tools are popular, many have limitations, including a limited role for family members in the assessment process, a limited allowance for individual variation among children as a result of standardization, and a limited predictability of later language and communication abilities. Perhaps the most important consideration for evaluation and assessment tools is **ecological**

TABLE 6.6

Speech–Language Pathologists' Ten Most Common Evaluation Tools

Instrument name	Instrument abbreviation	Author(s)
Preschool Language Scale—3	PLS–3	Zimmerman, Steiner, and Pond (1992)
Revised edition: Preschool Language Scale—4	PLS–4	Zimmerman, Steiner, and Pond (2002)
Sequenced Inventory of Communicative Development —Revised	SICD–R	Hedrick, Prather, and Tobin (1984)
Expressive One-Word Picture Vocabulary Test	EOWPVT	Gardner (1979)
Revised edition: Expressive One-Word Picture Vocabulary Test—2000 edition	EOWPVT–2000	Brownell (2000a)
Peabody Picture Vocabulary Test—Revised	PPVT–R	Dunn and Dunn (1981)
Revised edition: Peabody Picture Vocabulary Test—Third edition	PPVT–III	Dunn and Dunn (1997)
Revised edition: Peabody Picture Vocabulary Test—Fourth edition	PPVT–4	Dunn and Dunn (2006)
Receptive One-Word Picture Vocabulary Test	ROWPVT	Gardner (1990)
Revised edition: Receptive One-Word Picture Vocabulary Test—2000 edition	ROWPVT–2000	Brownell (2000b)
Birth to Three Developmental Scales	—	Bangs and Dodson (1986)
Revised edition: Birth to Three Assessment and Intervention System—Second edition	BTAIS–2	Ammer and Bangs (2000)
Clinical Evaluation of Language Fundamentals—Preschool	CELF–P	Wiig, Semel, and Secord (1992)
Revised edition: Clinical Evaluation of Language Fundamentals—Preschool, second edition	CELF–Preschool–2	Wiig, Secord, and Semel (2004)
Receptive–Expressive Emergent Language Scale—Second edition	REEL–2	Bzoch and League (1991)
Revised edition: Receptive–Expressive Emergent Language Test—Third edition	REEL–3	Bzoch, League, and Brown (2003)
Rossetti Infant–Toddler Language Scale	—	Rossetti (1990)
Early Language Milestone Scale—Second edition	ELM Scale–2	Coplan (1993)

Source: Adapted from "Expanding the Repertoire of Tools and Techniques for Assessing the Communication Skills of Infants and Toddlers," by E. R. Crais, 1995, *American Journal of Speech–Language Pathology, 4,* pp. 47–59.

validity, or the extent to which the data resulting from these tools can be extended to multiple contexts, including the child's home and day care settings. Crais advised practitioners to examine the evaluation and assessment tools they use and to identify ways to include more ecologically valid tools and techniques as they work with children.

TABLE 6.7

Speech–Language Pathologists' Ten Most Common Assessment Tools

Instrument name	Instrument abbreviation	Author(s)
Preschool Language Scale—3	PLS–3	Zimmerman, Steiner, and Pond (1992)
Revised edition: Preschool Language Scale—4	PLS–4	Zimmerman, Steiner, and Pond (2002)
Expressive One-Word Picture Vocabulary Test	EOWPVT	Gardner (1979)
Revised edition: Expressive One-Word Picture Vocabulary Test—2000 edition	EOWPVT–2000	Brownell (2000a)
Rossetti Infant–Toddler Language Scale	—	Rossetti (1990)
Receptive One-Word Picture Vocabulary Test	ROWPVT	Gardner (1990)
Revised edition: Receptive One-Word Picture Vocabulary Test—2000 edition	ROWPVT–2000	Brownell (2000b)
Sequenced Inventory of Communicative Development—Revised	SICD–R	Hedrick, Prather, and Tobin (1984)
Peabody Picture Vocabulary Test—Revised	PPVT–R	Dunn and Dunn (1981)
Revised edition: Peabody Picture Vocabulary Test—Third edition	PPVT–III	Dunn and Dunn (1997)
Revised edition: Peabody Picture Vocabulary Test—Fourth edition	PPVT–4	Dunn and Dunn (2006)
Clinical Evaluation of Language Fundamentals—Preschool	CELF–P	Wiig, Semel, and Secord (1992)
Revised edition: Clinical Evaluation of Language Fundamentals—Preschool, second edition	CELF–Preschool–2	Wiig, Secord, and Semel (2004)
Birth to Three Developmental Scales	—	Bangs and Dodson (1986)
Revised edition: Birth to Three Assessment and Intervention System—Second edition	BTAIS–2	Ammer and Bangs (2000)
MacArthur Communicative Development Inventories	CDI	Fenson et al. (1991)
Revised edition: MacArthur–Bates Communicative Development Inventories	CDI	Fenson et al. (2003)
Receptive–Expressive Emergent Language Scale—Second edition	REEL–2	Bzoch and League (1991)
Revised edition: Receptive–Expressive Emergent Language Test—Third edition	REEL–3	Bzoch, League, and Brown (2003)

Source: Adapted from "Expanding the Repertoire of Tools and Techniques for Assessing the Communication Skills of Infants and Toddlers," by E. R. Crais, 1995, *American Journal of Speech–Language Pathology, 4,* pp. 47–59.

Here is a checklist that you can follow to determine if your child's speech and language skills are developing on schedule. You should talk to your child's doctor about anything that is checked "no."

12–17 months	Yes	No
Attends to a book or toy for about 2 minutes.	○	○
Follows simple directions accompanied by gestures.		
Answers simple questions nonverbally.	○	○
Points to objects, pictures, and family members.	○	○
Says two to three words to label a person	○	○
or an object (pronunciation may not be clear).	○	○
Tries to imitate simple words.	○	○

FIGURE 6.6
Language screen for toddlers ages 12–17 months.
Source: From *Milestones in Your Child's Speech and Language Development,* by National Institute on Deafness and Other Communication Disorders, n.d., Bethesda, MD: Author. Copyright 2006 by National Institute on Deafness and Other Communication Disorders.
http://www.nidcd.nih.gov/health/voice/the basics_speechandlanguage.asp

Informal Language Screens.

Informal language screens in toddlerhood, like those in infancy, use common early language milestones. Checklists that allow clinicians and parents to determine whether children exhibit each behavior in question are a common type of informal language screen. The National Institute on Deafness and Other Communication Disorders (www.nidcd.nih.gov) distributes a series of developmental language screens that parents and clinicians can use informally. See Figure 6.6 for an example of a screen for toddlers ages 12–17 months.

Using informal language screens, parents can complete a checklist to assess their toddler's language abilities.

(*Photo Source:* Anne Vega/Merrill.)

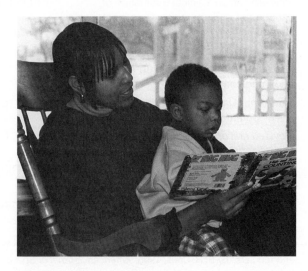

SUMMARY

In this chapter, we open with a discussion of the major language milestones that toddlers achieve. These milestones include not only the transition from prelinguistic to linguistic communication as toddlers utter their first word, but also toddlers' increasingly sophisticated use of gestures.

In the second section, we describe toddlers' achievements in language content, form, and use during the second and third years—which are numerous. With respect to language content, toddlers' receptive and expressive lexicons continue to grow, and these children use overextension, underextension, and overlap as they learn new words. In our discussion of these achievements, we describe the Quinean conundrum and explore two possible ways children overcome this conundrum as they attempt to narrow the nearly infinite number of referents for novel words. We also examine toddlers' ability to fast map new words.

With respect to language form, we explore major achievements in phonology, including acquiring new phonemes, phonological processes, and phonological perception. We define grammatical morphemes and explain how toddlers transition from using one-word utterances to using two-word utterances. With respect to language use, we explore some of the new discourse functions and conversational skills that become available to toddlers.

In the third section of this chapter, we explain that intraindividual and interindividual differences in language achievements continue throughout toddlerhood. *Individual* toddlers vary in their language acquisition rate and in their expressive and receptive lexical development. Three major factors that influence differences in language development *among a group* of toddlers are gender, birth order, and familial socioeconomic status.

In the final section of this chapter, we describe how researchers and clinicians measure language development in toddlerhood. We detail six specific paradigms researchers use to measure language development—naturalistic observation, elicited imitation tasks, elicited production tasks, the picture selection task, the act-out task, and truth value judgment tasks—and three ways clinicians measure it—assessments, evaluations, and informal screens.

KEY TERMS

age of mastery, p. 197

agent, p. 196

assessment, p. 213

assimilation, p. 197

categorical scope, p. 193

conventionality, p. 193

customary age of production, p. 197

ecological validity, p. 214

evaluation, p. 213

event-related potentials, p. 194

extendibility, p. 192

fronting, p. 198

goal, p. 196

location, p. 196

novel name–nameless category (N3C), p. 193

object scope, p. 193

overextension, p. 189

For online resources related to chapter content, including audio samples, valuable Web sites, suggested readings, and self-quizzes, please go to the Companion Website at http://www.prenhall.com/pence

7

Preschool

Building Literacy on Language

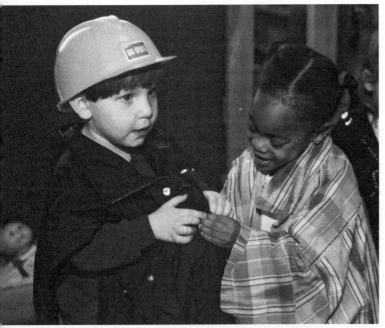

FOCUS QUESTIONS

In this chapter, we answer the following four questions:

1. What major language development milestones occur in the preschool period?
2. What major achievements in language content, form, and use characterize the preschool period?
3. What factors influence preschoolers' individual achievements in language?
4. How do researchers and clinicians measure language development in the preschool period?

In the United States, the preschool period is the 2 years before a child enters elementary school, or between about ages 3 and 5 years. Children experience many remarkable "firsts" during the preschool period. For example, they begin to use language to talk about objects, events, and thoughts that are not in the immediate context. Preschoolers also begin to gain important abilities in emergent literacy, which marks their transition to comprehending and expressing language in multiple modalities: oral and written. In the preschool years, children's language becomes even more sophisticated than in the toddler years as children begin to master form, content, and use in new ways. In this chapter, we begin with an overview of the major milestones in language development that preschoolers achieve, including decontextualized language and emergent literacy. Next, we explore achievements in language content, form, and use. We also discuss ways in which preschoolers differ both individually and from one another in their language development. Finally, we detail the ways in which researchers and clinicians measure the language development of preschool-age children.

WHAT MAJOR LANGUAGE DEVELOPMENT MILESTONES OCCUR IN THE PRESCHOOL PERIOD?

Compared with their younger toddler counterparts, preschoolers accomplish a lot in a day. No longer having to concentrate on keeping their footing, preschoolers have plenty of time for building towers out of blocks (and knocking them down), drawing and coloring, engaging in pretend play, riding bikes, and digging in the dirt. With exposure to so many different objects and activities, preschoolers (even those who do not attend preschool programs) have many more opportunities to hear new words, grammatical constructions, and language functions. One significant milestone of the preschool period is the acquisition of a specific type of language that does not rely on the immediate context for interpretation: decontextualized language. Preschool-age children reared in literate households or who attend preschool are also exposed to written language and begin to acquire important emergent literacy skills, which is probably the crowning achievement of the preschool period.

Decontextualized Language

As preschoolers continue to add to the *quantity* of words they understand and produce, a noticeable shift can also be seen in the *quality* of words they understand and use. During the preschool years, children begin to incorporate *decontextualized language* in their conversations in addition to the *contextualized language* they began using in infancy and toddlerhood. **Contextualized language** is grounded in the immediate context, or the here and now. Such language relies on the background knowledge that a speaker and a listener share, and on gestures, intonation, and immediately present situational cues. A child using contextualized language might say "Gimme that" while pointing to something in the listener's hands or might describe a lion as "big and furry" while standing in front of the lion's cage at the zoo.

In contrast, when a child wants to discuss people, places, objects, and events that are not immediately present, decontextualized language becomes appropriate and necessary. **Decontextualized language** relies heavily on the language itself in the construction of meaning. Such language may not contain context cues and does not assume that a speaker and a listener share background knowledge or context. A boy who uses decontextualized language might call for his mother in the kitchen when he is in the living room, remembering that they do not share the same physical context ("Mom, I spilled milk on the couch!") or might describe an event to someone after the event occurs ("We watched fireworks on the Fourth of July"). In both situations, the child realizes he cannot rely on the immediate physical context to help him communicate to the listener. As with all types of decontextualized discourse, the child must use highly precise syntax and vocabulary to represent events beyond the here and now.

The ability to use decontextualized language is fundamental to academic success because nearly all the learning that occurs in schools focuses on events and concepts beyond the classroom walls. For example, when teaching about the life cycle of a plant, a teacher might use the words *seed, dirt, water, sunlight, sprout,* and *grow,* even though he or she and the students cannot witness all these components and processes of the cycle simultaneously in the context of their conversation.

DISCUSSION POINT

What kind of task might a researcher design to determine whether a preschooler is using decontextualized language?

Emergent Literacy

During the preschool period, children develop several important literacy skills that allow them to begin to comprehend and use written language. They learn how print works, they begin to play with the sound units that compose syllables and words, and they develop an interest in reading and writing. Researchers refer to the earliest period of learning about reading and writing as **emergent literacy.** Although at this time children are not yet reading and writing in a conventional sense, their emerging knowledge about print and sounds forms an important foundation for the reading instruction that begins when they enter formal schooling (Justice & Pullen, 2003). Children's literacy abilities depend heavily on the **oral language** skills they began to acquire in infancy and toddlerhood. For example, children need not only well-developed phonological systems before they can make sense of grapheme-to-phoneme (letter-to-sound) correspondences but also well-developed vocabularies to derive meaning from text. For this reason, preschoolers are said to "build literacy on language."

Emergent literacy achievements depend largely on children's **metalinguistic ability,** or the ability to view language as an object of attention. Preschoolers may view language as an object of scrutiny as they pretend to write, look at words in a

DISCUSSION POINT

Adults rely on metalinguistic abilities in certain circumstances as well. Can you think of some occasions when you had to focus on language as an object of attention?

storybook, or make up rhyming patterns (Chaney, 1998). This ability to engage with language at a metalinguistic level is an important achievement of the preschool period that correlates well with children's success with writing and reading instruction, both of which depend on the ability to focus on language as an object of attention (Justice & Ezell, 2004).

Three important achievements in emergent literacy for preschoolers are alphabet knowledge, print awareness, and phonological awareness. **Alphabet knowledge** is children's knowledge about the letters of the alphabet. **Print awareness** is children's understanding of the forms and functions of written language, and *phonological awareness* is children's sensitivity to the sound units that make up speech (phonemes, syllables, words).

Alphabet Knowledge

Children who grow up in households in which book reading is common begin to show emerging knowledge of the alphabet during the first 3 years of life. Some children even know a letter or two before their second birthday. During the preschool years, children will typically recognize some of the letters in their names, show interest in specific letters occurring in the environment on signs or labels, and begin to write some letters with which they are especially familiar (Chaney, 1994). By age 5 years, children are often familiar with the letters that make up their names, a phenomenon referred to as the *own-name advantage* (Treiman & Broderick, 1998). In an informative study, Treiman and Broderick showed that 79% of preschoolers from middle-class homes were able to identify the first letter in their name. Also interesting is that children's acquisition of letter names appears to be related to the order of the alphabet (McBride-Chang, 1999). This phenomenon is likely the result of

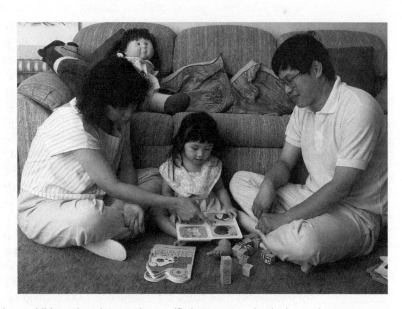

Preschool-age children show interest in specific letters occurring in the environment.

(*Photo Source:* Laura Dwight/PhotoEdit Inc.)

children's increased exposure to the beginning letters of the alphabet. Results of a separate study confirmed that the order in which children learn alphabet letters is not random and that multiple forces interact to influence this order. Specifically, researchers found that four complementary hypotheses aptly characterize the order in which preschool children learn the names of individual alphabet letters. These hypotheses are as follows (Justice, Pence, Bowles, & Wiggins, 2006):

1. *Own-name advantage:* Children learn the letters of their names earlier than other letters.

2. *Letter-name pronunciation effect:* Alphabet letters for which the name of the letter is in its pronunciation are learned earlier than letters for which this is not the case (e.g., letter *B* is pronounced /bi/, but letter *X* is pronounced /ɛks/).

3. *Letter-order hypothesis:* letters occurring earlier in the alphabet string (e.g., *A, B, C*) are learned before letters occurring later in the alphabet string (e.g., *X, Y, Z*).

4. *Consonant-order hypothesis:* Letters for which corresponding consonantal phonemes are learned early in development (e.g., *B, M*) are learned earlier than letters for which corresponding consonantal phonemes are learned later (e.g., *J, V*).

Print Awareness

Print awareness describes a number of specific achievements that children generally acquire along a developmental continuum (Justice & Ezell, 2004): development of *print interest,* recognition of *print functions,* understanding of *print conventions,* understanding of *print forms,* and recognition of *print part-to-whole relationships* (see Figure 7.1). First, young children develop an interest in and appreciation for print. They recognize that print exists in the environment and in books. Second, they begin to understand that print conveys meaning and has a specific function. Third, children develop an understanding of specific print conventions, including reading print from left to right and from top to bottom. Fourth, children learn the language that describes specific print units, including *words* and *letters.* Fifth, children learn the relationship among different print units, including how letters combine to form words.

Children's oral language abilities and the interactions they have with print influence how they develop print awareness. For example, when adults refer to print during storybook-reading sessions, children ask more questions and make more comments about print (Ezell & Justice, 2000). Furthermore, children show marked improvement in important early literacy abilities when adults question about and point to print during book-reading sessions (Justice & Ezell, 2002b).

CD VIDEO CLIP
To watch a preschooler participate in a study that measures attention to print during shared storybook reading, see the CD video clip *Research 4.*

Phonological Awareness

Phonological awareness, another important metalinguistic skill, is children's sensitivity to the sound structure of words. This awareness emerges incrementally, beginning around age 2 years and moving from a "shallow" level of awareness to a "deep" level of awareness (see Table 7.1; Stanovich, 2000). Children with shallow levels of phonological awareness show an implicit and rudimentary sensitivity to large units of sound structure. They can segment sentences into words and multisyllabic words into

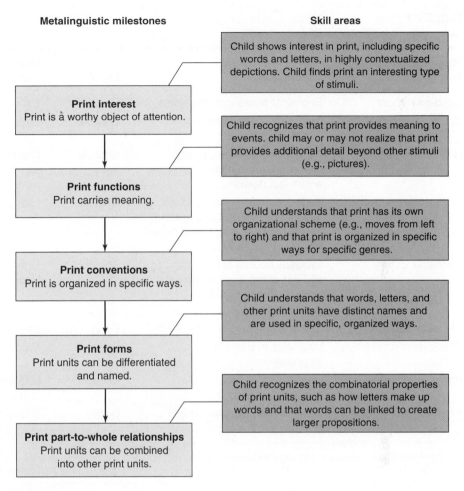

FIGURE 7.1

Achievements in print awareness.

Source: From "Print Referencing: An Emergent Literacy Enhancement Technique and Its Clinical Applications," by L. M. Justice and H. K. Ezell, 2004, *Language, Speech, and Hearing Services in Schools, 35,* p. 188. Copyright 2004 by American Speech–Language–Hearing Association. Reprinted with permission.

syllables. They can also detect and produce rhymes, combine syllable onsets with the remainder of the syllable to produce a word (e.g., /b/ + /ɪt/ = *bit*), and detect beginning sound similarities among words (e.g., _sing, sack, sun_). Children develop these shallow sensitivities during the preschool years, from about 3 to 5 years of age. In contrast, children with a deep level of phonological awareness demonstrate an explicit and analytical knowledge of the smallest phonological segments of speech (phonemes). They can count the number of phonemes in words (e.g., *bit* has three sounds, and *spit* has four sounds), can segment words into their constituent phonemes (e.g., *bit* can be broken into /b/ + /ɪ/ + /t/), and can manipulate the phonological segments within words (e.g., delete the first sound in _spit_ and move it to the end of the word to

TABLE 7.1
Achievements in Phonological Awareness

Phonological awareness skill	Description	Level	Developmental expectation
Word awareness	Segments sentences into words	Shallow	Early to middle preschool
Syllable awareness	Segments multisyllable words into syllables	Shallow	Early to middle preschool
Rhyme awareness	Recognizes when two words rhyme; produces pairs of words that rhyme	Shallow	Early to middle preschool
Onset awareness	Segments the beginning sound (onset) from the rest of a syllable; blends the beginning sound (onset) with the rest of a syllable	Shallow	Late preschool
Phoneme identity	Identifies sounds at the beginning and end of the word; identifies words that start with the same sound	Shallow	Late preschool, early kindergarten
Phoneme blending	Blends phonemes to make a word	Deep	Early kindergarten
Phoneme segmentation	Segments a word into its phonemes	Deep	Middle to late kindergarten
Phoneme counting	Identifies the number of phonemes in a word	Deep	Late kindergarten to end of first grade
Phoneme manipulation	Deletes, adds, and rearranges phonemes in a word	Deep	Elementary grades

Source: From "Embedded-Explicit Emergent Literacy. II: Goal Selection and Implementation in the Early Childhood Classroom," by J. N. Kaderavek and L. M. Justice, 2004, *Language, Speech, and Hearing Services in Schools, 35,* p. 218. Copyright 2004 by American Speech–Language–Hearing Association. Reprinted with permission.

make *pits; Justice & Schuele, 2004). See Developmental Timeline: Preschool for an overview of more milestones children achieve during the preschool years.

WHAT MAJOR ACHIEVEMENTS IN LANGUAGE CONTENT, FORM, AND USE CHARACTERIZE THE PRESCHOOL PERIOD?

As we first mentioned in Chapter 1 and then reviewed in Chapters 5 and 6, the three rule-governed domains that together compose language are *content,* or the words people use and their meanings; *form,* or the way in which people organize sounds, words, and sentences to convey content; and *use,* or how people use language in interactions with other individuals to express personal and social needs. As you may suspect, the preschool period ushers in even more achievements in each of these three areas.

DEVELOPMENTAL TIMELINE: PRESCHOOL

Phonology

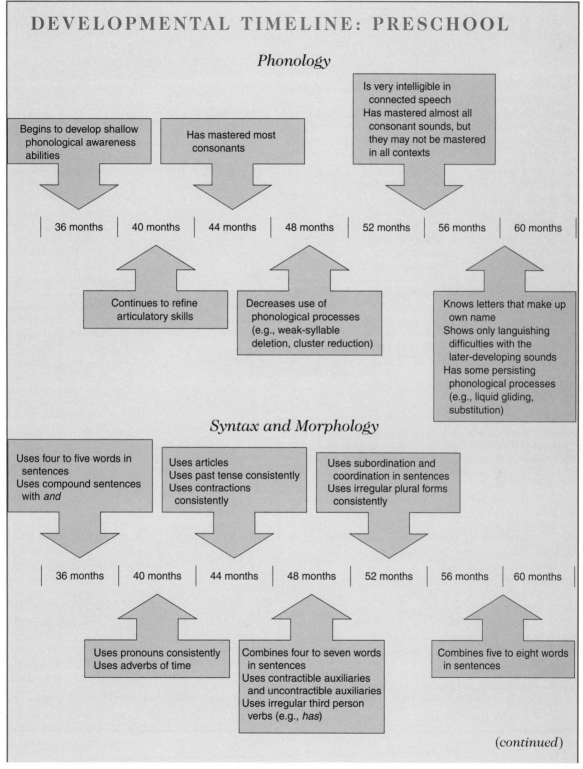

Is very intelligible in connected speech
Has mastered almost all consonant sounds, but they may not be mastered in all contexts

Begins to develop shallow phonological awareness abilities

Has mastered most consonants

| 36 months | 40 months | 44 months | 48 months | 52 months | 56 months | 60 months |

Continues to refine articulatory skills

Decreases use of phonological processes (e.g., weak-syllable deletion, cluster reduction)

Knows letters that make up own name
Shows only languishing difficulties with the later-developing sounds
Has some persisting phonological processes (e.g., liquid gliding, substitution)

Syntax and Morphology

Uses four to five words in sentences
Uses compound sentences with *and*

Uses articles
Uses past tense consistently
Uses contractions consistently

Uses subordination and coordination in sentences
Uses irregular plural forms consistently

| 36 months | 40 months | 44 months | 48 months | 52 months | 56 months | 60 months |

Uses pronouns consistently
Uses adverbs of time

Combines four to seven words in sentences
Uses contractible auxiliaries and uncontractible auxiliaries
Uses irregular third person verbs (e.g., *has*)

Combines five to eight words in sentences

(continued)

DEVELOPMENTAL TIMELINE: PRESCHOOL *(continued)*

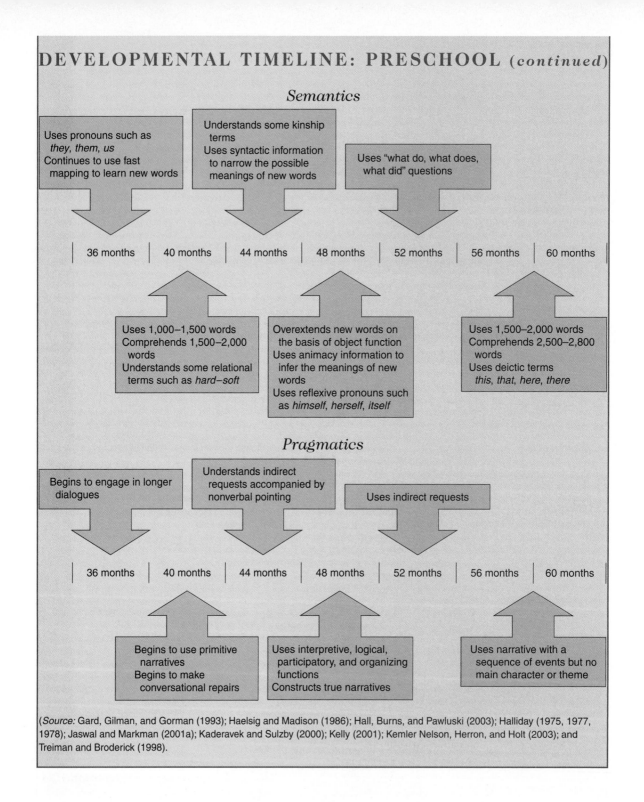

Semantics

Uses pronouns such as *they*, *them*, *us*
Continues to use fast mapping to learn new words

Understands some kinship terms
Uses syntactic information to narrow the possible meanings of new words

Uses "what do, what does, what did" questions

| 36 months | 40 months | 44 months | 48 months | 52 months | 56 months | 60 months |

Uses 1,000–1,500 words
Comprehends 1,500–2,000 words
Understands some relational terms such as *hard–soft*

Overextends new words on the basis of object function
Uses animacy information to infer the meanings of new words
Uses reflexive pronouns such as *himself*, *herself*, *itself*

Uses 1,500–2,000 words
Comprehends 2,500–2,800 words
Uses deictic terms *this*, *that*, *here*, *there*

Pragmatics

Begins to engage in longer dialogues

Understands indirect requests accompanied by nonverbal pointing

Uses indirect requests

| 36 months | 40 months | 44 months | 48 months | 52 months | 56 months | 60 months |

Begins to use primitive narratives
Begins to make conversational repairs

Uses interpretive, logical, participatory, and organizing functions
Constructs true narratives

Uses narrative with a sequence of events but no main character or theme

(*Source:* Gard, Gilman, and Gorman (1993); Haelsig and Madison (1986); Hall, Burns, and Pawluski (2003); Halliday (1975, 1977, 1978); Jaswal and Markman (2001a); Kaderavek and Sulzby (2000); Kelly (2001); Kemler Nelson, Herron, and Holt (2003); and Treiman and Broderick (1998).

Language Content

Even before children enter formal schooling, they acquire skills that ease their transition into the academic realm and the language that accompanies this transition. For example, preschoolers continue to acquire new words at lightning pace—about 860 words per year—averaging about 2 new words per day during this period (Biemiller, 2005). However, the strategies preschoolers use for acquiring new words and the kinds of words they learn are different from those in the infancy and toddler periods. We next discuss how preschoolers use fast mapping to add words to their lexicons, use their knowledge of semantics and syntax to infer the meanings of new words, and learn new words through shared storybook reading. We also describe some specific types of new language content preschoolers acquire, including deictic terms and relational terms.

Fast Mapping

Many researchers view word learning as a gradual process in which word representations progressively develop from immature, incomplete representations to mature, accurate, and precise representations. Recall that children are able to acquire a general representation of a new word with as little as a single exposure through *fast mapping* (Carey, 1978). After fast mapping occurs, children engage in **slow mapping,** during which they gradually refine representations with time and multiple exposures to the word in varying contexts. In fact, children may be refining meanings for as many as 1,600 words at any given time (Carey & Bartlett, 1978).

E. Dale (1965) described vocabulary knowledge development as a four-stage process:

Stage 1	No knowledge of a word	"I never saw it before."
Stage 2	Emergent knowledge	"I've heard of it but don't know what it means."
Stage 3	Contextual knowledge	"I recognize it in context—it has something to do with . . ."
Stage 4	Full knowledge	"I know it."

During the preschool period, children's vocabularies include words at each of these levels. Children may require multiple exposures to words in varying contexts to attain what Carey (1978) called **extended mapping,** or a full and complete understanding of the meaning of a word.

Preschoolers, like toddlers, use the principle of *novel name–nameless category* (N3C) to select nameless objects as the recipients of novel labels and can then fast map novel words through this process. For example, if you were to show a preschooler three novel objects (an apple, a chair, and a ball) and one novel object (a corkscrew) and ask him or her, "Find the dax," the child should be able to eliminate the familiar objects from contention and select the novel object as the "dax." Furthermore, using fast mapping, he or she should have a general understanding of what a dax is and will refine his or her understanding of daxes with time and additional exposures to the word and the object. See Figure 7.2 for an example of a fast-mapping task during which a preschooler selects an unfamiliar object as the referent of a novel label.

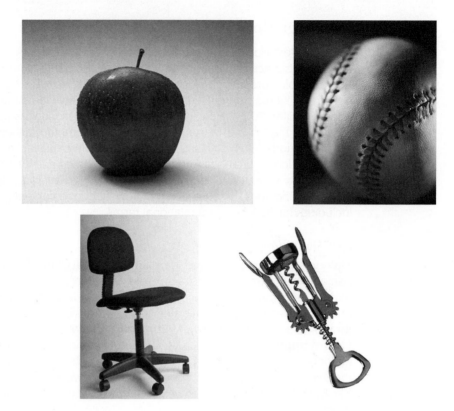

FIGURE 7.2
A fast-mapping task.

ADULT:	Find the *dax.*
PRESCHOOLER:	Right here. (*points to corkscrew, the novel item*)

Knowledge of Semantics and Syntax

In the preschool years, children know many vocabulary words and have a well-developed syntax, so when they learn new words, they rely on their knowledge of semantics and syntax to incorporate (or assimilate) the new words into their vocabulary. As we discuss in Chapter 6, toddlers learning new words may over-generalize as many as one third of word meanings on the basis of categorical, analogical, and relational similarities. The perceptual features of objects weigh heavily in toddlers' overgeneralizations (e.g., calling all round objects "balls"). In the preschool years, children continue to overextend object names on the basis of information they have about other objects, but they weigh the *function* of an object more heavily than its perceptual appearance. For example, if children know the name for a certain tool, they might call other tools that perform similar functions by the same name. In one study, 4-year-old children invented names for new artifacts on the basis of the functions of the objects rather than their perceptual properties. The children used the perceptual features to invent names only when they did not know the functions (Kemler Nelson, Herron, & Holt, 2003).

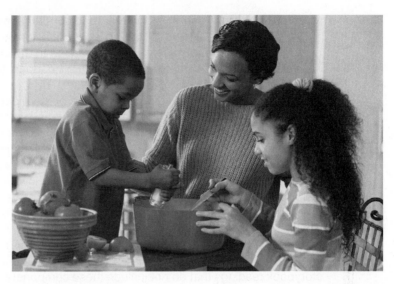

Preschoolers might use the principle of novel name–nameless category *(N3C) to infer that a novel label refers to a novel object.*

(*Photo Source:* © Ariel Skelley/Corbis.)

DISCUSSION POINT

What language development theory (from Chapter 2) could best explain children's ability to use knowledge of the animacy of an object to infer the meaning of a new word?

Preschool-age children also use knowledge about the *animacy* of objects when inferring the meaning of new words. Preschoolers select animate objects as referents for novel proper names and inanimate objects as referents for common nouns (Jaswal & Markman, 2001a). For example, if given the choice of a novel inanimate object and a novel animate object, preschoolers will select the inanimate object when you tell them "Find *the dax*" and will select the animate object when you tell them "Find *Dax.*"

Another way preschoolers infer the meanings of new words is by recruiting syntactic cues that signal the form class (e.g., noun, verb, adjective) of a novel word to narrow the possibilities for the referent of the word. For example, children who hear "This is *a* dax" interpret *dax* to be a *count noun,* whereas children who hear "This *is* Dax" interpret *Dax* to be a *proper name.* Likewise, children who hear "This is a *dax one*" interpret *dax* to be an *adjective* (Hall, Burns, & Pawluski, 2003). Children are also more likely to assume that a novel word is an adjective when it is applied to more than one object (e.g., "This is *round,* and that is *round,* too") because count nouns and proper names rarely take more than a single label (Hall, 1996).

Shared Storybook Reading

In addition to learning words through single and multiple incidental exposures, preschoolers acquire new words as they participate in shared storybook interactions with other people. The language contained within storybook readings is exceptionally rich. In fact, maternal language in storybook-reading activities contains a more diverse array of syntax and vocabulary and typically has a higher level of abstraction than that in other language contexts, including play (Sorsby & Martlew, 1991). DeLoache (1984) considered it a "happy coincidence" that the techniques parents use in storybook-reading situations to attract and maintain children's attention—including talking about familiar things, presenting a limited amount of new information, relating information to the child's experience, and assisting the child to respond correctly—"also happen to be especially effective teaching tools" (p. 94).

Although storybook-reading interactions present opportunities for word learning, individual differences in the frequency of these interactions and the quality of the language children hear as they engage in such interactions can affect children's language development. For example, variations in reading interactions with young children are related to children's receptive and expressive vocabulary abilities (Whitehurst et al., 1988). Research results show that children can learn new words through incidental exposure to words during storybook-reading sessions in which the meanings of target words are not discussed (Robbins & Ehri, 1994). However, storybook readings that include repeated and elaborated exposures to new words as well as an active (or dialogic) reading style on the adult's part improve children's learning of new words from storybooks more so than shared storybook readings that do not include these components (Arnold, Lonigan, Whitehurst, & Epstein, 1994; Lonigan & Whitehurst, 1998; Sénéchal, 1997; Sénéchal, Thomas, & Monker, 1995; Valdez-Menchaca, Marta, & Whitehurst, 1992; Whitehurst et al., 1988, 1994).

Deictic Terms

Now that we have discussed some strategies that preschoolers use to acquire new words, we introduce some of the specific kinds of language content preschoolers acquire. One such set of words is deictic terms. **Deictic terms** are words whose use and interpretation depend on the location of a speaker and listener within a particular setting. Examples of English deictic terms include the words *here* and *this,* which indicate proximity to the speaker, and the words *there* and *that,* which indicate proximity to the listener. To use deictic terms correctly, children must be able to adopt their conversational partner's perspective. Therefore, using deictic terms signals more advanced cognitive and pragmatic processes than those in earlier developmental phases. Children master proximal deictic terms such as *this* and *here* more easily than they master distal deictic terms such as *that* and *there.* Generally children master the contrast between deictic terms by the time they enter school (Clark & Sengul, 1978).

Relational Terms

Relational terms—including interrogatives (questions), temporal terms, opposites, locational prepositions, and kinship terms—are additional achievements in content for preschoolers. Children at this age become able to understand and use relational terms once they can grasp the concepts underlying the terms. For example, to understand and use temporal terms, children must first have a concept of time.

Interrogatives. Preschoolers become increasingly adept at answering and asking questions. These children understand and use question words, such as *what,* *where, who, whose,* and *which,* before they understand and use other interrogatives, such as *when, how,* and *why.* Preschoolers may respond inappropriately to questions they do not understand, as in the following example of a conversation between a teacher and a preschool-age child:

TEACHER: Why did the girl get so many presents?

CHILD: She got a bike, a doll, and coloring books.

Temporal Terms. Temporal terms describe the order of events (*before, after*), the duration of events (*since, until*), and the concurrence of events (*while, during*). Preschoolers understand temporal terms describing order before they understand temporal terms describing concurrent events. When preschoolers do not understand the meaning of temporal terms, they often interpret sentences according to word order (e.g., Weist, 2002). For example, preschoolers might interpret the sentence *Before you eat breakfast, take your vitamin pill* to mean "Eat breakfast, then take your vitamin pill." Preschool-age children might also interpret temporal terms according to their experience, so a child who takes a vitamin *before* breakfast each day might interpret the preceding example correctly.

Opposites. Opposites are another aspect of language content that preschoolers learn to understand and use. Some opposite pairs that preschoolers learn include *hard–soft, big–little, heavy–light, tall–short, long–short,* and *large–small.* Preschoolers learn opposites that they can perceive physically (such as *big–small*) before they learn more abstract opposites (such as *same–different*).

Locational Prepositions. Although children begin to use some locational prepositions as toddlers (e.g., *in, on*), they do not begin to use many other prepositions until preschool age. Locational prepositions, which describe spatial relations, include *under, next to, behind, in back of,* and *in front of* (Grela, Rashiti, & Soares, 2004; Tomasello, 1987). By the end of the preschool period, most children have a solid understanding of these terms.

Kinship Terms. Children initially interpret kinship terms such as *mommy, daddy, sister,* and *brother* to refer to specific individuals. Preschoolers eventually fathom the general meaning of these and other kinship terms, including *son, daughter, grandfather, grandmother,* and *parent.* The relative complexity of each kinship term has the most impact on the order in which children learn them, followed by children's familiarity with the family member to which each kinship term refers (Haviland & Clark, 1974). Thus, children learn the words *mother* and *father* before they learn the words *aunt* and *uncle* because the concepts of mother and father are simpler. Children who see their aunts and uncles regularly should also learn these kinship terms before children who are not familiar with their aunts and uncles. Interestingly, preschoolers have difficulty with the reciprocity of some kinship terms (Deák & Maratsos, 1998; Edwards, 1984). For example, children understand when they *have* a brother or a sister, but they have more difficulty understanding that they can *be* a brother or sister to someone else.

Language Form

During the preschool years, children refine their morphology, syntax, and phonology in significant ways. Preschoolers make noteworthy advances in grammatical and derivational morphology, sentence forms, and speech production abilities.

Grammatical and Derivational Morphology

We introduced grammatical morphemes in Chapter 1; they are the units of meaning added to a word to provide additional grammatical precision, such as the plural morpheme (*bird–birds*) and the verb inflection for present progressive actions (*fly–is flying*). *Derivational* morphology is similar to grammatical morphology in that it modifies the structure of words. However, derivational morphemes are the prefixes and suffixes added to a word to change its meaning and sometimes its part of speech. For instance, the suffix -*er* can be added to *write* to change its meaning and its part of speech from a verb to a noun (*writer*). The prefix *re-* can be added to *write* to change its meaning (*rewrite*). Additional common derivational morphemes include *pre-* (*preschool*), -*est* (*smallest*), -*ness* (*sweetness*), and -*ly* (*slowly*). As children learn new morphemes, they can manipulate word structure to become more precise and specific in their communication. Children can increase their possibilities for communicating exponentially once they master a few important morphemes. For example, a child who knows the word *read* can use the variations *reading, reread, reader,* and so forth.

As we discussed in Chapter 6, children acquire grammatical and derivational morphemes in about the same order, even among different languages. Six factors influence the order in which children acquire these types of morphemes (O'Grady, Dobrovolsky, & Arnoff, 1997):

1. *Frequent occurrence in utterance-final position:* Infants and children are most sensitive to sounds and words at the ends of utterances. Children first learn morphemes occuring as suffices.

2. *Syllabicity:* Children first learn morphemes that constitute their own syllables (e.g., present progressive -*ing*) and later learn morphemes that contain only a single sound (e.g., third person singular -*s*).

3. *Single relation between morpheme and meaning:* Children first learn morphemes with only one meaning (e.g., the morpheme *the* functions only as a definite article) before they learn morphemes that express multiple meanings (e.g., -*s* denotes present tense, third person, and singular number).

4. *Consistency in use:* Children learn the names of morphemes that are used consistently (e.g., possessive nouns always end in '*s*) more easily than morphemes that vary in their use (e.g., past tense verbs sometimes end in -*ed* but other times take an irregular form).

5. *Allomorphic variation:* Children learn morphemes that have a consistent pronunciation (e.g., -*ing*) before they learn morphemes that have allomorphic variation (e.g., the plural morpheme has three variations: /s/, /z/, and /ɪz/).

6. *Clear semantic function:* Children first learn morphemes that have a clear meaning (e.g., plural morpheme) before they learn morphemes with less clear meaning (e.g., third person singular morpheme).

The most signifant area of morpheme development in the preschool period is *verb morphology*. One way English speakers inflect verbs is with tense (e.g., past, present, future) to provide information about time. Often, the verb *to be* is an important marker of time. When the verb *to be* or any of its derivatives (*am, is, are, was, were*) is the main verb in a sentence—as in *I am Doug*—it is called a *copula*. When the verb *to be* or one of its derivatives is a helping verb in a sentence—as in *I am hugging Doug*—it is called an *auxiliary*. The *to be* copula and auxiliary forms can be made into contractions (*Doug's funny; I'm bouncing the ball*) or left in their uncontracted forms (*Doug is funny; I am bouncing the ball*). Preschoolers master the verb *to be* in its copula and auxiliary forms, representing a major syntactic achievement of these years.

Sentence Forms

In addition to these major morphological achievements, preschoolers make significant advances in using complex sentences. Preschoolers move from simple declarative subject–verb–object constructions ("Daddy drives a truck") and subject–verb–complement constructions ("Truck is big") to more elaborate sentence patterns, such as the following three (Justice & Ezell, 2002a):

1. *Subject–verb–object–adverb:* "Daddy's hitting the hammer outside."
2. *Subject–verb–complement–adverb:* "Daddy is hungry now."
3. *Subject–auxiliary–verb–adverb:* "Daddy is eating now."

CD VIDEO CLIP
To watch a 4-year-old boy use a series of complex and compound sentences, see the CD video clip *Language 6*.

Children also begin to embed multiple phrases and clauses into their utterances to create complex and compound sentences and to use coordinating conjunctions (e.g., *and, or, but*) and subordinating conjunctions (e.g., *then, when, because*) to connect clauses. By the end of the preschool period, children produce compound sentences, such as *I told Daddy and Daddy told Mommy,* as well as complex sentences with embedded clauses, such as *I told Daddy who told Mommy* (Justice & Ezell, 2002a).

Achievements in Speech Production

During the preschool years, children continue to refine their speech sound repertoires. By the end of the preschool period, most children have mastered nearly all the phonemes of their native language. Four- and 5-year-old children generally show only languishing difficulties with a few of the later-developing phonemes, including /r/ (*row*), /l/ (*low*), /s/ (*sew*), /tʃ/ (*cheese*), /ʃ/ (*show*), /z/ (*zoo*), /θ/ (*think*), and /ð/ (*though*). Children may also exhibit persistent difficulties with some of the earlier-acquired phonemes when they appear in complex multisyllabic words (e.g., /s/ in *spaghetti*) or in words with consonant clusters (such as the first three sounds in *split*). Despite a few ongoing challenges, preschoolers are highly intelligible and have an adultlike expressive phonemic repertoire.

The *phonological processes* (or systematic errors children make in their speech) continue to diminish during the preschool years as children's phonological systems stabilize; in the age 3–4 period, children have the fastest suppression rate (Haelsig & Madison, 1986). Four-year-olds may still exhibit weak-syllable deletion and cluster reduction, but these processes usually disappear by age 5 years. Two patterns that may persist past the fifth birthday are as follows:

Pattern	Description	Examples
1. **Liquid gliding**	When a liquid consonant (/r/ or /l/) is replaced by a glide consonant (/w/ or /j/—the first sound in *yellow*)	*rabbit* = "wabbit" *land* = "yand"
2. **Stopping**	When a fricative (such as /θ/—the "th" sound in *think*—or /ð/—the "th" sound in *though*) or an affricate (such as the first sound in *jeep*) is replaced by a stop consonant (such as /t/ or /d/)	*think* = "tink" or "dink" *though* = "dough" or "tow" *jeep* = "deep"

See Figure 7.3 for a list of phonological processes that persist into the preschool period.

Receptive phonology also continues to develop during the preschool years, which becomes important to children's early reading development. As discussed previously, reading requires a child to have robust phonological representations to make sense of the **alphabetic principle,** or the relationship between letters or combinations of letters (graphemes) and sounds (phonemes). Environmental and biological factors can affect children's development of adequate phonological representations. For instance, children who receive little linguistic stimulation and those who have ongoing middle ear infections are at risk for having delays in the development of phonological representations (Nittrouer, 1996).

Language Use

Use describes the ways in which language is used to meet personal and social needs. Preschool-age children implement many new discourse functions, improve their conversational skills, and begin to use narratives.

Discourse Functions

Recall from Chapter 6 that toddlers who are combining words can use language to satisfy six communicative functions: instrumental, regulatory, personal-interactional, heuristic, imaginative, and informative. Preschoolers begin to use language for even more complex discourse functions, including interpretive, logical, participatory, and organizing functions (Halliday, 1975, 1977, 1978). *Interpretive functions* make clear the whole of a person's experience. *Logical functions* express logical relations between ideas. *Participatory functions* express wishes, feelings, attitudes, and judgments, and *organizing functions* manage discourse.

Besides expressing additional pragmatic functions, preschool children continue to detect and use the pragmatic information other people convey. Such information

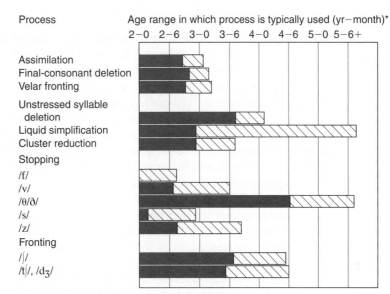

Process   Age range in which process is typically used (yr−month)*

*Solid bar represents use by average children; striped bar represents use by some normal children.

FIGURE 7.3
Phonological processes that persist into the preschool period.

Source: Reprinted from *Language Disorders from Infancy Through Adolescence* (2nd ed.), R. Paul, p. 310. Copyright 2001, with permission from Elsevier.

helps preschoolers better understand messages. For example, research results show that children understand an indirect request better when the speaker uses nonverbal pointing in addition to the request. Preschoolers who watched researchers point to an open door (nonverbal cue) while saying "It's going to get loud in here" (indirect request) were more likely to close the door than were preschoolers who heard only the indirect request to close the door (Kelly, 2001). This example demonstrates the importance of pragmatic information to language comprehension, even for preschoolers who can already use an array of pragmatic functions when communicating with other people.

Conversational Skills

CD VIDEO CLIP
To watch a 5-year-old girl repair a conversation by providing feedback to an adult, see the CD video clip *Language 7.*

Preschoolers begin to improve their conversational skills as they learn how to take turns in a conversation. Most preschoolers can maintain a conversation for two or more turns, particularly when they select the topic for discussion. Although they still have some difficulty realizing when communication breakdowns occur and giving listeners the appropriate amount of feedback to facilitate understanding, preschoolers are becoming increasingly sophisticated conversationalists. They understand that they should respond to questions and discover that speaking at the same time as another person results in ineffective communication.

Narrative Skills

A **narrative** is a child's spoken or written description of a real or a fictional event from the past, the present, or the future. W. Labov (1972) defined a narrative to minimally contain two sequential independent clauses about the same past event. "Hey, Mom, guess what we did in gym today" is one way a preschooler might begin a narrative, followed by "We got to play with a big parachute."

Preschool children's narratives serve as a showcase for multiple language achievements, including those in syntax, morphology, semantics, phonology, and pragmatics. Children must use syntax to arrange words and ideas, verb morphology to signal the time of events, vocabulary to represent events and persons precisely, phonology to pronounce words clearly and with proper intonation, and pragmatics to share an appropriate amount of information with the listener. Narratives use decontextualized language to describe people or characters not immediately present and events removed from the current context. Narratives differ from conversations because conversations are carried on by two or more persons, whereas narratives are largely uninterrupted streams of language. Children who produce narratives must take responsibility for the effectiveness of the communication.

To produce a narrative, the child introduces a topic and organizes the information pertaining to the topic in such a way that the listener can assume a relatively passive role, providing only minimal support to the speaker. Two important types of narratives are the **personal narrative,** in which an individual shares a factual event, and the **fictional narrative,** in which an individual shares an imaginary event. Both types of narratives generally thread a sequence of events together in a causal or temporal manner. A *causal* sequence unfolds following a cause-and-effect chain of events or provides a reason or rationale for some series of events (e.g., "Kathy locked her keys inside her house, so she had to call a neighbor"). A *temporal* sequence unfolds with time (e.g., "First we rode our bikes around the lake. Next we fed the ducks").

Although narrative skills begin to develop as early as age 2 years, most children cannot construct true narratives with a problem and resolution (or high point) until around age 4 years (Kaderavek & Sulzby, 2000; Peterson, 1990). Children who have not yet mastered narrative discourse might try to describe an event for a listener without providing a clear introduction, middle, or end to their story. Children's early narratives may include only a minimal description of the participants, time, and location relevant to the event, and may contain only a series of events, as in the following example:

CHILD: Cody brought a rabbit and left it on the porch. Then Mom said he should go hunting with Dad.

ADULT: Just one second. Who is Cody?

CHILD: My dog.

ADULT: Where did this happen?

CHILD: At home.

ADULT: So, your dad likes to hunt and he thinks Cody could help him to catch some rabbits because he brought a rabbit home?

CHILD: Yep.

THEORY TO PRACTICE

Effects of Telephone Conversations on Preschoolers' Narrative Skills

During telephone conversations, many of the cues that support face-to-face conversation (e.g., facial expressions, gestures) are absent and conversation that is more precise must be used to convey meaning. In one study, researchers suggested that talking on the telephone can boost children's narrative skills (Hutchison, 2001). Elementary school–age children who were part of a 6-week language intervention that incorporated telephone conversations included more utterances, words, and different words in their narratives than those of children who did not participate in the telephone intervention. Furthermore, children who participated in the telephone intervention included more advanced narrative characteristics in their stories, such as more explicit descriptions, more clauses and phrases to identify objects and locations, and more extensive elaboration of characters' emotional states.

DISCUSSION POINT
Why do you think the telephone intervention described above helped develop children's narrative skills?

Preschoolers' narratives become clearer as their ability to consider the listener's perspective emerges. Children's repertoire of linguistic devices, including adverbial time phrases (e.g., *yesterday, this morning*) and verb morphology (signaling the time of activities), grows during the preschool period, which helps increase the comprehensibility of their narratives. See Theory to Practice: *Effects of Telephone Conversations on Preschooler's Narative Skills* to read about another way in which preschoolers might hone their narrative skills in an everyday activity.

Because narratives are a complex, multidimensional language activity, narrative skills are a good predictor of later school outcomes for preschoolers exhibiting difficulties in developing language skills (Paul & Smith, 1993). The decontextualized language inherent in narratives likely plays a crucial role in the acquisition of early literacy skills and in subsequent school achievement (Peterson, Jesso, & McCabe, 1999).

WHAT FACTORS INFLUENCE PRESCHOOLERS' INDIVIDUAL ACHIEVEMENTS IN LANGUAGE?

As is true of infancy and toddlerhood, in the preschool period language development varies both individually and among any given group of children. Because language comprises different domains (syntax, semantics, morphology, phonology, and pragmatics) that children learn to comprehend and produce, language development is not an all-or-nothing phenomenon. Instead, a child will acquire competence in different domains at slightly different times and will be strong in some areas and weak in others. In addition, among a group of preschoolers, patterns of language and literacy will vary, and influences such as familial socioeconomic status and gender will continue to exert effects on language development.

Intraindividual Differences

Variation in Receptive and Expressive Language

Just as an *individual* infant or toddler understands more language than he or she produces, so do individual preschoolers. This disparity between receptive and expressive language continues into the preschool period and beyond.

Variation in Language Profiles

The individual preschooler usually grows more rapidly in some areas and more slowly in other areas. As such, a preschooler will exhibit one of many *language profiles* (Fey, 1986; J. Miller, 1981)—simultaneous patterns of language in multiple domains. A language profile encompasses only the language domains (phonology, syntax, semantics, or pragmatics) and not competencies (such as narrative discourse). Within his or her language profile, the individual child will have strengths and weaknesses in different areas. For instance, in Figure 7.4, Child B exhibits good language comprehension skills but relatively poor language production skills.

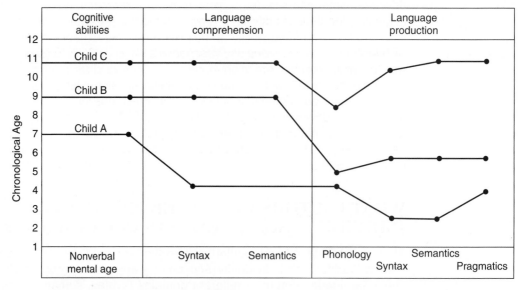

FIGURE 7.4
Three language profiles.

Source: From *Assessing Language Production in Children: Experimental Procedures* (p. 169), by J. Miller, 1981, Baltimore: University Park Press. Copyright 1981 by University Park Press. Adapted with permission.

Variation in Early Literacy Profiles

An individual preschooler may also differ in terms of his or her early literacy abilities. *Literacy profiles* are simultaneous patterns of literacy, including competencies such as narrative discourse and metasemantics. Knowing what a preschooler's strengths and weaknesses are with regard to his or her early literacy abilities can help educators tailor early literacy instruction to the child's individual needs.

Interindividual Differences

If you observe a *group* of preschoolers, they will also exhibit a variety of language and early literacy profiles. Likewise, they will differ in language achievements as a result of their families' socioeconomic status and of gender.

Variation in Language Profiles

When a group of preschoolers are compared, they will exhibit a variety of language profiles. For example, in Figure 7.4, Child A exhibits poor language comprehension and language production abilities relative to those of his or her peers of the same chronological age, whereas Child C's performance matches that of his or her on-target peers in all areas except phonology.

Variation in Early Literacy Profiles

Groups of preschoolers also differ in terms of their early literacy abilities. Such differences can also be illustrated in terms of profiles. In one study, children were classified into one of four literacy-ability clusters (low average—LA, high average—HA, high narrative—HN, low overall—LO) according to their abilities in five domains (semantics, syntax, phonemic awareness, metasemantics, and narrative discourse); see Figure 7.5 (Speece, Roth, Cooper, & De La Paz, 1999). These clusters are similar to language profiles in that they illustrate how a group of same-age children can exhibit varying performance levels across early literacy domains.

Effects of Socioeconomic Status

As in toddlerhood, familial socioeconomic status (SES) continues to exert an influence on children's language development in the preschool years. Differences may become even more prominent in the preschool years because not all children attend preschool programs, and those who do are subject to varying levels of program quality. Because the United States does not have universal prekindergarten, parents who can afford to send their children to quality preschool programs often do, and parents who cannot afford preschool may take advantage of nationally funded programs such as Head Start. Fortunately, research results suggest that the quality of teacher–child interactions in the classroom and the quality of teacher language can positively affect children's language growth in preschool and that teachers can be trained to incorporate high-quality language interactions (e.g., Girolametto & Weitzman, 2002; J. Huttenlocher, Vasilyeva, Cymerman, & Levine, 2002).

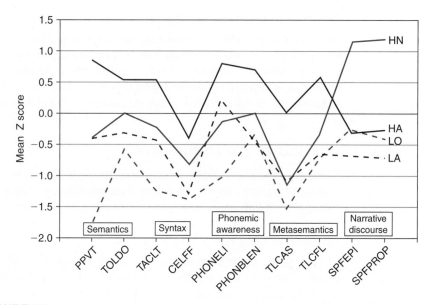

FIGURE 7.5

Four literacy profiles.

CELFF = Clinical Evaluation of Language Fundamentals: Formulated Sentences; HA = high average; HN = high narrative; LA = low average; LO = low overall; PHONBLEN = Phonemic Awareness: Blending; PHONELI = Phonemic Awareness: Elision; PPVT = Peabody Picture Vocabulary Test—Revised; SPFEPI = Story Production: Episodes; SPFPROP = Story Production: Propositions; TACLT = Test of Auditory Comprehension of Language—Revised; TLCAS = Test of Language Competence—Expanded: Ambiguous Sentences; TLCFL = Test of Language Competence—Expanded: Figurative Language; TOLDO = Test of Language Development—Primary:2: Oral Vocabulary.

Source: From "The Relevance of Oral Language Skills to Early Literacy: A Multivariate Analysis," by D. L. Speece, F. P. Roth, D. H. Cooper, and S. De La Paz, 1999, *Applied Psycholinguistics, 20,* p. 181. © 1999 Cambridge University Press. Reprinted with the permission of Cambridge University Press.

DISCUSSION POINT

How might a researcher study the quality of teachers' language use within the preschool classroom?

Children from low SES backgrounds might also benefit from attending classrooms in which children have mixed SES backgrounds. For example, Bagby, Rudd, and Woods (2005) suggested that children in heterogeneous classrooms (low SES and high SES) experience more language interactions, fewer negative interactions, and fewer physical interactions than do children in homogeneous classrooms (low SES only). This study thus provides some preliminary evidence on the positive effects of mixed-SES grouping on children's language, cognitive, and socioemotional development.

Effects of Gender

Recall from Chapter 6 that boys and girls differ in terms of their language development in toddlerhood. The results of longitudinal studies confirm that differences between girls and boys remain stable through the preschool years. Bornstein,

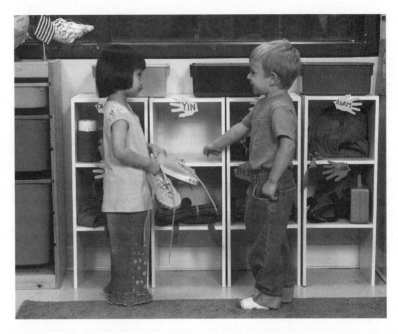

Boys and girls tend to differ from one another in their language development throughout the preschool-age years.

(*Photo Source:* Pearson Learning Photo Studio.)

DISCUSSION POINT

In what ways does the influence of gender on language development support both positions in the nature–nurture debate?

Hahn, and Haynes (2004) hypothesized that several issues account for gender differences in language development, including maturation rates, neurological development, interests, opportunities to learn because of gender role stereotypes, and boys' and girls' role models for their language (i.e., girls usually model their language on that of their mothers, who are typically more verbal than are fathers).

HOW DO RESEARCHERS AND CLINICIANS MEASURE LANGUAGE DEVELOPMENT IN THE PRESCHOOL PERIOD?

Researchers

Language Sample Analysis

One method researchers continue to use throughout the preschool years to study children's language achievements is language sample analysis. Although the general premise is the same as in toddlerhood, researchers investigating preschoolers' language development have a wider range of analysis tools at their disposal, and, more important, a larger amount of language to analyze. Researchers who measure preschoolers' language development can analyze children's language

RESEARCH PARADIGMS

Developmental Sentence Scoring

Developmental sentence scoring (DSS) is a tool that researchers can apply to language samples to quantify children's expressive syntax development (Lee, 1974). DSS involves examining structures from eight grammatical categories and assigning points to each category, on a scale from 1 point for the simplest developmental form to 8 points for the most complex developmental form. DSS is used to assess the following categories: indefinite pronouns, personal pronouns, main verbs, secondary verbs, negatives, conjunctions, interrogative reversals, and *wh-* questions. A sentence may also receive an additional point if it is syntactically and semantically adultlike. For example, if a child said, "He ate the cookie," the child would be awarded 1 point for personal pronoun use (*he*), 1 point for primary verb use (*ate*), and 1 point for a syntactically and semantically adultlike sentence. The researcher then calculates the average number of points for each utterance to derive the developmental sentence score. Norm references are available for DSS, so some researchers may want to compare children's scores before and after a particular language intervention.

form, content, and use in many ways. Some common measures of semantics include total number of words (TNW), number of different words (NDW), and type–token ratio (TTR, or NDW/TNW). Popular measures of syntax include mean length of utterance (MLU) and developmental sentence scoring (see Research Paradigms: *Developmental Sentence Scoring*). Researchers can also assess preschoolers' pragmatic abilities by coding language samples for the communicative functions the child uses—such as requesting, commenting, responding to questions—and by coding for communication acts—such as repair strategies, interruptions, and false starts. See Table 7.2 for examples of measures applied to spontaneous language samples.

When collecting a language sample from a child, researchers must follow some general rules of thumb to obtain the most representative sample possible. Language samples should be representative in terms of both their reliability and their validity. *Reliable* language samples are similar across multiple recording contexts for the same child. *Valid* language samples accurately represent the quantity and quality of language a child can produce.

J. Miller and Chapman (2000) recommended that the researcher or examiner who is collecting a language sample should try to establish rapport with the child as soon as the session begins by introducing himself or herself and describing his or her job. J. Miller and Chapman also recommended introducing the recording equipment to the child and explaining what will be discussed during the recording session (e.g., "We're going to talk about your family and the kinds of things that you like to do"). Once the researcher establishes rapport with the child, introduces the recording equipment, and describes the purpose of the session to the child, the researcher should begin obtaining the language sample,

TABLE 7.2

Measures Applied to Spontaneous Language Samples

Measure	General goal	Specific goal	Calculation
Mean length of utterance (MLU) in morphemes	To measure syntactic complexity	To determine the average length in morphemes in utterances	Total no. of morphemes/Total no. of utterances
Percentage of complex sentences	To measure syntactic complexity in later stages of syntactic development	To determine the percentage of sentences in a sample containing more than one clause	No. of complex sentences/No. of complete sentences
Total number of words (TNW)	To measure lexical productivity	To determine the total number of words used in a sample	Raw frequency of no. of main-body words
Number of different words (NDW)	To measure lexical diversity	To determine the number of different words used in a sample	Raw frequency of different main-body word roots
Type–token ratio (TTR)	To measure lexical diversity	To determine the ratio of different words used to total words used in a sample	NDW/TNW
Conjunction use	To measure syntactic complexity and the ability to organize discourse	To determine the number of coordinating conjunctions (e.g., *and, or, but, so*) and subordinating conjunctions (e.g., *because, still, although*) in a sample	Raw frequency of conjunctions used in a sample *or* Percentage of utterances containing conjunctions
Percentage of responses to questions	To measure discourse abilities	To determine the percentage of questions responded to in a sample	No. of questions responded to immediately following the question/No. of questions asked by another speaker
Percentage of intelligible utterances	To measure intelligibility (i.e., phonological abilities)	To determine the percentage of complete utterances that are intelligible	No. of complete and intelligible utterances/No. of complete utterances
Number of mazes (language disruptions)	To measure fluency	To determine the extent to which a speaker uses false starts, filled pauses (e.g., *um, uh*), repetitions, and reformulations	Raw frequency of mazes in a sample *or* Percentage of utterances containing mazes

Researchers and clinicians can use props, such as photo albums, to elicit language samples from preschoolers.

(*Photo Source:* © Laura Dwight/PhotoEdit Inc.)

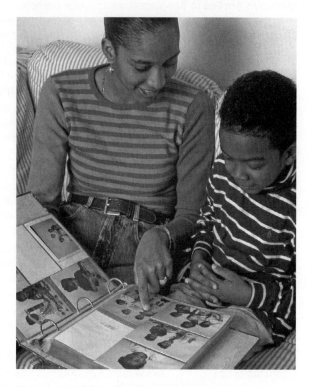

using the following three strategies to establish shared interests with the child (J. Miller & Chapman, 2000):

1. For children who are particularly reticent or who appear to be self-conscious about their speech, try not to say anything beyond the initial greetings for the first 5 minutes.

2. Engage in parallel play by directing talk toward the toys rather than toward the child (e.g., "These Play-Doh cookies look delicious!").

3. Engage in interactive play, but ensure that the activity does not preclude talking. Encourage discussion once the activity is under way.

Once the interaction begins, the following six strategies can be used to maintain a productive interaction (J. Miller & Chapman, 2000):

1. Be enthusiastic by using eye contact, by using vocal inflection, and by smiling.

2. Be patient by allowing the child plenty of time to initiate conversation and to respond to your questions and directions.

3. Listen and follow the child's lead by encouraging the child to elaborate on his or her ideas, by adding new information when appropriate, and by maintaining the child's pace.

4. Demonstrate that you value the child's communication efforts by giving the child your undivided attention, maintaining eye contact, and nodding to indicate agreement and interest.

5. Treat the conversation as if it were a genuine adult conversation by refraining from asking questions with obvious answers.

6. Keep the child's perspective in mind and adapt your language to the child's needs—for example, by shortening the length of utterances, simplifying vocabulary, and reducing sentence complexity.

Grammaticality Judgment Tasks

Researchers can use grammaticality judgment tasks to investigate various kinds of syntactic development in the preschool period. Grammaticality judgment tasks are metalinguistic in the sense that they require children to think about language and make judgments about the appropriateness of specific forms or interpret sentences. Two types of grammaticality judgment tasks are used: well-formedness judgments and judgments about interpretation (McDaniel & Smith Cairns, 1998). To make a *well-formedness judgment,* the child must decide whether a sentence is syntactically acceptable. For example, Sentence A, which follows, would be syntactically acceptable, but Sentence B would not:

A.   "What is your favorite movie?"
B.   "What your favorite movie is?"

In the case of Sentences A and B, the researcher would ask the child whether each sentence is appropriate by asking "Does this sentence sound good or bad?"

Judgments about interpretation are different. To make a judgment about interpretation, the child must interpret one or more parts of a sentence—for example, he or she might have to determine reference. In Sentence A, which follows, the child would need to indicate that *herself* refers to the baby, and in Sentence B, that *her* refers to someone other than the mother (the baby in this case):

A.   "The baby is feeding *herself.*"
B.   "The mother is feeding *her.*"

The researcher could introduce props or pictures to facilitate this interpretation task. In Sentence A, the researcher could say "We have a baby and a mother here and the baby is eating. Would it be ok to say the baby is feeding *herself*?" In this case, a child who understands that the referent is the baby would say "Yes." In Sentence B, the researcher might say "Ok, now the mother is eating. Would it be ok to say the mother is feeding *her*?" In this case, a child who understands that the mother is the referent would say "No."

Because preschoolers may not be accustomed to metalinguistic tasks such as the grammaticality judgment task, the researcher must introduce the task and be certain the child understands it and has had sufficient practice with it before the researcher proceeds (McDaniel & Smith Cairns, 1998). For example, the researcher should tell the child that they will be thinking about language together and explain that the child's job is to listen for things that "sound funny." After providing examples, the researcher should introduce some practice items about which a preschooler can reasonably be expected to make grammaticality judgments (e.g., number: "That boy *are* running"). Only after the researcher establishes that the child understands the task, by attending to language form rather than language content, should the researcher proceed to the target items.

Clinicians

Preschoolers, who better understand and produce language than their toddler and infant counterparts do, can participate in considerably more assessments to directly measure many oral language components. Standardized and normed assessments, as well as screenings that educators can use to tailor instruction, are popular ways to measure children's abilities and progress in many areas. Clinicians can use standardized assessments in educational settings to screen children for potential delays in language as they enter preschool, for example. Clinicians can also use standardized assessments to gain a deeper understanding of children's language abilities and possibly make a formal diagnosis of a speech or language problem if they suspect that a child may be lagging behind his or her peers in particular areas.

DISCUSSION POINT

In the previous section, we described some strategies for obtaining a representative language sample. What are some repercussions of *not* using these strategies? How might a language sample be affected?

Standardized assessments and screenings are also becoming an important tool in the preschool classroom. Teachers and early childhood educators can use such tools to evaluate their students' skills upon entry into preschool, monitor these students' progress, and tailor instruction to meet the language and early literacy needs of these children. Next, we provide descriptions of several language and literacy assessments that clinicians (and sometimes early childhood educators) may use to measure English-speaking preschoolers' language and early literacy achievements. We end with a brief discussion of assessment of children who are bilingual.

Formal Assessment of English-Speaking Children

Preschool Language Scale—Fourth Edition. The Preschool Language Scale—Fourth Edition (PLS–4; Zimmerman, Steiner, & Pond, 2002) is a norm-referenced measure of vocabulary, grammar, morphology, and language reasoning that contains two scales. The Auditory Comprehension scale measures children's language comprehension abilities, including receptive vocabulary, comprehension of concepts and grammatical markers, and the ability to make comparisons and inferences. The Expressive Communication scale measures children's language production abilities, including using expressive vocabulary, using grammatical markers, segmenting words, completing analogies, and telling a story in sequence.

Test of Language Development—Primary, Third Edition. The Test of Language Development—Primary, Third Edition (TOLD–P:3; Hammill & Newcomer, 1997) contains nine subtests that measure different oral language components. Picture Vocabulary, Relational Vocabulary, and Oral Vocabulary assess children's comprehension and meaningful use of spoken words. Grammatic Understanding, Sentence Imitation, and Grammatic Completion assess differing aspects of children's grammar. Word Articulation, Phonemic Analysis, and Word Discrimination are supplemental subtests that measure children's abilities to pronounce words correctly and to distinguish between words that sound similar.

Peabody Picture Vocabulary Test—Third Edition. The Peabody Picture Vocabulary Test—Third Edition (PPVT–III; Dunn & Dunn, 1997) is a norm-referenced measure of receptive vocabulary. The examiner presents sets of four pictures on a page and then asks the child to point to one of the pictures. The PPVT–3 is a popular tool because it provides normative references of receptive vocabulary for children and adults of all ages. Although delays in receptive vocabulary can signal a language difficulty or impairment, receptive vocabulary is only one component of language, so clinicians generally use the PPVT–3 along with other measures of language ability to assess children's language competencies.

The most current revision of the PPVT is the PPVT–4. Additions to the fourth edition include color pictures, updated illustrations, a larger easel, more vocabulary items (228 items), and wireless technology.

Clinical Evaluation of Language Fundamentals—Preschool, Second Edition. The Clinical Evaluation of Language Fundamentals—Preschool, Second Edition (CELF–Preschool–2; Semel, Wiig, & Secord, 2004) is a norm-referenced assessment of language abilities for children from ages 3 to 6 years. The CELF–Preschool–2 contains eight subtests: Sentence Structure, Word Structure, Expressive Vocabulary, Concepts & Following Directions, Recalling Sentences, Basic Concepts, Word Classes—Receptive, and Word Classes—Total. Three subtests (Sentence Structure, Word Structure, Expressive Vocabulary) form a *core language score* that clinicians can use to obtain a snapshot of children's key language abilities.

Phonological Awareness Literacy Screening—PreK. The Phonological Awareness Literacy Screening—PreK (PALS–PreK; Invernizzi, Sullivan, Meier, & Swank, 2004) is a screening instrument that early childhood educators can use to identify children's strengths and weaknesses in early literacy to plan instruction for the school year. The PALS–PreK measures children's knowledge of phonological awareness and print knowledge in six subtests: Name Writing, Alphabet Recognition and Letter Sounds, Beginning Sound Awareness, Print and Word Awareness, Rhyme Awareness, and Knowledge of Nursery Rhymes.

Test of Early Reading Ability—Third Edition. The Test of Early Reading Ability—Third Edition (TERA–3; Reid, Hresko, & Hammill, 2002) is a norm-referenced measure of children's mastery of early developing reading skills. Three subtests include Alphabet Knowledge (measures children's knowledge of the alphabet and its uses), Conventions (measures knowledge of print conventions), and Meaning (measures children's ability to construct meaning from print). The three subtests combine to form an overall reading quotient.

DISCUSSION POINT
What types of information about a child's language might be gathered from an interview that could not be obtained from standardized assessments or language samples?

Formal Assessment of Bilingual Children

Assessing the language and early literacy skills of children who are bilingual presents a unique challenge, and, in most cases, norm-referenced measures developed for English-speaking children may fail to paint an accurate picture of these children's competencies. See Multicultural Focus: *Informal Interviews with Caregivers and Teachers* for an alternative to formal assessment for these children.

MULTICULTURAL FOCUS

Informal Interviews with Caregivers and Teachers

An alternative way to assess children's language abilities is to use structured interviews with parents, caregivers, or teachers (Gutiérrez-Clellen, Restrepo, Bedore, Peña, & Anderson, 2000). These persons, who know children well, can provide valuable information on children's English proficiency. The person conducting the interview should inquire about the length of time the child has been speaking his or her native language, the length of time the child has been speaking English, the context in which the child acquired English, and the relative proficiency of both languages across situations. Parent interviews are also useful for determining whether language performance is related to patterns of language loss by comparing the child's language development and loss to that of siblings or other family members. The interviewer can then explain the child's performance in each language in terms of the child's prior learning experience and language history.

SUMMARY

This chapter begins with a discussion of the major language milestones preschoolers achieve, including the use of decontextualized language and important emergent literacy skills such as alphabet knowledge, print knowledge, and phonological awareness. In the next section of this chapter, we discuss preschoolers' achievements in language content, form, and use. Preschoolers' achievements in language content include fast mapping and slow mapping as a means of acquiring new words, using knowledge of semantics and syntax to acquire new words, learning new words through shared storybook reading, and acquiring new and more complex language content, including deictic terms and relational terms.

Preschoolers' achievements in language form include grammatical and derivational morphology and new sentence forms. Preschoolers also add to their speech sound repertoires and begin to demonstrate suppression of several phonological processes that began in toddlerhood. Preschoolers' achievements in language use include new discourse functions, improved conversational skills, and narrative skills.

We then describe some of the intraindividual and interindividual differences in preschoolers' language development, including different types of language and early literacy profiles and the effects of SES and gender on language development. Finally, we describe some of the ways in which researchers and clinicians measure preschoolers' language development. Some methods that researchers use include language sample analysis and grammaticality judgment tasks. Clinicians use standardized language assessments and language screenings.

KEY TERMS

alphabetic principle, p. 236
alphabet knowledge, p. 223
contextualized language, p. 222
decontextualized language, p. 222
deictic terms, p. 232
emergent literacy, p. 222
extended mapping, p. 229
fictional narrative, p. 238

liquid gliding, p. 236
metalinguistic ability, p. 222
narrative, p. 238
oral language, p. 222
personal narrative, p. 238
print awareness, p. 223
slow mapping, p. 229
stopping, p. 236

For online resources related to chapter content, including audio samples, valuable Web sites, suggested readings, and self-quizzes, please go to the Companion Website at http://www.prenhall.com/pence

8

School-Age Years and Beyond

Developing Later Language

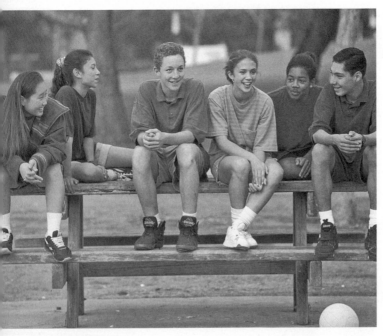

FOCUS QUESTIONS

In this chapter, we answer the following four questions:

1. What major language development milestones occur in the school-age years and beyond?

2. What major achievements in language content, form, and use characterize the school-age years and beyond?

3. What factors influence school-age children's, adolescents', and adults' individual competencies in language?

4. How do researchers and clinicians measure language development in the school-age years and beyond?

Now that we have discussed language development in infancy, toddlerhood, and the preschool years, you may wonder what language and communication achievements remain for school-age children and adolescents to master. After all, by the time children leave preschool, they can pronounce almost all the sounds of their native language, they can produce sentences that include complex clauses and phrase structures, and they can use language for a number of communicative functions. In actuality, substantial development and refinement of syntax, pragmatics, and semantics occurs throughout the school-age years and adolescence. In this chapter, we begin with an overview of some of the major language development milestones that school-age children and adolescents achieve. Then, we discuss accomplishments in language form, content, and use that occur in the school-age years and beyond. We also explore factors that affect the language competencies of individual school-age children, adolescents, and adults. In the final section, we describe methods for measuring these individuals' language development.

WHAT MAJOR LANGUAGE DEVELOPMENT MILESTONES OCCUR IN THE SCHOOL-AGE YEARS AND BEYOND?

In infancy and toddlerhood, identifying language milestones is fairly straightforward. Researchers can note when children typically speak their first word or begin to combine words into short sentences. However, pinpointing language milestones in the school-age years and adolescence is not as simple. During these years, language development is more subtle than it is in early childhood. People do not usually notice the *products* of language development unless they know what to look for. Therefore, this section on major language development milestones focuses on the *process* of language development in the school-age years and beyond. Two processes that differentiate school-age children from their younger counterparts are the shifting sources of language input and the acquisition of metalinguistic competence.

Shifting Sources of Language Input

Before the school-age years, children's sole source of language input is oral. However, once children learn to read, they can acquire language input from the written text as well. Beginning around age 8–10 years, children shift to gaining more and

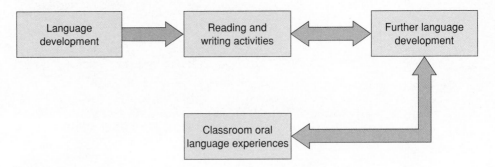

FIGURE 8.1

Relation among language development, reading and writing development, and oral language experiences in the classroom.

Source: From *Reading and Linguistic Development* (p. 26), by P. Menyuk, 1999, Cambridge, MA: Brookline Books. Copyright 1999 by Brookline Books. Adapted with permission.

more of their language input from text. As a result of increased exposure to language through reading, children develop language in an increasingly individualized manner (Nippold, 1998). For example, a child who is interested in cars and reads books about cars will likely acquire a set of car-related vocabulary words, including *carburetor, transmission,* and *spark plugs.*

Reading not only helps build children's lexical knowledge, but also has a role in developing the phonological, semantic, and pragmatic aspects of oral language. Menyuk (1999) suggested that reading allows children opportunities to reflect on language because, unlike oral language, reading allows children to review and think about written words that remain in front of them. Because oral language plays a crucial role in reading and writing abilities, and vice versa, oral language must develop both independently of reading and writing activities *and* in symbiotic relationship with reading and writing development (Menyuk, 1999). This symbiotic relationship is evident in the classroom when you consider the reading and writing activities that take place and the opportunities for oral language exchanges between students and teachers, and between peers (see Figure 8.1).

Being able to read requires the child's successful understanding of grapheme-to-phoneme (letter-to-sound) correspondence. Children's success at understanding this correspondence rests on how well they have established print and phonological awareness in the preschool period. (Recall from previous chapters that *print awareness* is the child's knowledge of print forms and functions, whereas *phonological awareness* is the child's sensitivity to the sound structure of language.) Children who enter school with skills in these areas are more likely to succeed at beginning reading (Chaney, 1998).

Between the preschool years and adulthood, children learning to read generally progress through a predictable series of qualitatively distinct developmental stages (Chall, 1996). Chall presented these stages in what she termed a "model" or "scheme" instead of a theory of reading development. She organized her scheme for understanding reading development in much the same way that Piaget organized his theory of stages and his stages of cognitive development (Inhelder & Piaget, 1958; Piaget, 1970). The **prereading stage,** which spans from birth until the beginning of formal education, is witness to some of children's most critical developments, including oral language, print awareness, and phonological awareness. An abundance of research results demonstrate the importance of prereading achievements to later reading success (e.g., Burgess, Hecht, & Lonigan, 2002; Bus, van IJzendoorn, & Pellegrini, 1995; Oliver, Dale, & Plomin, 2005; Whitehurst & Lonigan, 1998). After the prereading stage, children progress through five stages that build on this early foundation (Chall, 1996):

1.   *Initial reading, or decoding, stage:* Stage 1 covers the period of kindergarten through first grade, when children are 5–7 years old. During this stage, children begin to decode words by associating letters with corresponding sounds in spoken words. During Stage 1, children usually move sequentially through three phases (Biemiller, 1970, cited in Chall, 1996). In the first phase, when children read, they make word substitution errors in which the substituted word is semantically and syntactically probable. For example, they might read the sentence *The dog is growling* as *The dog is barking,* substituting the semantically and syntactically plausible word *barking* for a word they do not know (*growling*). In the second phase, when children read, they make word substitution errors in which the substituted word has a graphic resemblance to the original printed word. They might read the sentence *The dog is growling* as *The dog is green,* substituting the word *growling* with a word that looks similar but does not make sense semantically. In the third phase, when reading, children make word substitution errors in which the substituted word has a graphic resemblance to the original printed word but is also semantically acceptable. For example, they might read the sentence *The dog is growling* as *The dog is growing* or *The dog is going,* either of which involves substituting a semantically plausible and perceptually similar word. Children who are more proficient at reading move through these phases more quickly than do children who are less proficient.

2.   *Confirmation, fluency, and ungluing from print:* Stage 2 covers the period of second to third grade, when children are 7–8 years old. During this stage, children hone the decoding skills they learned in Stage 1. As children read familiar texts, they become particularly proficient with high-frequency words and use the redundancies of language to gain fluency and speed in reading. *Fluency* refers to reading that is efficient, well paced, and free of errors. It improves as children practice reading with texts that are familiar to them and that closely match their reading abilities. In Stage 2, children gradually begin to transition from *learning to read* to *reading to learn.*

3.   *Reading to learn the new—a first step:* Stage 3 lasts from Grade 4 to Grade 8 or 9, when children are ages 9–14 years. During Stage 3, children read to gain new information and are solidly reading to learn by the end of this stage. Chall suggested thinking about Stage 3 in two distinct phases. In the first phase, Stage 3A (Grades 4–6, or ages 9–11 years), children develop the ability to read beyond egocentric purposes so that they can read about and learn conventional information about the world. By the end of Phase 3A, children can read works of typical adult length, but not at the adult level of reading difficulty. In Phase 3B (Grades 7–8 or 9

Between ages 9 and 14 years, children refine their reading abilities so that they are able to read text to learn new information. Most children are no longer "learning to read" but are "reading to learn."

(*Photo Source:* Michael Newman/ PhotoEdit Inc.)

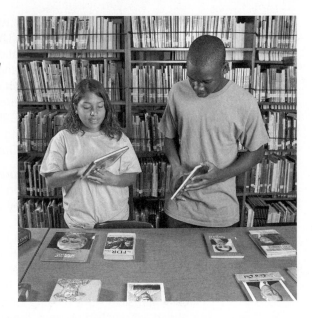

and ages 12–14 years), children can read on a general adult level. Reading during Stage 3 helps expand children's vocabularies, build background and world knowledge, and develop strategic reading habits. See Multicultural Focus: *Reading to Learn* for an example of how to encourage children learning English as a second language to read to learn.

MULTICULTURAL FOCUS

Reading to Learn

Students learning English as a second language may struggle not only with oral language but also with aspects of reading comprehension. V. Anderson and Roit (1996) presented 10 easy-to-implement strategies for using students' native language, social skills, and cognitive abilities to help them learn to read in English. One strategy involves using culturally familiar informational texts in the classroom that provide a balance of familiar information and new information. A *culturally familiar text* contains culturally familiar content about animals, foods, events, activities, and experiences. Using culturally familiar informational texts has three advantages. First, children can read about something that sparks their interest. Second, students can demonstrate their intelligence by providing new knowledge to their peers and by relating their personal experiences to the class. Third, and most important, this strategy allows students to identify with text, react to text, and connect text to their prior knowledge.

DISCUSSION POINT
Do you see any similarities between Chall's Stage 4 and one of Piaget's stages of cognitive development? If so, how are they similar?

4. *Multiple viewpoints—High school:* Stage 4 covers the high school period, between ages 14 and 18 years. During Stage 4, students learn to handle increasingly difficult concepts and the texts that describe them. The most important difference between reading in Stage 3 and reading in Stage 4 is that in Stage 4, children can consider multiple viewpoints. Stage 4 necessarily builds on the knowledge in Stage 3, when children read to learn, because without the background knowledge from Stage 3, children would not be able to read more difficult texts with multiple sets of facts, theories, and viewpoints.

5. *Construction and reconstruction—A world view: College:* Stage 5 occurs from age 18 years onward. During Stage 5, readers read selectively to suit their purposes. Reading selectively involves knowing which portions of the text to read—whether the beginning, middle, or end of the text, or some combination thereof. Readers also make judgments about what to read, how much to read, and in what level of detail to achieve comprehension. Readers at Stage 5 use advanced cognitive processes, such as analysis, synthesis, and prediction, to construct meaning from text. The difference between Stage 5 reading and reading in Stages 3 and 4 is illustrated by the following responses to the question *Is what you just read true?*

STAGE 3: Yes, I read it in a book. The author said it was true.

STAGE 4: I don't know. One of the authors I read said it was true; the other said it was not. I think there may be no true answers on the subject.

STAGE 5: There are different views on the matter. But one of the views seems to have the best evidence supporting it, and I would tend to go along with that view. (Chall, 1996, p. 58)

Acquisition of Metalinguistic Competence

Although children begin to acquire some **metalinguistic competence**—or the ability to think about and analyze language as an object of attention—in the preschool years, their competence increases significantly in the school-age years and beyond. One important reason children's metalinguistic abilities undergo dramatic growth in the school-age years is that many of the activities children engage in during these years draw on language analysis. For example, children in first-grade classrooms may have to identify the number of phonemes in a word, and children in seventh-grade classrooms might have to determine the meaning of an unfamiliar word by using their knowledge of the root of the word. Some specific types of metalinguistic competence that children in the school-age years achieve are phonological awareness and figurative language.

Phonological Awareness

In Chapter 7, we defined *phonological awareness* as children's sensitivity to the sound structure of words. Although children generally master some early developing phonological awareness abilities in the preschool years (segmenting words from sentences, segmenting multisyllabic words, detecting and producing rhymes), they usually do not master some of the later developing abilities until kindergarten or first grade. The later developing abilities in phonological awareness involve awareness of the smallest units of sound (phonemes) and include blending sounds, segmenting sounds from words, and manipulating sounds. This level of phonological awareness is termed *phonemic awareness* to delineate that the child must attend to the individual speech sounds in syllables and words.

The ability to be aware of the distinct sounds in syllables and words usually develops by kindergarten or first grade (around age 5–6 years). Blending tasks might take the following form: "What word is /b/ /æ/ /t/?" "What word is /p/ /ɪ/ /n/?" The ability to blend sounds to make words supports a child's reading development, particularly his or her decoding skills. However, this relationship between phonemic awareness skills, such as blending, and reading development is bidirectional in that learning to read also improves a child's phonemic awareness.

The ability to segment sounds from words also develops by kindergarten or first grade. Segmentation tasks might involve asking the following questions: "What is the first sound in *car*?" "What is the last sound?" and "What are the three sounds in *cat*?" The ability to segment words into their onset-rime segments (/b/ /ot/ for *boat;* /k/ /ot/ for *coat*) and their individual phonemes (/b/ /o/ /t/; /k/ /o/ /t/) is related to children's awareness of spelling sequences in words and their reading development (Goswami, 1990, 1991; Goswami & Mead, 1992). Children can use their knowledge of spelling patterns in words to help them read new words they encounter in texts. For example, if a child knows the spelling pattern of words such as *boat* and *coat,* he or she should be able to use this knowledge to infer how to pronounce the word *moat.*

Sound manipulation is the most complex phonological awareness ability and usually develops by second grade (around age 7 years). A sound manipulation task might resemble the following: "Say *rate* without the /r/." "What word do you have if you switch the /p/ and /t/ sounds in *pat*?" Such tasks require children to intensively analyze and manipulate the sound structures of individual words.

Figurative Language

Language that people use in nonliteral and often abstract ways is called **figurative language.** Using figurative language is a metalinguistic ability because children must recognize that language is an arbitrary code (Westby, 1998). People use figurative language to evoke mental images and sense impressions in other people. Figurative language includes metaphors, similes, hyperboles, idioms, irony, and proverbs.

Metaphors. A **metaphor** is a type of figurative language that conveys similarity through an expression that refers to something it does not denote literally (See Figure 8.2 for an example). Metaphors consist of a term called the *topic,* which is compared to another term called the *vehicle.* The topic and the vehicle share features and form the basis of comparison called the *ground.* Two types of metaphors are used: predictive and proportional (Table 8.1). Children begin to understand metaphors in the preschool years, and their comprehension improves throughout the school-age years and into adulthood as their ability with figurative language increases.

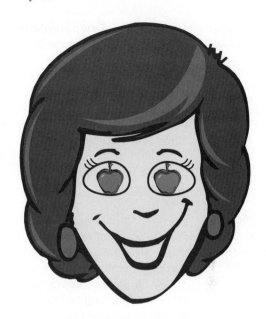

FIGURE 8.2
Literal interpretation of the
metaphor *She's the apple of my
eye.*

Similes. **Similes** are similar to predictive metaphors in that they contain a topic, a vehicle, and the ground. They are different in that they make the comparison between the topic and vehicle explicit by using the word *like* or *as.* Common similes using *like* include *like water off a duck's back* and *sitting like a bump on a log.* Common similes using *as* include *quiet as a mouse* and *flat as a pancake.* Nippold (1998) summarized research results indicating that the extent to which children use similes (and metaphors) relates to situational factors, including whether the children are engaging in a formal writing task or comparing dissimilar objects. Children's ability to understand and produce similes and metaphors is related to their performance on measures of general cognition, language, and academic achievement. However, whether these abilities are prerequisites to understanding and producing metaphors and similes is unclear.

TABLE 8.1
Types of Metaphors

Type	Definition	Example	Explanation
Predictive	Contains one topic and one vehicle	*All the world's a stage.*	*World* is the topic and *stage* is the vehicle.
Proportional	Contains two topics and two vehicles and expresses an analogical relationship	*The artist was an apple tree with no fruit* (Nippold, 1998, p. 89).	The analogy is "apple tree is to fruit as artist is to artwork."

Source: Adapted from *Later Language Development: The School-Age and Adolescent Years* (2nd ed.), by M. A. Nippold, 1998, Austin, TX: PRO-ED.

DISCUSSION POINT

Do you think school-age children use hyperboles more or less than other types of figurative language? Why or why not?

Hyperboles. A **hyperbole** is a particular form of figurative language that uses exaggeration for emphasis or effect. Examples of hyperbole include *I'm so hungry, I could eat a horse* and *I nearly died laughing.* Research examining children's understanding of hyperbole (and other forms of figurative language) is somewhat inconclusive. For example, Creusere (1999) summarized research results showing that salient intonation patterns may help 8- and 10-year-olds' comprehension of hyperbole, or children may make use of the discrepancy between the literal and intended meanings of an utterance to determine the speaker's intent. In the first case, to understand the hyperbole, children would exploit paralinguistic cues (intonation patterns), whereas in the second case they would exploit pragmatic cues.

DISCUSSION POINT

How might you assess a school-age child's understanding of idioms?

Idioms. **Idioms** are expressions that contain both a literal and a figurative meaning. *I've put that on the back burner* and *We're in the same boat* are examples of idioms. Illustrations of two common idioms are provided in Figure 8.3. People use two major types of idioms: opaque and transparent (Gibbs, 1987, cited in Nippold, 1998). *Opaque idioms* demonstrate little relationship between the literal interpretation and the figurative interpretation (e.g., *drive someone up the wall*), whereas the figurative meaning of a *transparent idiom* is an extension of the literal meaning (e.g., *hold one's tongue*). Gibbs' study showed that children ages 5, 6, 8, and 9 years could explain transparent idioms more easily than opaque idioms. Furthermore, children could interpret the meanings of idioms more correctly in multiple-choice tasks than in explanation tasks and had more success interpreting idioms

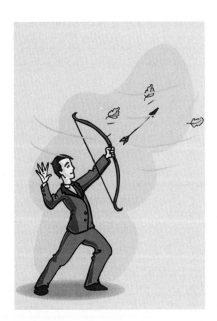
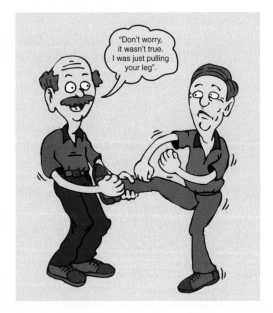

FIGURE 8.3
Literal interpretations of the idioms (A) *shoot the breeze* and (B) *pull someone's leg.*

when they received contextually supportive information than when they did not. Children's ability to comprehend the text they read predicts their understanding of idioms presented in context (Levorato, Nesi, & Cacciari, 2004). In general, understanding of idioms improves throughout the school-age years and adolescence and into adulthood. Opaque and less frequently used idioms are the most difficult to understand. In Nippold's (1998) study, adolescents and adults rated how familiar they were with certain idioms and how transparent the idioms were. Table 8.2 provides a sample of their mean ratings.

Irony. Irony is a type of figurative language that involves incongruity between what a speaker (or writer) says and what actually happens. Many puns make use of irony, as does sarcasm. Shakespeare used two main forms of irony in his plays: verbal and dramatic. With *verbal irony,* the speaker says one thing but means another. Exclaiming "What a beautiful day!" when the weather is cold and rainy is an example of verbal irony. With *dramatic irony,* the audience is aware of facts of which the characters are unaware. Some research results suggest that people use both acoustic cues and contextual information to infer ironic intent in other persons' spontaneous speech (Bryant & Tree, 2002).

Proverbs. **Proverbs** are statements that express the conventional values, beliefs, and wisdom of a society (Nippold, 1998). Nippold reported that of the types of figurative language, proverbs are one of the most difficult to master. Proverbs serve a variety of communicative functions, such as the following:

Commenting: *Blood is thicker than water.*
Interpreting: *His bark is worse than his bite.*
Advising: *Don't count your chickens before they hatch.*
Warning: *It's better to be safe than sorry.*
Encouraging: *Every cloud has a silver lining.*

TABLE 8.2
Mean Idiom Familiarity and Transparency Ratings for Adolescents and Adults

Idiom	Familiarity		Transparency	
	Adolescents	Adults	Adolescents	Adults
Go through the motions	2.35	1.70	1.90	1.65
Skating on thin ice	1.30	1.30	1.35	1.55
Take down a peg	4.30	3.30	2.60	2.70
Vote with one's feet	4.55	4.35	2.65	2.80

Familiarity measures how often a person has heard or read the idiom before: 1 = many times, 2 = several times, 3 = a few times, 4 = once, 5 = never. *Transparency* measures how closely the literal and nonliteral meanings of the idiom compare: 1 = closely related, 2 = somewhat related, 3 = not related.
Source: From *Later Language Development: The School-Age and Adolescent Years* (2nd ed., pp. 118–120), by M. A. Nippold, 1998, Austin, TX: PRO-ED. Copyright 1998 by PRO-ED. Adapted with permission.

Nippold reported that proverb understanding improves gradually during the adolescent years and that the presence of a supportive linguistic environment can facilitate adolescents' understanding of proverbs. The degree to which adolescents understand proverbs has been correlated with measures of academic success in literature and mathematics (Nippold, 2000), likely because proverb understanding requires the student to be able to contend with abstract and metalinguistic aspects of language.

WHAT MAJOR ACHIEVEMENTS IN LANGUAGE CONTENT, FORM, AND USE CHARACTERIZE THE SCHOOL-AGE YEARS AND BEYOND?

As children mature to school age and into adolescence, they continue to make significant gains in language content, form, and use. In doing so, they increase—among other things—their receptive and expressive vocabularies, their ability to clarify language ambiguities, their use of decontextualized language, the number of functions for which they use language, their conversational skills, and their narrative abilities. We discuss such gains next. (See Developmental Timeline: *School-Age Years* for a summary of specific achievements.)

Language Content

The typical school-age child makes considerable gains in several language content areas. Most of these gains occur as a result of reading text, which provides students with access to words and concepts that are not typically the topic of everyday conversations. Gains in content during the school-age years also occur as a result of the classroom environment, where the topic of conversation is generally decontextualized. Four areas of notable content development for school-age students are (a) lexical development, (b) understanding of multiple meanings, (c) understanding of lexical and sentential ambiguity, and (d) development of literate language.

Lexical Development

School-age students' receptive and expressive vocabularies expand so much that upon graduation from high school students have command over about 60,000 words (Pinker, 1994). According to Nippold (1998), school-age children learn new words in at least three ways: through direct instruction, contextual abstraction, and morphological analysis.

Direct Instruction. *Direct instruction* involves learning the meaning of a word directly from a more knowledgeable source. This source may be another person or a dictionary. Throughout a person's life span, other people teach him or her words, either because the person asks them for definitions or because they presuppose that the person should learn the definitions. Children do not begin to use dictionaries to learn the meanings of words until about second grade (age 7 or 8 years). They continue to use this method throughout middle school and high school.

DEVELOPMENTAL TIMELINE: SCHOOL-AGE YEARS

Phonology

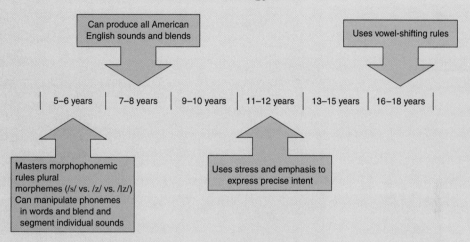

Can produce all American English sounds and blends

Uses vowel-shifting rules

| 5–6 years | 7–8 years | 9–10 years | 11–12 years | 13–15 years | 16–18 years |

Masters morphophonemic rules plural morphemes (/s/ vs. /z/ vs. /ɪz/) Can manipulate phonemes in words and blend and segment individual sounds

Uses stress and emphasis to express precise intent

Syntax and Morphology

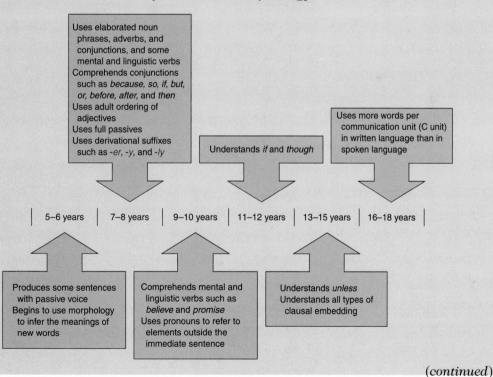

Uses elaborated noun phrases, adverbs, and conjunctions, and some mental and linguistic verbs
Comprehends conjunctions such as *because, so, if, but, or, before, after,* and *then*
Uses adult ordering of adjectives
Uses full passives
Uses derivational suffixes such as *-er, -y,* and *-ly*

Understands *if* and *though*

Uses more words per communication unit (C unit) in written language than in spoken language

| 5–6 years | 7–8 years | 9–10 years | 11–12 years | 13–15 years | 16–18 years |

Produces some sentences with passive voice
Begins to use morphology to infer the meanings of new words

Comprehends mental and linguistic verbs such as *believe* and *promise*
Uses pronouns to refer to elements outside the immediate sentence

Understands *unless*
Understands all types of clausal embedding

(continued)

DEVELOPMENTAL TIMELINE: SCHOOL-AGE YEARS *(continued)*

Semantics

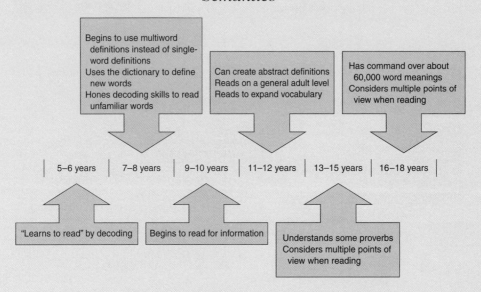

Begins to use multiword definitions instead of single-word definitions
Uses the dictionary to define new words
Hones decoding skills to read unfamiliar words

Can create abstract definitions
Reads on a general adult level
Reads to expand vocabulary

Has command over about 60,000 word meanings
Considers multiple points of view when reading

| 5–6 years | 7–8 years | 9–10 years | 11–12 years | 13–15 years | 16–18 years |

"Learns to read" by decoding

Begins to read for information

Understands some proverbs
Considers multiple points of view when reading

Pragmatics

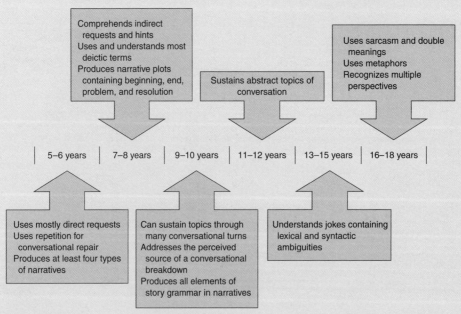

Comprehends indirect requests and hints
Uses and understands most deictic terms
Produces narrative plots containing beginning, end, problem, and resolution

Sustains abstract topics of conversation

Uses sarcasm and double meanings
Uses metaphors
Recognizes multiple perspectives

| 5–6 years | 7–8 years | 9–10 years | 11–12 years | 13–15 years | 16–18 years |

Uses mostly direct requests
Uses repetition for conversational repair
Produces at least four types of narratives

Can sustain topics through many conversational turns
Addresses the perceived source of a conversational breakdown
Produces all elements of story grammar in narratives

Understands jokes containing lexical and syntactic ambiguities

Source: Chall (1996); Curenton and Justice (2004); Gard, Gilman, and Gorman (1993); Nippold (1998); Owens (2001, 2005); Paul (1995); Pinker (1994); and Westby (1998).

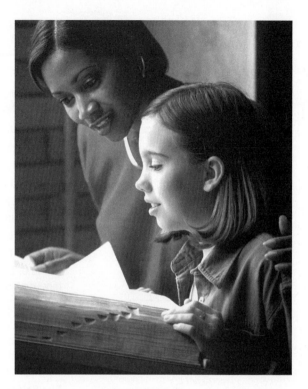

During the elementary grades, children begin to use dictionaries to learn the meanings of new words directly.

(*Photo Source:* © Gabe Palmer/Corbis.)

Contextual Abstraction. *Contextual abstraction* involves using context clues in both spoken and written forms of language to determine the meanings of unfamiliar words. In Chapter 7, we discussed the process by which children learn new words in context: Children form an initial representation of a word through *fast mapping*. After repeated exposure, children refine the representation of the word through the process of *slow mapping*. School-age children, adolescents, and adults all learn the meanings of words in the same way when they encounter unfamiliar words in context. They make either pragmatic inferences or logical inferences about the meanings of the words (Westby, 1998). *Pragmatic inferences* about the meaning of a word bring an individual's personal world knowledge or background knowledge to the text. *Logical inferences* use only the information provided by the text and are more difficult to make. Westby explained that people make pragmatic inferences more often when they are reading narrative texts and logical inferences when they are reading expository texts. See Table 8.3 for examples of context clues that readers can draw on to abstract the meanings of new words from a text.

Morphological Analysis. *Morphological analysis* involves analyzing the lexical, inflectional, and derivational morphemes of unfamiliar words to infer their meanings. For instance, a child who encounters the word *homophone* in a language arts text can use knowledge of the morphemes *homo-* (meaning "same") and *-phone* (meaning "sound") to make an educated guess about the meaning of the word.

TABLE 8.3
Examples of Context Clues for Abstracting the Meanings of Words from Text

Syntactic cues	Example
Appositives	*Quinoa,* the seed of a leafy plant native to the Andes, is often mistaken for a grain because of its taste and appearance.
Relative clauses	The *Incas,* who were people indigenous to the Andean region, fed quinoa to their armies.
The conjunction *or*	The Incas were *indigenous,* or native, to the country of Ecuador.
Direct explanation	If you visit Ecuador, you can visit Incan ruins known as *Ingapirca.*
Linked synonyms	While driving through Ecuador, you will experience scenic views of the rolling, meandering, *undulating* countryside.
Participial phrases	The travelers, exhausted from a long day at the Otavalo market, vowed to practice their *bargaining* strategies.
Categorical sequence	Some of Ecuador's popular produce items include mangoes, pineapples, papayas, and *plantains.*

Semantic cues	Example
Restatement	Persons in some regions of Ecuador must be careful of *landslides.* They must guard themselves against the downward sliding of earth and rock.
Illustrations or examples	The flag of Ecuador is *multicolored.* For example, it contains the colors yellow, blue, and red.
Similes	The *thermal baths* in Ecuador are like outdoor hot tubs.
Metaphors	The Andes mountains are a colorful *tapestry*.
Personification	Clouds *scatter* rain over the region on some afternoons.
Summary	When traveling, be especially cautious in or avoid areas where you are likely to be *victimized.* These areas include crowded subways, train stations, elevators, tourist sites, marketplaces, festivals, and marginal areas of cities.
Cause and effect	Because the Galapagos Islands are so *isolated,* they are home to species of animals and plants that are not found anywhere else in the world.

Source: From *Later Language Development: The School-Age and Adolescent Years* (2nd ed., p. 18), by M. A. Nippold, 1998, Austin, TX: PRO-ED. Copyright 1998 by PRO-ED. Adapted with permission.

Although younger children (ages 6–10 years) become proficient at using morphemes to infer the meanings of new words, their older counterparts (ages 9–13 years) are proficient at using both morphological information and context clues to arrive at meanings of unfamiliar words. Examples of morphemes with clear lexical meaning that older children (age 9 years and onward) might use to decipher the meanings of unfamiliar words include the common prefixes *un-, re-, dis-, en-, em-,* non-, over-, mis-, sub-, fore-, de-, trans-, super-, semi-, anti-, mid-, and under-, as well as the "not" prefixes (in-, im-, ir-, il; White, Sowell, & Yanagihara, 1989).

Understanding of Multiple Meanings

As the lexicons of school-age children grow and the children encounter more and more words, they realize that many words are **polysemous** (have more than one meaning). As students develop, they become able to provide multiple definitions for words with several similar meanings, but they have particular difficulty understanding the secondary meanings of words that bear little or no relation to the primary meaning. Being able to supply multiple meanings for words requires not only lexical knowledge but also metalinguistic knowledge, both of which are necessary to achieve full competence at the literate end of the oral–literate language continuum, which we discuss in the subsequent section entitled "Literate Language."

Understanding of Lexical and Sentential Ambiguity

Understanding of lexical and sentential ambiguity is another related area of notable content achievement for school-age children. **Lexical ambiguity** occurs for words and phrases with multiple meanings, such as *That was a real bear,* in which *bear* has several meanings. Lexical ambiguity at the level of the word may take one of three forms:

1. *Homophones:* **Homophones** are words that sound alike and may be spelled alike (*brown bear* vs. *bear weight*) or may be spelled differently (*brown bear* vs. *bare* hands).
2. *Homographs:* **Homographs** are words that are spelled the same and may sound alike (*row a boat* vs. *row of homes*) or may sound different from each other (*record player* vs. *record a movie*).
3. *Homonyms:* **Homonyms** are words that are alike in spelling and pronunciation but differ in meaning (*brown bear* vs. *bear weight*). They are a specific type of homophone.

Lexical ambiguity regularly fuels the humor in jokes, riddles, comic strips, newspaper headlines, bumper stickers, and advertisements, such as the joke *Is your refrigerator running? . . . You'd better go catch it!* (Nippold, 1998). When students encounter ambiguous words, they must first notice the ambiguity, then scrutinize the words to arrive at the appropriate meaning. Students with weak oral language skills are often not adept at noticing when lexical ambiguities are present and are less likely than other students to seek clarification for the ambiguity, both of which can result in a communication breakdown (Paul, 1995).

Sentential ambiguity involves ambiguity within different components of sentences. It includes not only lexical ambiguity but also phonological ambiguity, surface-structure ambiguity, and deep-structure ambiguity. **Phonological ambiguity** occurs with varying pronunciations of a word (*She needs to visit her psychotherapist* vs. *She needs to visit her psycho therapist*). **Surface-structure ambiguity** results from varying stress and intonation (*I fed her bird seed* vs. *I fed her bird seed*). With

deep-structure ambiguity, a noun serves as an agent in one interpretation and as an object in another (e.g., *The duck is ready to eat* can mean "The duck is hungry" or "The duck is ready to be eaten"; Nippold, 1998, p. 140).

Development of Literate Language

Recall that in Chapter 7 we described the difference between contextualized and decontextualized language. When children enter school, the language they hear and use becomes increasingly decontextualized, or removed from the here and now. **Literate language** is the term used to describe language that is highly decontextualized. The literate language style characterizes language used to "monitor and reflect on experience, and reason about, plan, and predict experiences" (Westby, 1985, p. 181). *Literate language* refers to the child's ability to use language without the aid of context cues to support meaning. The child must rely on language itself to make meaning. Developing a literate language style, or progressing from contextualized to decontextualized language, is crucial for children's participation in the type of discourse used in school settings. Imagine the following conversation taking place between 4-year-old Hattie and her 8-year-old sister, Elizabeth:

HATTIE: That's my toy!

ELIZABETH: No, remember we have to share this toy? Mom and Dad bought it for both of us to play with.

Children's discourse development moves along a continuum reflecting oral language on the one end and literate language on the other (Westby, 1991). In the preceding example, Hattie's and Elizabeth's utterances represent opposite ends of this continuum. At the lower level of the discourse continuum is *oral language,* or the linguistic aspects of communicative competence necessary for communicating basic desires and needs (phonology, syntax, morphology, and semantics). Westby described children at this end of the continuum as "learning to talk." Children learning to talk can satisfy some basic language functions, including requesting and greeting. They can also produce simple syntactic structures. For example, English speakers can form yes-or-no questions by inserting *do* before the subject of the sentence (*You like ice cream* becomes *Do you like ice cream?*) and can mark the past tense by adding *-ed* or by retrieving the appropriate irregular past tense verb. The most salient characteristic of oral language is its highly contextualized style. Highly contextualized language depends heavily on the immediate context and environment. Markers of highly contextualized language include *referential pronouns,* or pronouns that refer to something physically available to the speaker ("I want *that*"), as well as gestures and facial expressions. Only when children have mastered oral language can they begin to "talk to learn" or to use language to reflect on past experiences and reason about, predict, and plan for future experiences using decontextualized language (Westby, 1991).

Children who "talk to learn" are at the literate language end of the discourse continuum. At this end, children use language to communicate but also to engage in higher order cognitive functions, such as reflecting, reasoning, planning, and hypothesizing. Highly specific vocabulary and complex syntax that expresses ideas, events, and objects beyond those of the present typify literate language. Four specific features of literate language that children learn to use are as follows (Curenton & Justice, 2004):

1. *Elaborated noun phrases:* An elaborated noun phrase is a group of words consisting of a noun and one or more modifiers providing additional information about the noun, including articles (*a, an, the*), possessives (*my, his, their*), demonstratives (*this, that, those*), quantifiers (*every, each, some*), *wh-* words (*what, which, whichever*), and adjectives (*tall, long, ugly*).

2. *Adverbs:* An adverb is a syntactic form that modifies verbs and enhances the explicitness of action and event descriptions. Adverbs provide additional information about time (*suddenly, again, now*), manner (*somehow, well, slowly*), degree (*almost, barely, much*), place (*here, outside, above*), reason (*therefore, since, so*), and affirmation or negation (*definitely, really, never*).

3. *Conjunctions:* Conjunctions are words that organize information and clarify relationships among elements. *Coordinating conjunctions* include *and, for, or, yet, but, nor*, and *so. Subordinating conjunctions* are more numerous and include *after, although, as, because,* and *therefore,* as well as others.

4. *Mental and linguistic verbs:* Mental and linguistic verbs refer to various acts of thinking and speaking, respectively. *Mental verbs* include *think, know, believe, imagine, feel, consider, suppose, decide, forget,* and *remember. Linguistic verbs* include *say, tell, speak, shout, answer, call, reply,* and *yell.*

Consider the extent to which these four literate language features are present in the following example of decontextualized language:

Yesterday, after I arrived at work, I was about to sit down at my desk, when I decided that I would make a cup of coffee first. You see, I was desperate for some caffeine, given that I had not had a cup of coffee at home. I started to grab some coffee from the machine, at which point I heard a familiar voice in the hallway. Now, before I tell you who it was . . .

DISCUSSION POINT

Describe in writing something you did yesterday. Document the use of literate language features in this written sample. Which features occur most frequently? least frequently?

The way this speaker paints a picture for the listener is by using a variety of techniques that go well beyond using the correct vocabulary and syntax. The speaker provides lexical specificity by using elaborated noun phrases (*my desk, a cup of coffee*), adverbs (*yesterday, now*), and mental and linguistic verbs (*decided, tell*). The speaker also spreads conjunctions liberally throughout the story to weave together events in a causal (*given*) and temporal *(at which point)* manner. These devices provide the listener with context that would not otherwise be available. As children move through the elementary grades into adolescence and high school, they should be able to use literate language structures—both when they speak and when they write—to create context for other individuals.

Language Form

As students move through the elementary grades into high school, their achievements in form progress in a slow and subtle manner. Three notable areas of school-age development in language form are (a) complex syntax development, (b) morphological development, and (c) phonological development.

Complex Syntax Development

CD VIDEO CLIP

To watch a 7-year-old boy, who is beginning to use the passive voice construction, tell a story about being adopted from China, see the CD video clip *Language 8*.

The most important achievements in form for school-age children involve complex syntax. *Complex syntax* refers to developmentally advanced grammatical structures that mark a literate language style (Paul, 1995). These structures occur relatively infrequently in spoken language, but when students use them in written language, such use indicates the students have achieved more advanced levels of grammar. Examples of complex syntax include noun-phrase postmodification with past participles (*a dance called the waltz*), complex verb phrases using the perfective aspect (*Stephanie has arrived from Vancouver*), adverbial conjunctions (*only, consequently*), and passive voice construction (*The fish were caught by an experienced fisherman).*

Many of these complex syntactic skills children exhibit are rarely used in conversation, such as the passive voice, so these form accomplishments can be difficult to witness. Rather, the development of syntax during the school-age years is more easily visible in students' writing. Persuasive writing in particular is a vehicle for the expression of more complex syntax. According to Nippold (2000), persuasive writing is a challenging communicative task that students develop during the school-age period. It requires an awareness of what other people believe and value and the ability to present personal ideas in a logical sequence. Syntactic complexities arise in persuasive writing because children must produce "longer sentences that contain greater amounts of subordination and stronger linkages between sentences, attainments that are partially achieved through the proper use of adverbial connectors" (p. 20).

Morphological Development

Children's morphological development is closely related to their syntactic development. Major morphological developments in the school-age years include the use of derivational prefixes and derivational suffixes. *Derivational prefixes* are added to the beginnings of words to change their meanings. For example, when the derivational prefix *un-* is added to the word *healthy,* to make *unhealthy,* the meaning of the word is changed to its negative counterpart. Other derivational prefixes include *dis-, non-,* and *ir-.*

Derivational suffixes include *-hood, -ment, -er, -y,* and *-ly,* among others. Derivational suffixes are added to the ends of words to change their form class, their meaning, or both. For example, the verb *encroach* can be changed to a noun by adding the derivational suffix *-ment, (encroachment).* Some of the more difficult derivational suffixes include *-y* (to form adjectives such as *squishy* and *tasty*), which children acquire around age 11 years, and *-ly* (to form adverbs such as *correctly* and *aptly*), which children learn in adolescence.

Phonological Development

A few developments in phonology also remain to be achieved during the school-age years. Previously in this chapter, we described school-age children's accomplishments in phonological awareness, including their ability to segment syllables from multisyllabic words and their ability to blend and manipulate the sounds in words. In addition, children make progress in their **morphophonemic development.**

One type of morphophonemic development concerns the use of sound modifications when certain morphemes are joined. For example, around age 5 or 6 years, children correctly use the plural ending /ɪz/, as in *matches* and *watches*, which differs phonologically from sound modifications in other pluralized words (e.g., hat_s_, dog_s_).

A second type of morphophonemic development involves vowel shifting, which takes place when the form class of a word is changed by adding a derivational suffix. Examples of vowel shifting include /aɪ/ to /ɪ/ (*decide–decision*), /eɪ/ to / æ / (*sane–sanity*), and /i/ to /ɛ/ (*serene–serenity*). Most children do not master vowel shifting until about age 17 years (Owens, 2005). Finally, a third type of morphophonemic rule school-age children learn is how to use stress and emphasis to distinguish phrases from compound words (*hot dog* vs. *hotdog, green house* vs. *greenhouse*) and to distinguish nouns from verbs (*record* vs. *record, present* vs. *present*). Children usually master stress and emphasis by 12 years of age (Ingram, 1986, as cited in Owens, 2005).

Language Use

During the school-age years and beyond, individuals develop the ability to use language for many reasons. People also further refine their conversational and narrative abilities during this period. Three important achievements in language use attained during this time are (a) functional flexibility, (b) conversational abilities, (c) and narrative development.

Functional Flexibility

Functional flexibility refers to the ability to use language for a variety of communicative purposes, or functions. This flexibility is increasingly important for school-age children, who must be able to compare and contrast, to persuade, to hypothesize, to explain, to classify, and to predict in the context of their classroom activities. Figure 8.4 provides a more complete list of language functions that school-age children must use in the classroom, which attests to the importance of the language flexibility required of such children. Each function requires a distinct set of linguistic, social, and cognitive competencies, all of which develop during the school-age years.

In addition to using these individual functions, children must be able to integrate these functions to achieve certain purposes. For example, according to Nippold (1998), students must be able to integrate at least seven skills in order to use language to persuade:

1. Adjust to listener characteristics (e.g., age, authority, familiarity)

2. State advantages as a reason to comply

3. Anticipate and reply to counterarguments

4. Use positive techniques such as politeness and bargaining as strategies to increase compliance

---

1. *To instruct:* To provide specific sequential directions
2. *To inquire:* To seek understanding by asking questions
3. *To test:* To investigate the logic of a statement
4. *To describe:* To tell about, giving necessary information to identify
5. *To compare and contrast:* To show how things are similar and different
6. *To explain:* To define terms by providing specific examples
7. *To analyze:* To break down a statement into its components, telling what each means and how they are related
8. *To hypothesize:* To make an assumption to test the logical or empirical consequences of a statement
9. *To deduce:* To arrive at a conclusion by reasoning; to infer
10. *To evaluate:* To weigh and judge the relative importance of an idea

---

FIGURE 8.4

Ten higher level functions of language required of school-age children.

Source: From *Teaching Disadvantaged Children in the Preschool,* by C. Bereiter and S. Engelmann, 1966, Upper Saddle River, NJ: Prentice Hall. Copyright 1966 by Prentice Hall. Adapted with permission.

5. Avoid negative strategies such as whining and begging
6. Generate a large number and variety of arguments
7. Control the discourse assertively

Students who cannot use language flexibly are more likely than other students to have difficulties with the academic and social demands of elementary, middle, and high school.

Conversational Abilities

During the school-age years and into adolescence, children gradually improve their conversational abilities—for example, by doing the following (Nippold, 1998):

1. Staying on topic longer
2. Having extended dialogues with other people that last for several conversational turns
3. Making a larger number of relevant and factual comments
4. Shifting smoothly from one topic to another
5. Adjusting the content and style of their speech to the listener's thoughts and feelings

Children also become more proficient at understanding and using indirect requests as they develop. By about age 7 years, they begin to use indirect language, including hints, and they recognize other people's indirect requests for action (e.g., "Do you know what time it is?"). Likewise, children become more adept at detecting conversational breakdowns and repairing them. Whereas younger children favor using repetition to provide additional information during breakdowns, at around age 9 years, school-age children begin to use more

THEORY TO PRACTICE

Structured Peer Relationships

Asperger's syndrome (AS) is a pervasive developmental disorder on the autism spectrum; people with AS have challenges in social interaction and communication. In new studies, researchers are investigating how speech–language pathologists (SLPs) and educators can assist school-age children with AS with social interaction and communication. For example, Safran, Safran, and Ellis (2003) provided practical recommendations for assisting children with AS in the areas of academics, behavior, and communication. One strategy for improving the communicative abilities of children with AS is creating *structured peer relationships.* In these relationships, a few peers commit to interacting with the student and to providing him or her with social support. Specific goals for the student include learning how to have fun with other people, how to experience a sense of togetherness, how to fix interpersonal problems, and how to enjoy other individuals' input. The role of educators and the SLP in encouraging and supporting the student's "peer group" as they implement strategies with the student with AS is important to the success of this strategy.

DISCUSSION POINT

What other kinds of strategies could an educator or SLP use to improve the pragmatic abilities of a student with AS?

sophisticated strategies, such as providing additional background information and defining terms to repair breakdowns when they occur. See Theory to Practice: *Structured Peer Relationships* for an example of an intervention for children who are not developing pragmatic abilities in the same manner as their peers.

Narrative Development

School-age children and adolescents use narration in both classroom and social settings. Narration is more complex than conversation because the speaker carries the linguistic load and the listener or audience takes a relatively passive role; by contrast, in conversation the multiple participants share responsibility for the give-and-take of information.

Types of Narratives. Younger children (about 5–6 years old) can produce at least four types of narratives (Stein, 1982, as cited in Owens, 2001):

1. *Recounts* involve telling a story about personal experiences or retelling a story that has been read. An adult who has shared an experience with a child usually prompts a recount. Because the experience is shared, the adult can provide additional detail when the child does not provide enough. These are also called personal narratives.

2. *Accounts,* like recounts, are also a type of personal narrative. However, they are spontaneous. Unlike a recount, in an account the adult has not shared the experience. Accounts are thus highly individualized because adults cannot prompt the child or supply missing information.

3. *Event casts* are similar to what sportscasters do during a sporting event. Event casts describe a current situation or event as it is happening. Children often use event casts while they play, to direct other people's actions.

4. *Fictionalized stories* are made up and usually have a main character who must overcome a challenge or a problem. These stories are also called *fictional narratives*.

CD VIDEO CLIP

To watch a boy tell a story that includes many of the advanced elements of mature narratives, see the CD video clip *Language 9*.

Elements of Mature Narratives. Early in the school-age years, children begin to manipulate the content, plot, and causal structure of their narratives. With respect to causality, school-age children learn how to move both forward and backward in time as they tell their narratives, whereas younger children can only move forward in time. Schoolchildren's narratives also begin to describe other individuals' physical and mental states and motivations for actions. As children mature, their narratives grow to include multiple episodes. An episode is the statement of a problem or challenge and all the elements that relate to the solution of the problem or challenge. Whereas children ages 5–6 years may include only one episode in their narratives, older children may include two or more.

Story grammar refers to the components of a narrative (e.g., characters, setting, episodes) as well as the rules that govern how these components are organized. Usually, story grammar in English consists of the setting and an episode structure. See Table 8.4 for a description of the components of story grammar. By the end of the elementary grades, children will often include many or all of these features in their narratives.

Expressive Elaboration. Ukrainetz and colleagues (2005) described the combination of narrative elements in an expressive or artful manner of storytelling as **expressive elaboration.** These features add to the story grammar contained in a narrative to enhance its overall expressive quality. These researchers examined the narratives of 293 children aged 5–12 years to study the development of children's expressive elaboration in three main categories:

1. *Appendages:* Cues to a listener that a story is being told or has ended (e.g., a formal introduction to the story, such as "Once upon a time . . ."; a summary of the story provided before beginning; a formal ending to the story, such as "The end")

2. *Orientations:* Elements that provide more detail to the setting and characters (e.g., character names, relations between characters, personal attributes of characters)

3. *Evaluations:* Ways in which the narrator can convey narrator or character perspectives (e.g., using interesting modifiers, repetition for emphasis, internal-state words, or dialogue)

The results of this study revealed that the presence of all three major categories of expressive elaboration increased with the children's age. When the children were divided into three age clusters, 5- to 6-year-olds consistently differed from 7- to 9-year-olds and 10- to 12-year-olds in their use of all three categories of expressive elaboration. However, 7- to 9-year-olds and 10- to 12-year-olds differed statistically only in their use of orientations.

TABLE 8.4
Components of Story Grammar

Component	Description	Example
Setting statement	Introduce the characters; describe their habitual actions and the social, physical, and/or temporal contexts; introduce the protagonist.	*There was this boy and*
Initiating event	Event that induces the character(s) to act through some natural act, such as an earthquake; a notion to seek something, such as treasure; or the action of one of the characters, such as arresting someone.	*. . . he got kidnapped by these pirates.*
Internal response	Characters' reactions, such as emotional responses, thoughts, or intentions, to the initiating events. Internal responses provide some motivation for the characters.	*He missed his dog.*
Internal plan	Indicates the characters' strategies for attaining their goal(s). Young children rarely include this element.	*So he decided to escape.*
Attempt	Overt action(s) of the characters to bring about some consequence, such as to attain their goal(s).	*When they were all eating, he cut the ropes and*
Direct consequence	Characters' success or failure at attaining their goal(s) as a result of the attempt.	*. . . he got away.*
Reaction	Character's emotional response, thought, or actions to the outcome or preceding chain of events.	*And he lived on an island with his dog. And they played in the sand every day.*

Source: From Owens, Robert E. *Language Development: An Introduction,* 5/e © 2001. Published by Allyn and Bacon, Boston, MA. Copyright © 2001 by Pearson Education. Reprinted by permission of the publisher.

WHAT FACTORS INFLUENCE SCHOOL-AGE CHILDREN'S, ADOLESCENTS', AND ADULTS' INDIVIDUAL COMPETENCIES IN LANGUAGE?

Like infants, toddlers, and preschoolers, school-age children, adolescents, and adults differ from their peers in certain ways with respect to language development. In this section, we focus on gender differences in language development and use in the school-age years and beyond.

In the school-age years and adolescence, gender differences become apparent between males and females in terms of vocabulary and conversational styles. Many people are aware of just how significant these differences are, in large part as a result of Deborah Tannen's (1991) book *You Just Don't Understand: Women and Men in Conversation* and John Gray's (1993) book *Men Are from Mars, Women Are from Venus: A Practical Guide for Improving Communication and Getting What You Want in Your Relationships.* These popular-press books illustrate how important gender differences in language are to relationships and day-to-day interactions with other people.

As discussed in previous chapters, differences in language development for males and females begin to emerge at an early age, perhaps from birth. Research results demonstrate that language socialization plays a large role in these differences. For example, parents refer more frequently to emotion with daughters than with sons, describing negative emotions such as sadness and dislike more often with daughters (Adams, Kuebli, Boyle, & Fivush, 1995). Differences in the emotional content of parent–child conversations are related to children's references to emotion by age 6 years as well; girls use more unique emotion terms than boys do (Adams et al., 1995). Next, we discuss two main areas of language in which gender differences may play a role: (a) vocabulary use and conversational style and (b) conversational pragmatics.

Gender Differences in Vocabulary Use and Conversational Style

The quantitative and qualitative evidence for differences between male and female vocabulary use and conversational style is dated. Research results from the 1960s through the early 1980s revealed larger differences in vocabulary use and conversational styles between genders than more recent research does. For example, previous research showed that women use more polite words, such as *please* and *thank you,* whereas men use coarser words and swear more often (Grief & Berko Gleason, 1980). Other previous research results demonstrated that men's language is more assertive than women's language and that certain features of women's language reflect this less assertive style, including the following three (Lakoff, 1975):

1. Use of more tag questions ("You like lasagna, don't you?")

2. Use of rising intonation in declarative sentences, so that declarative sentences sound more like questions

3. Use of polite requests more often than commands

However, more recent research results suggest that context and social status effects on language use may be stronger than gender effects are (e.g., Dixon & Foster, 1997; Hannah & Murachver, 1999; Koike, 1986; Robertson & Murachver, 2003). One example concerns *hedges,* or linguistic devices that soften utterances by signaling imprecision and noncommitment, such as *about, sort of, you know, possibly,* and *perhaps.* Dixon and Foster (1997) found no effect of gender on speakers' use of hedges in conversation, but these researchers did find effects of speaking contexts. Specifically, the research results revealed that both men and women used fewer hedges in competitive contexts than in noncompetitive contexts and more hedges when addressing males than when addressing females.

School-age children can also adjust their speech to a male-preferential or female-preferential style according to the content. Robertson and Murachver (2003) found that school-age children accommodate their speech to that of their conversational partner, regardless of the partner's gender. For example, children used more instances of tag questions and compliments (female-preferential speech style) when their conversational partner used this style and more negative comments, disagreements, and directives (male-preferential speech) when their conversational partner used this speech style.

Gender Differences in Conversational Pragmatics

Males and females differ not only in the *kinds* of language they use, but also in *how* they use language. For example, body posture and eye contact differ for men and women. Women usually face their conversational partners and make eye contact, whereas men are more likely to take a more distant stance and make less eye contact (Tannen, 1994). Men also change conversational topics more frequently than women do, whereas women exhaust conversational topics more thoroughly (Tannen, 1994). Women indicate their attention by using fillers such as *uh-huh* and *yeah* more often than men do, and women usually interrupt the speaker only to clarify the message and support the speaker. One large difference relates to the percentage of topics sustained in conversations. Although women introduce topics into conversations frequently, only about 36% of these topics are sustained, whereas 96% of the topics males introduce are sustained (Ehrenreich, 1981, cited in Owens, 2001). As with vocabulary use, men's and women's conversational pragmatics may be more a function of context than gender. See K. J. Anderson and Leaper (1998) for a meta-analysis of 43 studies comparing men's and women's conversational interruptions across a variety of situational contexts, as an excellent summary of these between-gender differences.

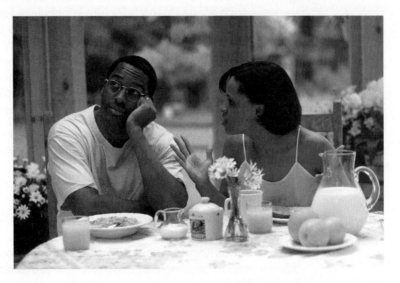

Men and women differ in the kinds of language they use as well as the ways in which they use language.

(*Photo Source:* © Michael Keller/Corbis.)

HOW DO RESEARCHERS AND CLINICIANS MEASURE LANGUAGE DEVELOPMENT IN THE SCHOOL-AGE YEARS AND BEYOND?

Researchers and clinicians measure school-age language development in various ways, such as by using standardized tests, naturalistic language situations for collecting language samples, and elicitation procedures. In this section, we describe different assessment types and then explore ways to measure the development of language form, content, and use during the school-age years and beyond.

Assessment Types

The way in which a clinician, researcher, or teacher measures language development usually depends on the person's reason for doing so. Practitioners use **formative evaluations** when they want guidance on the language-learning activities they should use and when they want to focus on the language development *process.* For example, before beginning a new curricular unit, a teacher might informally administer a formative assessment of a child's vocabulary knowledge by having the child try to define specific words he or she will encounter in the unit. The teacher could then focus on the words the child does not know as they progress through the unit.

Conversely, practitioners use **summative evaluations** when they want to focus on the *products* and final outcomes of language learning and development. For example, a clinician might administer a summative assessment of vocabulary knowledge—such as the Peabody Picture Vocabulary Test, third edition (PPVT–III; Dunn & Dunn, 1997) or fourth edition (PPVT–4; Dunn & Dunn, 2006)—to evaluate a child who has participated in a year-long vocabulary intervention designed to raise his or her vocabulary level to that of same-age peers.

Besides focusing on process versus product, practitioners may have more specific goals in mind for assessing school-age children's language development. To accomplish such goals, they use four types of assessments:

1. **Screenings** are brief assessments usually performed at the beginning of the school year (or another key developmental juncture) to help identify students who need extra assistance in certain areas.

2. **Diagnostic assessments** can be conducted any time during the school year to obtain an in-depth probe of a specific child's instructional needs. These assessments are typically used to identify the presence of a language disability.

3. **Progress-monitoring assessments** are conducted routinely (at least three times a year) to document a child's rate of improvement in an area and to monitor the efficacy of curricula and interventions.

4. **Outcome assessments** help determine the discrepancy between expected and observed outcomes in a particular area.

Assessment of Language Content

Researchers and clinicians can assess children's language content by analyzing spontaneously generated language samples and by using structured elicitation procedures. Standardized tests are also available for measuring school-age children's language content, including achievements in lexical meaning, abstract relational meaning, and figurative language.

Measurement of Lexical Meaning

Using language samples and elicitation procedures, researchers and clinicians can examine children's understanding of lexical meaning (Lund & Duchan, 1993). Lund and Duchan suggested the following procedure for analyzing language samples:

1. Examine transcripts for instances when the child used a word differently than an adult would use it (e.g., overextensions, underextensions, and incorrect referents).

2. Examine transcripts for gestures, pronouns, and indefinite and idiosyncratic terms that replace specific words, which may indicate that the child has a deficit in a particular class of meaning (e.g., verbs of motion, superordinate terms). Determine whether the deficit is in one class or multiple classes.

3. Examine transcripts for the absence of particular word classes, including noun modifiers and conjunctions.

Elicitation procedures for examining a child's lexical meaning include having a child define words (when you suspect he or she may be using them incorrectly) and playing games in which the child will need to use the word class of interest. For example, a Simon Says game might prompt children to use motion verbs, such as "Simon says leap forward; now kneel. . ."

Standardized tests that measure lexical meaning include the aforementioned Peabody Picture Vocabulary Test, third edition (PPVT–III; Dunn & Dunn, 1997) and fourth edition (PPVT–4; Dunn & Dunn, 2006), and the Test of Word Knowledge (TOWK; Wiig & Secord, 1992). We discussed the PPVT–III in Chapter 7 in the section on assessing preschoolers' language development. Of additional importance to school-age children and adolescents is that clinicians and researchers can continue to use the PPVT–III and PPVT–4 throughout adulthood. Recall that the PPVT is a norm-referenced measure of *receptive vocabulary,* or the words a person comprehends.

The TOWK is appropriate for children ages 5–17 years and is used to evaluate students' semantic and lexical knowledge through their ability to understand and use vocabulary. Compared to the PPVT, it provides a more comprehensive analysis of children's lexical abilities. Researchers and clinicians can use the TOWK as part of a complete diagnostic language battery. Level 1 of the assessment (for children ages 5–8 years) includes subtests that measure expressive vocabulary, word definitions, receptive vocabulary, and word opposites. An optional subtest for 5- to 8-year-olds measures synonyms. Level 2 of the assessment (for children ages 8–17 years) includes subtests that measure word definitions, multiple contexts, synonyms, and figurative language usage. Supplementary subtests cover word opposites, receptive vocabulary, expressive vocabulary, conjunctions, and transition words. Test developers also suggest that clinicians can use the TOWK as a resource for gifted and talented assessment to identify students who excel in semantic knowledge.

Measurement of Abstract Relational Meaning

Researchers and clinicians can also analyze children's understanding of abstract relational meaning by using language samples and elicitation procedures. With language samples, the researcher or clinician again examines language transcripts, this time paying particular attention to how children use relational terms such as prepositions. When children use relational terms, such as spatial prepositions (e.g., *among, between, through*), they understand not only something about the *properties* of an object but also something about the *state* of the object. Cognitive theorists would be particularly interested in children's use of such abstract relational terms.

Elicitation procedures can involve having the child follow directions, retell stories, and complete metalinguistic exercises. When having the child follow directions, the researcher or clinician can assess the child's comprehension of spatial prepositions (*Put the ball under the cup*) and dative relations (*Give the monkey the cat* vs. *Give the cat the monkey*).

In retelling stories, an examiner tells a child a story that features specific linguistic devices (e.g., time markers such as *first, second,* and *third*) to model how a story can be constructed using these features. Then, the child retells the story and the examiner listens for inclusion of the modeled features.

With metalinguistic exercises, the examiner presents the child with statements to reflect on, analyze, and interpret, such as the following (Lund & Duchan, 1993):

"John will go and Henry will go. Who will go?"

"John will go or Henry will go. Who will go?"

"John will go so Henry will go. Who will go?" (p. 262)

Measurement of Figurative Language

Because children may infrequently use figurative language in spontaneous speech, elicitation procedures are the best choice for assessing children's understanding of figurative language such as metaphors, idioms, and proverbs. To assess children's understanding of metaphors, researchers and clinicians can use an interview-style procedure in which they ask a child to first provide a literal meaning for a word and then ask the child to explain sentences in which words are used metaphorically.

An appropriate way to measure understanding of idioms is to use a picture selection task. In such a task, a child is asked to find a picture that matches an idiomatic expression. To measure older children's understanding of proverbs, the researcher or clinician can simply ask the child to explain the meaning of one or more proverbs (e.g., Explain to me the meaning behind "A stitch in time saves nine.").

CD VIDEO CLIP

To watch a 6-year-old participate in a study that examined understanding of metaphors involving verbs, see the CD video clip *Research 5.*

Assessment of Language Form

Assessment of language form involves measuring phonological and syntactic development. Some measurement procedures for these types of language development are described next.

Measurement of Phonological Development

To measure a school-age child's phonological development, clinicians can use a standardized assessment such as the Goldman–Fristoe Test of Articulation—2 (Goldman & Fristoe, 2000). This test is appropriate for children and adolescents through age 21 years. In this test, the examiner uses pictures and verbal cues to sample spontaneous and imitative sound production of consonants. The examiner can then determine whether the child or adolescent correctly produces specific speech sounds or sound sequences in different contexts (e.g., medial vs. final position of a word).

Measurement of Syntactic Development

To measure syntactic development in the school-age years and beyond, examiners can use language samples, elicitation procedures, and standardized measures. Language samples are useful for measuring advanced syntax. To do so, the researcher or clinician segments the transcript of spoken or written language into **communication units (C units)** or **terminable units (T units).** C units and T units both consist of an independent clause and any of its modifiers, such as a dependent clause. The difference between C units and T units is that C units are used for oral language analysis; they can include incomplete sentences and sentence fragments. T units are used to analyze written language transcripts (e.g., a written essay), and include only complete sentences. After a transcript is segmented into T or C units, the units are analyzed in various ways, such as calculating the mean length of the units in words or calculating the percentage of units containing dependent clauses. Simply counting the number of units a sample contains also provides an informative measure of *language productivity,* or the amount of language a child produces. The researcher or clinician who has collected a language sample might also be interested in examining the number and types of noun phrases, verb phrases, questions, and negation strategies a student uses in spoken or written language samples.

Elicitation procedures are also useful for examining advanced syntax, including complements, verb clauses, multiclause utterances, question forms, and negation. For example, presenting a student with improbable pictures is a good method for eliciting verb clauses because the student can tell you what is wrong with the picture (e.g., "The baby is holding an elephant!"). To elicit negative forms, the examiner can create the need for objects that are not present. For example, to elicit a negative form ("The pen doesn't work"), the examiner can present the student with a pen and paper and ask him or her to draw something. Other broken or non-functioning materials should also elicit negative forms.

One standardized test that measures syntactic development is the Test of Language Development—Intermediate, Third Edition (TOLD–I:3; Hammill & Newcomer, 1997). The TOLD–I:3 is appropriate for children ages 8 years through 12 years, 11 months. It is used to assess a student's understanding and meaningful use of spoken words as well as different aspects of grammar. The subtests of the TOLD–I:3 that measure syntax include Sentence Combining,

Word Ordering, and Grammatic Comprehension. The TOLD–I:3, like other standardized tests of language, is also used to identify students whose language skills are significantly depressed, which possibly indicates the presence of a language disorder.

Assessment of Language Use

Using language samples, researchers and clinicians can assess students' language use by measuring the extent to which students control conversational topics and produce appropriate and on-topic versus inappropriate and off-topic responses in a conversation. Justice and Kaderavek (2003) developed a coding system for examining discourse patterns between mothers and their preschoolers with language impairment; however, a researcher or clinician could adapt this system for school-age children and adolescents as well. See Table 8.5 for an explanation of the discourse codes, which could be used to examine a child's participation patterns in conversations.

DISCUSSION POINT

What are some other topics that could serve as prompts for a persuasive writing task?

One standardized assessment used to measure school-age children's language use abilities is the Test of Language Competence—Expanded edition (TLC–Expanded; Wiig & Secord, 1989). The following subtests of the TLC–Expanded are used to measure students' higher level language functions: Ambiguous Sentences, Listening Comprehension: Making Inferences, Oral Expression: Recreating Speech Acts, and Figurative Language. The TLC–Expanded also includes a supplemental memory subtest and a screening composite used to determine whether students would benefit from more in-depth testing. Level 1 of the test is appropriate for students between 5 and 9 years old, and Level 2 is appropriate for students between 10 and 18 years old. See Research Paradigms: *Assessment of Later Language Development* to read about a paradigm researchers use to assess development of later language acquisition, including language use.

TABLE 8.5
Coding System for Examining Control of Interaction in Discourse

Category and code	Description
NTO	*New topic:* A partner produces an utterance that introduces a new topic. The topic is considered new if it was not the focus of either partner's most recent utterance.
OTO	*Own topic:* A partner produces an utterance that maintains topic control following an own new topic (NTO) initiation or an extension of an established joint topic (JT).
PTO	*Partner topic:* One partner produces an utterance that is related to a preceding new topic (NTO) initiation or an own topic (OTO) continuation of the other partner. This situation represents joining in the topic of discourse by the new partner.
JT	*Joint topic:* A partner produces an utterance on the same topic as that of the partner's turn (PTO). The utterance may be brief or extended.
EXT	*Extension of topic:* A partner produces an utterance that extends the topic of his or her joint topic (JT).

Source: From "Topic Control During Shared Storybook Reading: Mothers and Their Children with Language Impairments," by L. M. Justice and J. N. Kaderavek, 2003, *Topics in Early Childhood Special Education, 23,* p. 142. Copyright 2003 by PRO-ED. Adapted with permission.

RESEARCH PARADIGMS

Assessment of Later Language Development

To assess later language development of syntax, semantics, and pragmatics, researchers can use written language measures in addition to spoken language measures. In one study, Nippold, Ward-Lonergan, and Fanning (2005) examined children's, adolescents', and adults' development in these areas by using a persuasive writing task. Participants handwrote a persuasive essay on the controversial topic of animals being trained to perform in circuses, then the researchers coded the essays for specific indicators of syntactic, semantic, and pragmatic development. These researchers suggested that the developmental information provided by the 11- to 24-year-old participants could serve as a starting point for establishing expected achievement levels in these areas of later language development. Nippold and colleagues also suggested that their research results may have implications for persons who experience difficulties with these areas of language, which are important for persuasive writing.

Later language development can also be assessed in the written modality.

(*Photo Source:* Scott Cunningham/ Merill.)

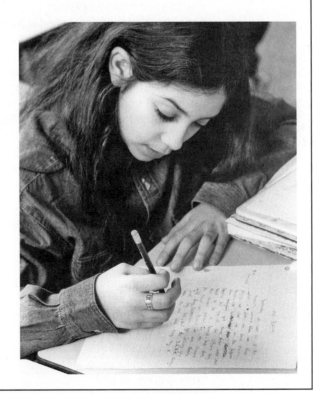

SUMMARY

We open this chapter with a discussion of the major language processes that differentiate school-age language development from earlier language development. These processes are the shifting sources of language input and the acquisition of metalinguistic competence. School-age children begin to gain increased language input from the written text and their metalinguistic competence improves as they engage in analyzing language as an object of attention, such as when they encounter figurative language.

In the second section, we describe important achievements in language content, form, and use in the school-age years and beyond. Specific achievements in language content include lexical development through direct instruction, contextual abstraction, and morphological analysis; understanding of multiple meanings; understanding of lexical and sentential ambiguity; and acquisition of a literate language style through the use of elaborated noun phrases, adverbs, conjunctions, and mental and linguistic verbs. Specific achievements in language form include the development of complex syntax, some of which is used mainly in the written modality; morphological forms, such as derivational prefixes and suffixes; and phonological forms, including morphophonemic changes and the use of stress and emphasis. Specific achievements in language use include functional flexibility; conversational abilities, such as detecting and repairing conversational breakdowns; and narrative development, including the use of expressive elaboration.

In the third section, we discuss how school-age children, adolescents, and adults differ in their individual language competencies, focusing on gender differences and contextual influences on language forms and use. Finally, we explore ways in which researchers and clinicians measure the development of language content, form, and use in the school-age years and beyond. In particular, we discuss the use of naturalistic language samples, elicitation procedures, and standardized tests to measure language development and competencies.

KEY TERMS

For online resources related to chapter content, including audio samples, valuable Web sites, suggested readings, and self-quizzes, please go to the Companion Website at http://www.prenhall.com/pence

9

Language Diversity

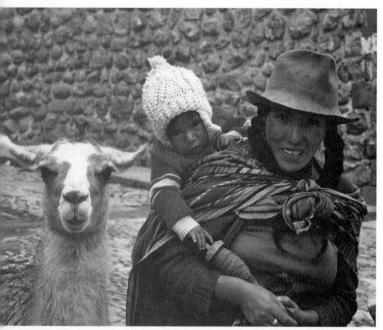

FOCUS QUESTIONS

In this chapter, we answer the following four questions:

1. What is the connection between language and culture?
2. How do languages evolve and change?
3. What are bilingualism and second language acquisition?
4. What are some prevailing theories of second language acquisition and their implications for practice?

Most people in the world acquire or learn more than one language during their lifetime (Grabe, 2002); in fact, an estimated 60–75% of the global population speaks more than one language (C. Baker, 2000). Multilingualism is even more prevalent in areas of the world where people in neighboring states speak different languages. For example, the European Union encourages multilingualism among its member states, specifically advocating that citizens learn two languages in addition to their native language. When people share a language, they have an important bond in common because language conveys more than the meanings behind individual words. With language comes history, tradition, and identity—in short, the culture of a group of people. In this chapter, we first discuss the connection between language and culture. Second, we examine the process of language change and evolution through dialectical variation, pidgins, and creoles. In the third section, we explore bilingualism and second language acquisition, and, finally, we examine some prevailing theories of second language acquisition and discuss their implications for practice.

WHAT IS THE CONNECTION BETWEEN LANGUAGE AND CULTURE?

The Interrelatedness of Language and Culture

Anthropologist Franz Boas viewed language as reflecting the conceptual ideas and forms of thinking characteristic of a culture (Lucy, 1992). Linguist and anthropologist Edward Sapir (1921) further stated that language does not exist apart from culture. These views expressing the interconnectedness between language and culture make sense on many levels. People learn about language through their culture (e.g., pragmatics such as interaction styles and speech registers) and about their culture through language (e.g., vocabulary to describe culturally specific phenomena).

The connection between language and culture is often evident in television shows and in interactions with other individuals, even those who speak the same language. Because the United States is a melting pot of cultures, Americans have borrowed words and phrases from many world cultures. Yiddish is one such example. Novelist and lecturer Michael Wex remarked on the National Public Radio program *Fresh Air* that despite the few fluent Yiddish speakers, many Yiddish words and expressions are commonly used in American English. Describing Yiddish words, Wex said,

> They convey something that the basic English translation doesn't have in it. . . . There's an emotional coloring that you just don't get. . . . Because so much of Yiddish life was devoted to dealing with frustration in a way that anticipated a lot of modern North American life, there's this open space for it to enter in and fill up those gaps that English, which was once a very polite language, just doesn't seem to have the words to fill. (Gross, 2005)

Accepting that language and culture are tied to each other seems natural, yet such acceptance raises the question "Which comes first?" One prominent view on the interrelatedness between language and culture is that from the time humans are born we are socialized both *through* the use of language and *to* the use of language (Schieffelin & Ochs, 1986). The ways in which we interact with infants and young children who are acquiring language provide a window into how we socialize other persons "through and to" language use.

Infant-Directed Speech

All cultures have specific ways of interacting with young language learners. In Western cultures, such as that in the United States, adults speak directly to infants from birth using a unique speech register called *infant-directed (ID) speech.* Noticeable characteristics of ID speech include a high overall pitch, exaggerated pitch contours, and slower tempos than those used in *adult-directed (AD) speech.* ID speech effectively attracts and maintains infants' attention, and infants seem to prefer it to AD speech (Cooper & Aslin, 1990; Fernald & Kuhl, 1987). In addition to eliciting attention, ID speech may facilitate language acquisition in several ways, such as clarifying vowels (Bernstein Ratner, 1986; Kuhl et al., 1997) and aiding acquisition of words (Fernald, 2000; Fernald & Mazzie, 1991; Golinkoff & Alioto, 1995). See Chapter 5 for more information on the role of ID speech in language acquisition.

Although incontrovertible evidence exists for this special speech register in many Western societies, Western ID speech is not universal. Evidence from southern working-class African Americans, Athapaskan Indians, Samoans, and Kaluli indicates that the simplifying characteristics of ID speech are not present in all cultures (Schieffelin & Ochs, 1986). Instead, Schieffelin and Ochs summarized that differences in the communicative interactions between adults and young children "socialize children into different cultural orientations toward communication, meaning, and the social status of children" (p. 174). For example, Athapaskan adults expect their children to repeat the adults' language without understanding the meaning behind it. Furthermore, rather than attempting to reformulate the underlying intentions of children's unintelligible utterances, Athapaskan adults provide a situational and culturally appropriate translation to familiarize children with conventional context-specific responses. In contrast, adults from African American, Samoan, and Kaluli cultures usually ignore unintelligible child speech rather than reformulate it or pursue the child's intentions. The ID speech of different cultures thus

DISCUSSION POINT
What might a culture's predominant style for interacting with infants tell us about that culture's perspective on early language development?

ranges in its **communicative accommodation** from highly child centered to highly situation centered.

The extent to which communicative accommodation leans toward the child-centered or situation-centered end of the continuum can vary according to the child's age as well. For instance, Kaluli and Samoan parents emphasize highly situation-centered communication throughout infancy and early childhood, whereas Mayan parents use situation-centered communication with young infants and child-centered communication with toddlers who are beginning to produce intelligible utterances.

HOW DO LANGUAGES EVOLVE AND CHANGE?

Dialects

Dialects are regional or social varieties of language that differ from one another in terms of their pronunciation, vocabulary, and grammar. In comparison, **accents** are varieties of language that differ solely in pronunciation. Dialects develop during a prolonged period in which people are separated by geographic barriers, such as mountains and rivers, or by social barriers, such as social-class differences. Almost all languages have dialects; therefore, everyone speaks some dialect, or variety, of a language. In general, people who speak different dialects of a language can understand one another. However, because of social-class differences, some dialects are held in higher esteem than other dialects are, and sometimes one particular dialect is considered the standard for a language. For example, Standard American English (SAE; also called General American English/GAE) has the highest status in the United States, as does Received Pronunciation (RP) in England.

American English Regional Dialects

American English regional dialects date to Colonial America, when people from different areas of the British Isles began to settle in different areas along the East Coast and then moved inland (Wolfram & Schilling-Estes, 2006). These early settlers brought geographically and regionally unique vocabulary and ways of speaking to the New World and began to incorporate and use vocabulary words from the Native American tribes in the areas where they settled. Several factors contributed to the creation and maintenance of American English regional dialects, including language contact, population movement, expanding transportation and communication networks, and shifting cultural centers (Wolfram & Schilling-Estes, 2006).

Language contact is the process whereby speakers of a language other than English shape the pronunciation, grammar, and vocabulary of English in the surrounding area. Examples include the Hispanic influences on English in areas bordering Mexico and the Native American influences on English in early American settlements (especially with respect to vocabulary).

Population movement, or the migration of persons from one dialect region to another, can affect the maintenance of a dialect in one of two ways. On the one

Dialects are regional or social varieties of language that differ from one another in their pronunciation, vocabulary, and grammar.

(*Photo Source:* Mark Scott/Getty Images Inc.—Taxi.)

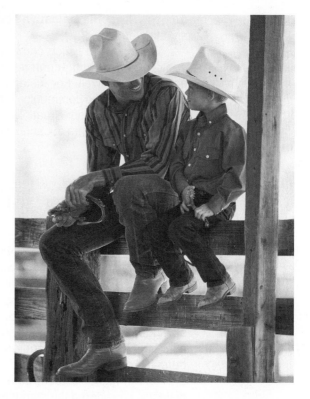

hand, the dialect may begin to vanish in a region that receives an influx of persons from other areas. Such is the case currently for some southern cities: for example, Atlanta, GA, Raleigh–Durham, and Charlotte, NC. On the other hand, the dialect may become more pronounced in an area where the cultural and regional identity is strong. For example, the term *fixin'*, which indicates an immediate future action, and the use of double modals, such as *might could* and *used to could,* remain acceptable grammatical constructions in southern U.S. dialects.

Expanding transportation and communication networks can also affect a regional dialect in the same two ways: It may vanish, or it may become more pronounced. Such networks have an impact on once-isolated regions, such as small islands along the eastern seaboard of the United States, which now host tourists from many dialect regions of the country.

Shifting cultural centers also influence dialect change in the United States. Suburban areas are now becoming influential in the development of dialects, just as large urban areas once were. One example of how a large nonurban cultural center can give life to a new regional variety is California English, whose speakers introduced such words as *dude* and *awesome,* as well as the conversational filler *like.*

Southern Dialects. Southern dialects are among the more recognizable varieties of English (see Figure 9.1, which illustrates the major dialect areas of the United States). Specific southern dialects include Appalachian English, Smoky Mountain

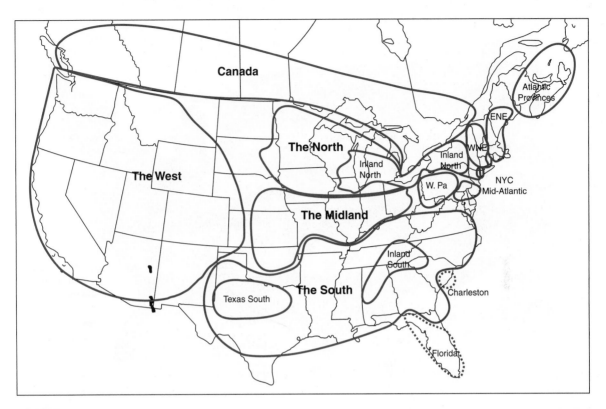

FIGURE 9.1
Dialect map of the United States.

ENE = Eastern New England; WNE = Western New England.
Source: From "Language Evolution or Dying Traditions? The State of American Dialects," by W. Wolfram and N. Schilling-Estes, in
American Voices: How Dialects Differ from Coast to Coast (p. 1), edited by W. Wolfram and B. Ward, 2006, Malden, MA: Blackwell.
Copyright 2006 by Blackwell Publishing. Reprinted with permission.

dialect, Charleston dialect, Texas English, New Orleans dialect, and Memphis dialect, although the general dialect of the region is Southern American dialect. Southern American dialect differs in its phonology, grammar, and lexicon from other dialects in several ways (Bailey & Tillery, 2006). For example, speakers of Southern American dialect pronounce the vowels /ɛ/ and /ɪ/ the same, which means that *pin* and *pen* sound identical (like *pin*). Speakers also use a *monophthong,* or pure vowel sound, in place of a diphthong at the ends of words and prior to voiced consonants such as /d/ and /z/, pronouncing /raɪd/ ("ride") as /raːd/ ("raaad") and /raɪz/ ("rise") as /raːz/ ("raaaz").

Southern dialects have unique grammatical constructions as well. Some speakers use the contraction *y'all* as a second-person plural pronoun and further use the phrase *all y'all* specifically to acknowledge each individual in a group, as in the sentences *I encourage y'all to visit next summer. I can't wait to see all y'all again.* As mentioned previously, some speakers of southern dialects also use multiple modals (*might could, might should, might should oughta*) and the construction *fixin' to,* which indicates an immediate future action, as in *I'm fixin' to call your mother.*

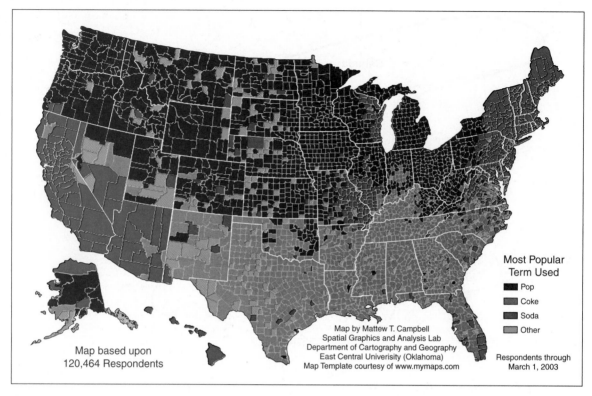

FIGURE 9.2

Names for carbonated beverages by U.S. county.

Source: From "Generic Names for Soft Drinks by County" [Map], by M. T. Campbell and G. Plumb, in *The Great Pop vs. Soda Controversy,* edited by A. McConchie, n.d. Copyright by Matthew T. Campbell and Greg Plumb. Reprinted with permission. Retrieved September 26, 2006, from http://www.popvssoda.com/countystats/total-county.html

    Vocabulary in southern dialects is also distinct. To illustrate, consider the results of McConchie's (n.d.) and Campbell and Plumb's (n.d.) surveys: these showed that speakers of southern dialects often use the word *Coke* to refer to a sweetened carbonated beverage (see Figure 9.2) and the word *sub* to refer to the type of sandwich served on a roll with meats, cheese, lettuce, tomato, and so forth (see Figure 9.3).

Northern Dialects.   Dialects of the North include Boston dialect, Maine dialect, Pittsburgh dialect, New York dialect, Philadelphia dialect, and Canadian English. Distinctive phonological features of northern dialects include dropping postvocalic *r* sounds, as in "cah" for *car* and "yahd" for *yard* (Roberts, Nagy, & Boberg, 2006). Although grammar in northern dialects is not significantly different from that of other regions, some dialects use combinations such as *you all, you guys, youse,* or *y'uns* for the second-person plural pronoun, and Philadelphians specifically eliminate the object of the preposition *with* ("Are you coming with?") (Newman, 2006; Salvucci, 2006). Vocabulary in northern dialects includes such words as *tonic* (Fitzpatrick, 2006) and *soda* (Campbell & Plumb, n.d.) for sweetened carbonated

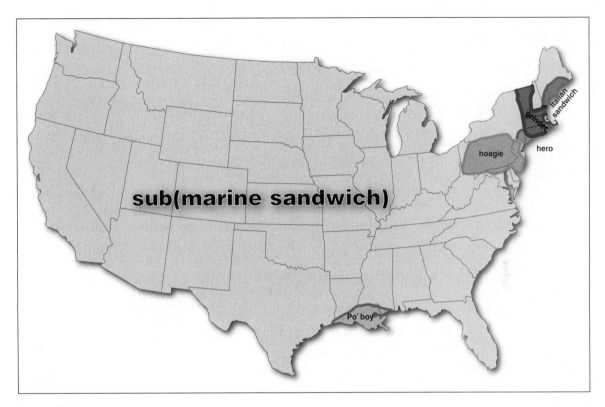

FIGURE 9.3

Sub, grinder, hoagie, or hero?

Source: From "American Dialects," by B. Vaux, in *Let's Go USA 2004,* edited by J. Todd, 2004, New York: St. Martin's Press. Copyright 2004 by Bert Vaux. Reprinted with permission.

beverages. People of northern dialect regions are also as likely to use the words *grinder, hoagie,* and *hero* as *sub* (see Figure 9.3).

Midwestern Dialects.   Persons from areas such as Chicago, IL, Ohio, St. Louis, MO, and Michigan speak midwestern dialects. These dialects, which some people erroneously claim to be accent free or most typical of a "standard" American dialect, actually have phonological, grammatical, and lexical features that differentiate them from other regional dialects. With respect to phonology, midwestern dialects tend to merge the /o/ and /ɔ/ vowel sounds (e.g., *Don–Dawn, hot–caught, dollar–taller, sock–talk*) into a single vowel, rendering the words "Don" and "Dawn" virtually indistinguishable, as shown in Figure 9.4 (W. Labov, Ash, & Boberg, 2005). In general, speech in the western Pennsylvania area demonstrates a consistent merging of these vowels, speech in the St. Louis corridor maintains the distinction between these two vowels, and speech in most of the midwestern region has vowels that are perceptually similar in most contexts. For other vowel sounds, rather than merging two sounds, speakers of midwestern dialects pronounce vowels with the tongue in a different place in the mouth than that in other dialects. This phenomenon is called the *Northern Cities Shift*

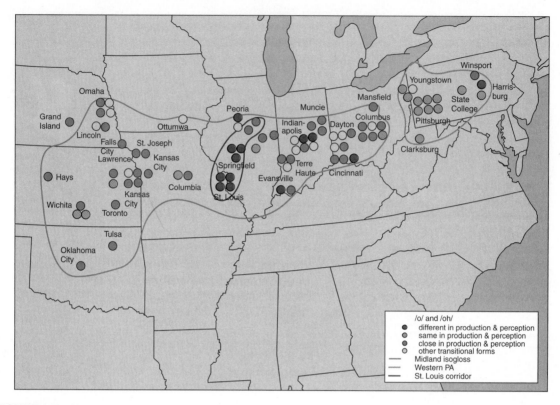

FIGURE 9.4
The merging of /o/ and /ɔ/ (oh) in midwestern English.

Source: From *The Atlas of North American English* (p. 264), by W. Labov, S. Ash, and C. Boberg, 2005, New York: Mouton/de Gruyter. Copyright 2005 by Mouton/de Gruyter. Reprinted with permission.

(NCS) because of the predominance of this pattern in large cities in the Midwest (Gordon, 2006; W. Labov et al., 2005). Figure 9.5 illustrates the NCS, whereby, for example, the vowel in the words *bit* and *bet* is pronounced like the vowel in *but*.

Midwestern dialect grammatical features include the *need/want/like + past participle* construction. For example, a mother leaving her young son with a babysitter for the evening might say "I'm so sorry that I have to run. Jeremy's diaper <u>needs changed</u>. Buster <u>wants fed</u> and if he jumps up on your lap, he <u>likes scratched</u> behind the ears."

In the Midwest, *pop* is the prevalent term for sweetened carbonated beverages (Campbell & Plumb, n.d.) and *sub* is the most common sandwich term, although in some areas the word *hoagie* is also used (see Figure 9.3).

Western Dialects. Because the western United States was settled more recently than other regions of the country were, the western dialect area remains largely undefined (Conn, 2006; W. Labov et al., 2005). In some respects, western dialects share features with their northern and southern counterparts. Phonologically, many western dialects have a single vowel for the words *caught* and *cot,* as do midwestern dialects. Some western dialects, particularly in California, exhibit *fronted back vowels,* so that *totally* sounds like "tewtally" and *dude* sounds like "diwd" (Conn, 2006).

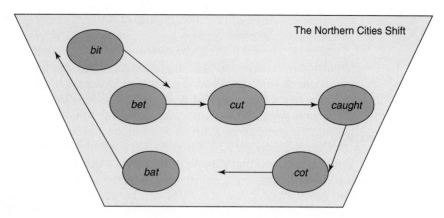

FIGURE 9.5
Vowel changes in the Northern Cities Shift.

Source: From "Straight Talking from the Heartland (Midwest)," by M. J. Gordon, in *American Voices: How Dialects Differ from Coast to Coast* (p. 109), edited by W. Wolfram and B. Ward, 2006, Malden, MA: Blackwell. Copyright 2006 by Blackwell Publishing. Reprinted with permission.

With regard to vocabulary, western dialects are divided on the *pop–soda–Coke* debate. Speakers of western dialects in the Northwest use the term *pop,* whereas speakers of western dialects in the Southwest use the term *soda.* The word *sub* is the most popular sandwich term in the West, and people use *hoagie* less often. People from the Northwest (Washington, Oregon) also use the word *coast* to refer to the beach.

American English Sociocultural Dialects

Sociocultural dialects differ from geographical dialects of the West, Midwest, North, and South in that they transcend region. Instead, persons from certain socioeconomic classes and cultural orientations speak these dialects. Three examples of sociocultural dialects are African American Vernacular English, Chicano English, and Jewish English.

African American Vernacular English (AAVE) comprises the English dialects many slave descendants speak. AAVE dialects emerged during the period when persons from Africa arrived in the United States as slaves. Slaves speaking the same African languages were often separated to prevent uprisings. In addition, once the slaves arrived in the United States, they were not permitted to attend schools. As a consequence of these practices, African Americans began to form *pidgins* (discussed later in the chapter), which were combinations of their African languages and the European languages they were exposed to, so that they could communicate with their owners and with other slaves.

AAVE contains many distinct phonological and grammatical regularities (e.g., Baugh, 2006; W. Labov, 1998). Speakers may reduce consonant clusters, so that *old* becomes *ol',* *west* becomes *wes',* and *kind* becomes *kin'.* Speakers of AAVE may also delete the suffix *-s*—whereby *50 cents* becomes *50 cent,* and *She drives* becomes *She drive*—and the possessive suffix 's—so that *my sister's car* becomes *my sister car.* Another common feature of AAVE dialects is phonological inversion, whereby *ask* becomes *aks.*

Special grammatical constructions in AAVE include the distinction between habitual and temporary forms of the present progressive and copula *be.* For example, the sentence *Anita be working* is habitual, meaning Anita works on a regular basis. In comparison, the sentence *Anita working* is temporary, meaning Anita is working at the time. Another grammatical construction that AAVE speakers sometimes use is syntactic alternation, such as "How much it is?"

Chicano English (ChE) is a dialect spoken in Hispanic communities in which Spanish is not normally the first language or dominant language of the persons living there. In addition to being used in communities such as the Los Angeles area and areas close to the U.S.–Mexican border, ChE has been documented in non-Spanish-speaking midwestern communities (Frazer, 1996). Some features of ChE include final /z/ devoicing in words such as *lies* and *toys,* using a tense-vowel /i/ in place of its lax counterpart in words ending in *-ing* (i.e., saying /ɪŋ/ instead of /ɪŋ/), and using intonation patterns characteristic of Spanish.

The Jewish English dialect is another type of sociocultural dialect. This dialect has characteristics of both the Yiddish and the Hebrew languages. Jewish English pronunciation includes a hard *g* sound in words like *singer* (sounds like *finger*), overaspiration of /t/ sounds, and a loud, exaggerated intonation and fast rate of speech (Bernstein, 2006). Many Jewish English vocabulary words have become a part of the mainstream American culture as well, including *schlep, bagel, schmooze, klutz,* and *kosher.*

DISCUSSION POINT

Can you think of some additional phonological, grammatical, and lexical features that characterize the dialect or dialects you speak?

Pidgins

A *pidgin* is a simplified type of language that develops when speakers who do not share a common language come into prolonged contact. Pidgins have no native speakers; instead, people use them as a second language, particularly when they are conducting business with one another (Southerland, 1997). Pidgins typically use the lexicon of the more dominant of the two languages and the phonology and syntactic structure of the less dominant language, as is the case for the Hawaiian Pigdin English that Philippine laborers in Hawaii spoke prior to the 1930s (Southerland, 1997). Hawaiian Pidgin English included lexical items of the more dominant language (English) and syntactic structure of the less dominant language (Philippine languages)—for example, by omitting the copula *to be* verb when describing a permanent attribute of a person or an object (e.g., "Da man tall"; "Da lady short").

Creoles

Pidgins become *creoles* when speakers pass them down through generations as a first language. Creoles continue to evolve and become more elaborate and stable with each new generation of native speakers. Some creoles remain nondominant in their community, whereas other creoles gain status as official languages. See Multicultural Focus: *Nicaraguan Sign Language* for a discussion of how Nicaraguan Sign Language evolved among a group of people who did not share a common language.

MULTICULTURAL FOCUS

Nicaraguan Sign Language

The emergence of Nicaraguan Sign Language since the 1970s has presented a unique opportunity to observe the process of language creation and evolution. Before the 1970s, individuals in Nicaragua who were Deaf had little contact with one another because of the lack of a unifying national educational system. When individuals who were Deaf were finally exposed to one another in the context of schools, they began to form a true Deaf community. Because children and adolescents had no common language, to communicate with one another they began to use gestures coupled with any home signs they had. These simple language systems, or *pidgins,* evolved into more complex creoles after new cohorts of children began signing with their older peers.

Evidence that Nicaraguan Sign Language is evolving into an increasingly more complex language comes in many forms. One way in which researchers can study this evolution is by examining the spatial modulations that speakers make. *Spatial modulations* are grammatical elements that appear in all sign and spoken languages and perform functions such as indicating number, location, time, and the subject or object of a verb (Senghas & Coppola, 2001). Senghas and Coppola found that newer cohorts of Nicaraguan Sign Language speakers use and understand spatial modulations in ways that earlier users of the language do not. For example, newer cohorts of speakers use spatial modulations to indicate shared reference, whereas their older counterparts do not. Thus, as more generations of children learn Nicaraguan Sign Language, the grammatical specificity and precision of the language improves. Such research provides evidence for the creative and transformational nature of human language, and demonstrates the notable role that children can play in language creation.

DISCUSSION POINT

Which language development theory could account for the creation of Nicaraguan Sign Language and how?

WHAT ARE BILINGUALISM AND SECOND LANGUAGE ACQUISITION?

According to the 2000 U.S. Census, 17.9% of people aged 5 years and older (46,951,595 people) speak a language other than English at home. Some of these people are also proficient in English, perhaps because they learned the two or more languages simultaneously or began to learn an additional language within a few years of being born. Other people may have learned English as a second language in school in the United States or as a foreign language in school in another country. Whatever the case, many people living in the United States acquire two or more languages during their lifetime. The generic term for this diverse group of persons is **dual language learners** (Genesee, Paradis, & Crago, 2004). In this section of the chapter, we describe the difference between bilingualism and second language acquisition, and we explore research on specific varieties of the two.

Many children learn more than one language from birth.

(*Photo Source:* Pearson Learning Photo Studio.)

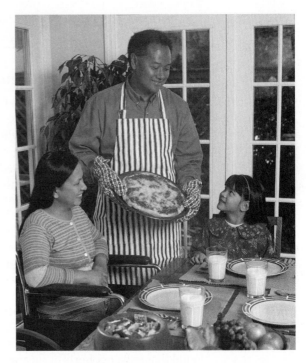

Bilingualism

Bilingualism is a term that describes the process whereby children essentially acquire *two* first languages. Many young children around the world acquire *more than two* first languages. The term used to describe this process is *multilingualism*. However, for the sake of simplicity, in this text we use the more common term *bilingualism* to describe children who acquire two or more first languages. Some children acquire two or more first languages from birth, whereas other children acquire them sequentially.

Simultaneous Bilingualism

With *simultaneous bilingualism,* the child acquires two or more languages from birth, or simultaneously. Simultaneous bilingual children usually receive language input in two or more forms from their parents, grandparents, other close relatives, or child care providers. Simultaneous bilingualism occurs in one of two contexts: The child is part of a majority ethnolinguistic community, or he or she is part of a minority ethnolinguistic community (Genesee et al., 2004). Bilingual children from these two types of communities may experience differential levels of success at acquiring and maintaining proficiency with their two first languages.

A **majority ethnolinguistic community** is a group that speaks a language that the majority of people in an area (e.g., country, state, province) value and assign high social status. The language that the majority ethnolinguistic community speaks may be an official language in the community, or it may be the unofficial standard in the community. In general, persons from a majority ethnolinguistic community share cultural and ethnic backgrounds. Examples of majority ethnolinguistic communities include Standard American English (SAE; also called *General American English,* or GAE), speakers in the United States, French speakers in France, and German speakers in Germany.

One example of simultaneous bilingualism in a majority ethnolinguistic community would be a young child acquiring both English and French in Montreal, Canada. In Montreal, both English-speaking and French-speaking cultural groups are valued by people in the community. Children learning both French and English simultaneously in Montreal would likely acquire and maintain equal proficiency with both languages because these children would have the opportunity to use both languages in school, at home, and in the community at such places as the grocery store and the doctor's office.

In contrast to a majority ethnolinguistic community, a **minority ethnolinguistic community** is a group that speaks a language that few people in the community speak or value. Languages that people in minority ethnolinguistic communities speak may have lower social status and may receive little or no institutional support. Examples of minority ethnolinguistic communities include Japanese speakers in the United States and French speakers in Germany.

Some children who are simultaneous bilingual individuals in a minority ethnolinguistic community may experience setbacks in acquiring or maintaining the minority language of the community. For instance, in the case of a German–English bilingual family in the United States, the child may hear and speak German only in the context of the home and not in the community, in child care, or in other situations. Without German language input from multiple sources in multiple contexts, the child will most likely begin to use the majority language, English, at the expense of the minority language, German. Shifting to the majority language is common among bilingual children in minority ethnolinguistic communities, especially when they enter formal schooling.

Other children who are simultaneous bilingual individuals in minority ethnolinguistic communities may have more success at maintaining the minority language. For example, although Spanish–English bilingual children in Southern California use English in school, they likely use Spanish at home and in their community, where other Spanish speakers live. Support from the other people in the minority ethnolinguistic community should increase the chances that the children will maintain their bilingualism throughout adulthood.

Sequential Bilingualism

Sequential bilingualism is similar to simultaneous bilingualism in that the child acquires two first languages. The difference is that the child learns his or her two first languages in succession, usually within the first 3 years of life, before developing proficiency with only one of the languages. Children may acquire two or more languages sequentially rather than simultaneously for two reasons. First, some parents prefer to use just one language from birth and wait to introduce an additional language. A second reason is because input from one language may not be available directly after birth. For example, the child may start to attend child care with a provider who speaks a different language, or the child's grandparents, who speak a different language, may move to the area after the child has begun to acquire one language. Children who acquire two or more languages sequentially experience the same kinds of advantages and setbacks as those experienced by children who acquire multiple languages simultaneously, depending on their status in a majority or minority ethnolinguistic community.

Two Systems or One?

Researchers disagree as to whether bilingual children have two separate language systems from the start or whether they begin with a single language system that eventually splits into two. Volterra and Taeschner (1978) proposed that bilingual children begin with a single language system that combines lexical items from both languages they are acquiring. Next, these children begin to differentiate between lexical items in the two languages but use a single grammatical system. Finally, between ages 3 and 3.5 years, the children begin to separate both the lexical and the grammatical systems of the two languages. According to this **unitary language system hypothesis**, then, children are not bilingual until they successfully differentiate between the two languages.

An opposing viewpoint is that bilingual children establish two separate language systems from the outset of language acquisition (Genesee, 1989; Genesee, Nicoladis, & Paradis, 1995). Unlike the unitary language system hypothesis, the **dual language system hypothesis** does not presuppose that children move through stages whereby they eventually differentiate between two languages.

Each hypothesis offers different predictions about how bilingual children's phonology, grammar, and vocabulary should develop. As a result, research into this controversy continues. Genessee and colleagues (2004) suggested that if the unitary language system hypothesis were correct, children would frequently mix words and phrases from both languages without considering the language context or their conversational partners. They would also mix grammatical rules from their two languages, and, most important, their language development would slow to a detrimental pace while they worked to differentiate their two languages.

Research results thus far favor the dual language system hypothesis. For example, a study of 24-month-old German–English bilingual toddlers revealed that their vocabulary size was not inferior to the vocabulary sizes of their monolingual English and monolingual German counterparts (Junker & Stockman, 2002). Furthermore, nearly half the bilingual toddlers' vocabulary was present in both German and English, which demonstrated that early language separation is possible.

In a previous investigation, other researchers had similar findings. In this study, bilingual and monolingual infants were observed. The two groups exhibited similar ages of onset for canonical babbling and used similar amounts of well-formed syllables and vowel-like sounds. These similarities applied to infants from middle and low socioeconomic status and to full-term and premature babies (Oller, Eilers, Urbano, & Cobo-Lewis, 1997).

In a separate study in which researchers examined bilingual acquisition across two modalities, three children acquiring Langues des Signes Québécoise (a sign language) and French, and three children acquiring French and English achieved their early linguistic milestones in each of their languages at the same time and similarly to monolingual children. From the time these bilingual children uttered

DISCUSSION POINT

Would proponents of the unitary language system hypothesis encourage simultaneous bilingualism? Why or why not?

their first words or used their first signs, they also produced a substantial number of semantically corresponding words in each of their two languages, which demonstrated language separation from an early age. Another way the bilingual children demonstrated language separation was by modifying their language choices depending on the listener (Petitto, Katerelos et al., 2001).

Code Switching

A common phenomenon among bilingual individuals is *code switching,* or *code mixing.* In this process, speakers who have more than one language alternate between the languages. When the alternation occurs within a single utterance, it is called **intrautterance mixing** (or within one sentence, *intrasentential mixing*). When the alternation occurs between utterances, it is called **interutterance mixing** (or between sentences, it is called *intersentential mixing*). When engaging in code switching, bilingual persons may mix smaller units of language, such as phonemes, inflectional morphemes, and lexical items, or they may mix larger items such as phrases and clauses. Children tend to use interutterance mixing more often than intrautterance mixing, especially in the one-word and two-word stages of development (Genesee et al., 2004). This pattern shifts as children develop because as utterances increase in length and grammatical complexity, children have more opportunities to engage in intrautterance mixing. See Table 9.1 for examples of code switching involving different elements of language.

Bilingual children may engage in code switching for three main reasons. One is that children code switch to fill in lexical or grammatical gaps. Evidence for such code switching comes in at least two forms (Genesee et al., 2004). First, children tend to code switch more often while using their less proficient language. Thus, they may code switch to draw on the strengths in their more proficient language when they lack a grammatical construction or lexical item in their less proficient

TABLE 9.1
Zentella's (1997) Examples of Bilingual Code Switching in Spanish and English

Mixed element of language	Example	Translation[a]	Page no. in Zentella (1997)
Phoneme	"*he*"	/xi/, like the *ch* sound in *Bach*	291
Lexical item	"It's already full, *mira.*"	"look"	119
Object noun phrase	*Tú estás metiendo* your big mouth."	"You're butting in"	118
Subject noun phrase	"*Tiene dos* strings, una chiringa."	"It has two"	118
Independent clause with coordinating conjunction	"My father took him to the ASPCA *y lo mataron.*"	"and they killed him"	118
Subordinate clause without subordinate conjunction	"Because *yo lo dije.*"	"I said it"	118

[a] Translation is of the italicized element in the Example column.

language. Second, children tend to code switch more when they do not know a translation equivalent for a word, no matter whether they are using their more proficient or less proficient language.

DISCUSSION POINT

How can you be sure that code switching is not evidence for the unitary language system hypothesis and that children who code switch are not mistakenly treating two languages as one?

A second reason bilingual children may code switch is for pragmatic effect (Genesee et al., 2004). For example, children may code switch to emphasize the importance of what they are saying, to convey emotion, or to quote what someone else said in another language.

Third, and finally, bilingual children may engage in code switching according to the social norms of their community. For instance, certain communities may engage in code switching to demonstrate their belonging to two cultures. Children learn to follow the code-switching patterns of the adults who surround them—for example, by engaging in code switching more often in casual and informal situations than in public and formal contexts.

Second Language Acquisition

Second language acquisition (SLA), or L2 acquisition, is the process by which children who have already established a solid foundation in their first language (L1) learn an additional language. Second language acquisition usually takes place in the context of a school, either as the majority language for a particular community or as a foreign language. As with bilingualism, success at acquiring a second language and maintaining an L1 or L2 depends on a number of factors, including whether an individual is part of a majority ethnolinguistic community or a minority ethnolinguistic community.

Interlanguage

During the process of L2 acquisition, speakers create a language system called an **interlanguage**. The interlanguage includes elements of the L1 and the L2, as well as elements found in neither of the two languages (Gass & Selinker, 2001). For example, evidence of L1 phonology and syntax in the L2 can often be seen (see Table 9.2). Depending on a person's exposure to and education in the L2, linguistic forms of the interlanguage may stabilize with time. **Language stabilization** occurs once the interlanguage stops evolving and L2 learners reach a plateau in their language development. Gass and Selinker (2001) cautioned that because of a lack of research on the extent to which L2 learners experience temporary or permanent plateaus in their development, practitioners should avoid using the term **language fossilization**, which means

> to become permanently established in the interlanguage of a second language learner in a form that is deviant from the target-language norm and that continues to appear in performance regardless of further exposure to the target language. (p. 12)

Regardless of whether an L2 learner stabilizes in his or her development, considering the notion of interlanguage is still important in order to understand the process by which L2 learners transition to a new system, including their potential struggles and errors. See Research Paradigms: *Methods for Studying Second Language Learning* for an overview of several methods for investigating L2 learning.

TABLE 9.2

Examples of L1 Influences on the L2

L1	L2	Example	Explanation
French	English	"I have ([aev]) no money."	French does not have the phoneme /h/, so the interlanguage of many speakers does not include it.
German	English	"I have ([haef]) no money."	German changes the /v/ in a syllable-final position to /f/, so the interlanguage of many speakers includes this feature.
English	Spanish	"Caro" ([karo]) "Carro" ([karo])	English has neither the tapped /r/ sound nor the trilled /r/ sound that Spanish has, so speakers usually substitute /r/.
German	English	"I bring not the children."	German places negative markers after the verb in the main clause of the sentence.
Italian	English	"How many years you have?"	Some languages (such as Spanish and Italian) describe age in terms of "how many years one has" instead of "how old one is."

L1 = first language; L2 = second language.

Attitudes and Policies Regarding Dual Language Instruction

Dual language instruction has been an important consideration throughout history. In ancient times, when written materials were scarce, students who wanted to read widely had to learn more than a single language (Lessow-Hurley, 1990). Ancient societies thus valued and endorsed dual language instruction. In later times, dual language instruction became important for religious purposes. For example, Latin remained the language of worship for Catholics, and Hebrew persisted as the language of worship for Jews, well after people ceased to use these languages in their homes and communities. In more modern times, dual language instruction has endured in most areas of the world, especially in countries with official bilingualism, such as Canada, Israel, and Belgium.

The United States, too, has a history of changing attitudes and policies regarding dual language instruction (Lessow-Hurley, 1990). For example, in the 19th century, Native American tribes often provided dual language instruction to their students. German communities in the Midwest also instituted dual language programs with success and support until the onset of World War I, when such programs began to collapse around the country as a result of intense feelings of nationalism. Consequently, dual language programs were virtually nonexistent between World

RESEARCH PARADIGMS

Methods for Studying Second Language Learning

As with measuring L1 acquisition, researchers who study L2 acquisition can measure productive language competence in qualitative ways, such as with naturalistic observations, and in quantitative ways, such as with normative tests and measures. Performance data can be elicited from L2 learners in at least a dozen ways, as summarized by Larsen-Freeman and Long (1991, pp. 27–30):

1. *Reading aloud:* Participants read aloud word lists, sentences, or passages containing sounds under investigation.
2. *Structured exercises:* Participants perform grammatical manipulations by completing fill-in-the-blank, sentence-rewrite, sentence-combining, or multiple-choice activities that contain the morphemes or syntactic patterns under investigation.
3. *Completion task:* Participants hear or read the beginning of a sentence and then complete the sentence in their own words.
4. *Elicited imitation:* Participants hear sentences containing the structure under investigation and then must repeat or reconstruct the sentence.
5. *Elicited translation:* Participants translate sentences from their L1 into their L2.
6. *Guided composition:* Participants tell a story or write a composition on the basis of a set of stimuli, such as pictures.
7. *Question and answer (with stimulus):* Participants look at pictures and then answer questions that elicit particular target forms.
8. *Reconstruction:* Participants read, listen to, or watch a story and then must retell the story in their own words.
9. *Communication games:* Participants play a game, sometimes with a native speaker. They may use materials designed to elicit particular language forms.
10. *Role-play:* Participants engage in a role-play with the researcher that focuses on target speech acts.
11. *Oral interview:* Researchers orally interview a participant. They may constrain the interview topic to elicit a particular structure or may allow the participant to choose the topic of conversation.
12. *Free composition:* The participant writes a composition on a given topic.

DISCUSSION POINT

What additional approaches could be used to gather language data from L2 learners?

War I and World War II. Not until the advent of the cold war and the civil rights movement did dual language instruction regain importance in the United States, although it remains controversial in many communities and school systems.

English as a Second Language

Learning *English as a second language* (ESL) is when a person who speaks *a first language* other than English then learns English in the context of an English-speaking country, such as England or the United States. Sometimes people refer

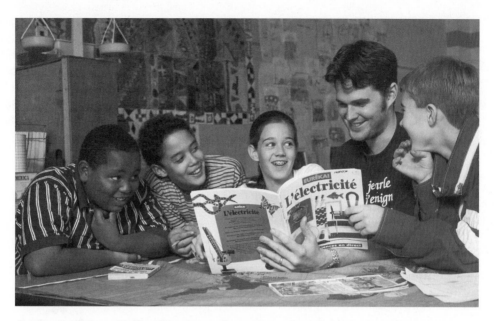

Some schools have dual language instruction programs in which students are schooled in two or more languages throughout the day.

(*Photo Source:* Billy E. Barnes/PhotoEdit Inc.)

to learning *English as an additional language* (EAL) when a person who speaks *two or more languages* subsequently learns English. However, many times the term *ESL* is used generically to describe either situation.

In the 2002–2003 school year, schools provided services to 4 million students learning ESL (8% of all students) in the United States. California and Texas reported the largest number of students receiving services (26% of students in California; 15% of students in Texas; U.S. Department of Education, National Center for Education Statistics, 2005). Current public policy initiatives that support teaching ESL include the No Child Left Behind Act, through which standards were developed and implemented to ensure success for children with limited English proficiency in the United States. A second public policy initiative is Title III, which is administered by the Office of English Language Acquisition, Language Enhancement and Academic Achievement for Limited English Proficient Students (OELA). Title III provides funding to states to implement language programs and scientifically based and effective professional development to help teachers provide effective ESL instruction. Under Title III, states may decide on the specific type of education program they want to implement, including the option to implement bilingual or dual language programs.

When children who have limited or no English proficiency arrive in classrooms where English is the language of instruction, they usually progress through four early stages in their L2 development (Tabors, 1997, cited in Genesee et al., 2004). In the first stage, the **home language stage**, children use their home language (L1) in the classroom with other children and adults. Children generally do not persist in using this language for long because they soon realize that doing so does not promote successful communication with other people.

In the second stage, the **nonverbal period**, children produce little to no language as they begin to acquire their L2 receptively. Some children in the nonverbal period use gestures, such as pointing, to communicate until they have acquired a sufficient number of words in their L2. Older children remain in the nonverbal period from a few weeks to a few months, but younger children usually remain nonverbal for longer periods.

In the third stage, the period of **telegraphic and formulaic use**, children begin to imitate other people, to use single words to label items, and to use simple phrases that

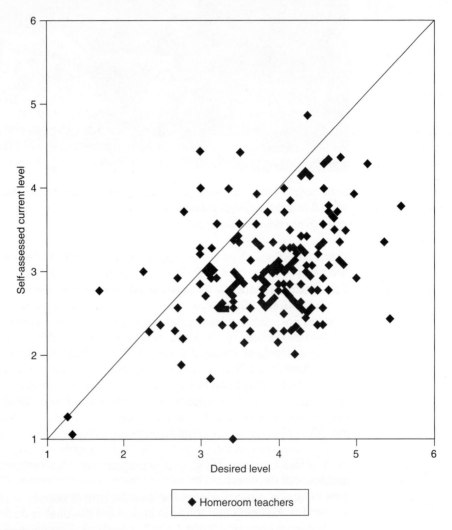

FIGURE 9.6
Differences in teachers' current and desired levels of English proficiency in Korea, Taiwan, and Japan.

Source: From "What Level of English Proficiency Do Elementary School Teachers Need to Attain to Teach EFL? Case Studies from Korea, Taiwan, and Japan," by Y. G. Butler, 2004, *TESOL Quarterly, 38,* p. 260. Copyright 2004 by Teachers of English to Speakers of Other Languages, Inc. Reprinted with permission.

they memorize. During this period, although children are producing language, they can not create sentences for a wide variety of communicative functions. Rather, they can express a limited variety of functions, such as requesting ("Please"), negating ("No, I don't know"), affirming ("Yes"), and commenting ("Very good"), among others.

In the fourth stage, the period of **language productivity**, children are not yet proficient speakers of their L2; however, their communicative repertoire continues to expand. During this stage, children begin to create simple S–V–O (subject–verb–object) sentences, and they rely heavily on the **general all-purpose verbs**, or *GAP verbs, make, do,* and *go.* For example, preschoolers learning ESL may say "I make picture," "I do that too," or "I go home."

English as a Foreign Language

English as a foreign language (EFL) differs from ESL in that children, adolescents, and adults learn English in a non-English-speaking country. Persons learning EFL have a number of reasons for doing so, including establishing oral proficiency in order to engage in business transactions with English-speaking counterparts and establishing grammatical proficiency to increase their chances of being accepted into an English-speaking institution of higher learning. In some countries, native English speakers are employed as EFL teachers, but many teachers have learned EFL themselves. Mixed opinions surround decisions to hire nonnative English speakers as EFL teachers.

To gauge the amount of discrepancy that exists between EFL teachers' perceived competence in English and their desired level of competence, Butler (2004) surveyed 522 teachers from Korea, Taiwan, and Japan. Her findings revealed that most teachers' current perceived level of competence was lower than their desired level. In Figure 9.6, such teachers are represented as dots *below* the diagonal line, and most of the EFL teachers fall into this category. The discrepancy between perceived English competence and desired competence can pose problems for teachers' confidence, pedagogical skills, and student motivation, which can in turn affect students' success at learning English (Butler, 2004).

WHAT ARE SOME PREVAILING THEORIES OF SECOND LANGUAGE ACQUISITION AND THEIR IMPLICATIONS FOR PRACTICE?

As with more general theories about language development, L2 acquisition theories consist of explanatory statements, accepted principles, and methods of analyzing the acquisition. However, L2 acquisition theories differ from L1 development theories in a unique way. Whereas humans begin to acquire their L1 from birth, they may not begin to learn a second language until several years later, possibly even as adults. Thus, theories of L2 acquisition must account for a host of additional variables, both internal to and external to the learner, that influence one's acquisition of second and foreign languages. In this section of the chapter, we provide an overview of some prevailing nurture-inspired and nature-inspired theories of L2 acquisition. We also describe the implications of these theories for L2 instruction.

Nurture-Inspired Theories

Recall that nurture-inspired theories of language development emphasize the notion that humans gain knowledge through experience—specifically through interactions with other people and with the environment. Following, we discuss two nurture-inspired theories of L2 learning: one that emphasizes cognitive factors necessary for learning, and one that focuses on the importance of social interactions to L2 learning.

Cognitive Theory with Attention-Processing Model

Principles.   The cognitive theory of L2 acquisition rests on five principles that relate to the learner's mental and intellectual functioning (H. D. Brown, 2001). The first principle is that *automaticity* helps account for how L2 learners can acquire language without truly "thinking" about it. According to this principle, L2 learners acquire language subconsciously by using it meaningfully; focusing not on the *forms* of language, but on its *uses;* processing an unlimited number of language forms efficiently and automatically; and resisting the temptation to analyze language forms. Overanalyzing language and consciously lingering on language rules may negatively affect automaticity.

The second principle is that by engaging in *meaningful learning,* L2 learners assimilate new information into their existing memory structures. Engaging in such learning is similar to the cognitive process Piaget called *assimilation.*

Some second language learners are particularly motivated to learn, such as travelers to a foreign country.

(*Photo Source:* Wilfried Krecichwost/Getty Images Inc.—Photodisc.)

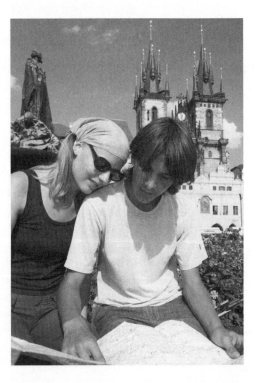

The third principle of cognitive theory stems from Skinner's behaviorist principle of operant conditioning (discussed in Chapter 2) and involves the *anticipation of reward*. That is, one factor that drives L2 learners to act or "behave" is anticipation of a reward—either tangible or intangible, and either immediate or long term.

In contrast to the anticipation-of-reward principle, the fourth principle of cognitive theory involves *intrinsic motivation:* The motivation stems from within the L2 learner. In other words, the process of learning an L2 can be rewarding in and of itself, so the learner does not need external rewards.

The fifth, and final, principle concerns *strategic investment*. According to this principle, the L2 learner personally invests time, effort, and attention to L2 learning by using the strategies for understanding and producing language that he or she brings to the learning process.

Implications for L2 Instruction.   On the basis of cognitive theory, L2 teachers should do the following (H. D. Brown, 2001):

Principle 1: Automaticity

- Do not avoid overt attention to language systems such as grammar, phonology, and discourse. Rather, when instructing in these areas, aim to avoid overwhelming students with these formal aspects of language so that the students can learn to process and use language automatically and fluently.
- Focus much of the lessons on language pragmatics, or how to use language purposefully in genuine contexts and with a variety of functions.
- Recognize that students require time to use language fluently and with automaticity, and exercise patience throughout this process.

Principle 2: Meaningful Learning

- Capitalize on meaningful learning by appealing to students' interests and academic and career goals.
- Strive to embed new material into students' existing background knowledge to facilitate the processes of assimilation and accommodation.
- Avoid rote-learning exercises, including drilling and memorization.

Principle 3: Anticipation of Reward

- Use an appropriate amount of oral praise so that students maintain their confidence.
- Encourage students to complement and support one another.
- Use short-term reminders of progress (such as progress charts), especially for younger learners, to help students recognize their personal development.
- Show excitement and enthusiasm in the classroom.
- Help learners understand the long-term benefits of learning their second language.

Principle 4: Intrinsic Motivation

- Consider students' intrinsic motives and design activities that feed into these motivations.

Principle 5: Strategic Investment

- Use what you know about students' learning styles when designing lessons.
- Use a variety of techniques (e.g., group work, individual work, visual presentation, auditory presentation) to accommodate all students' learning preferences.

Interaction Hypothesis

Principles. The *interaction hypothesis* for L2 learning is similar to Vygotsky's theory of L1 development (see Chapter 2) in that it rests on the communicative interactions between the L2 learner and other people. Both the sender and the receiver in communicative interactions are responsible for the success of their communication, and this hypothesis accounts for the importance of this communication dynamic. The interaction hypothesis emphasizes the L2 learner's opportunities to negotiate for meaning during conversations by, for example, making modifications to speech, using repetition, and clarifying often during a conversation.

Implications for L2 Instruction. Advocates of the interaction hypothesis would recommend a focus on communicative strategies that speakers use to carry out specific language functions during interactions with others. Teachers should have students practice selecting and using language forms that are appropriate for specific communicative situations. Teachers should also have students practice using language with both peers and nonpeers (e.g., adults, teachers) in a range of contexts to support language development.

Nature-Inspired Theories

Recall that nature-inspired theories of language development assert that an individual's underlying language system is in place at birth and that he or she extracts rules about his or her native language apart from other cognitive abilities. Next, we describe two nature-inspired theories of L2 learning that emphasize how humans have relatively little influence over the process and order by which they learn the rules of their L2.

Universal Grammar

Principles. Recall from Chapter 2 that universal grammar (UG) is the system of grammatical rules and constraints that are consistent among all world languages. UG is a nature-inspired theory of L2 acquisition because its underlying premise is that an innate, species-specific module is dedicated solely to language and not other forms of learning. Proponents of UG argue that as with L1 acquisition, L2 learners acquire elements of language that other people cannot teach and that input alone cannot provide. For example, native speakers use sentence fragments, false starts, and other forms of language that are "imperfect," yet L2 learners can still demonstrate adequate performance in many cases. UG theory also suggests that adolescents and adults may experience difficulty in acquiring their L2. Lenneberg (1967, as cited in Danesi, 2003) made this claim explicit in his **critical period hypothesis**, which states that the critical period for language acquisition spans the period between birth and puberty.

Implications for L2 Instruction. UG probably has the fewest instructional implications of all L2 acquisition theories. Unlike the nurture-inspired theories of L2 acquisition, UG does not have implications for communication context, student motivation, or external input that is gained through interactions with other people. Instead, UG has implications for understanding the errors that L2 learners make as they acquire their second language and for the natural order by which they acquire specific language structures.

Monitor Model

Principles.   The *monitor model* of L2 acquisition (Krashen, 1985) consists of five underlying hypotheses: (a) the acquisition-learning hypothesis, (b) the monitor hypothesis, (c) the natural order hypothesis, (d) the input hypothesis, and (e) the affective filter hypothesis:

1.   The *acquisition-learning hypothesis* states that two independent systems are crucial to L2 learning performance: the acquired system and the learned system. The *acquired system* is an unconscious system by which L2 learners acquire language through natural communicative interactions with other people, similar to the way in which young children acquire their L1. In comparison, the *learned system* is the result of a conscious process through which L2 learners gain knowledge of the rules of their L2.

2.   The *monitor hypothesis* explains the relation of the learned system to the acquired system. The monitor plans, edits, and corrects utterances that the acquired system initiates when the L2 learner has sufficient time to think, focuses on correctness, and knows the rule he or she is trying to express. Krashen (1985) suggested that L2 learners should make only minimal use of the monitor and instead rely as much as possible on the acquired system.

3.   The *natural order hypothesis* suggests that L2 learners acquire grammatical structures in a natural and predictable sequence. This order does not vary according to instruction but is the result of the acquired system.

4.   The *input hypothesis* states that L2 learners move forward in their competence by receiving input that is just slightly ahead of their current state of grammatical knowledge, or **comprehensible input**. Krashen's (1985) theory suggests that language that contains structures an L2 learner has already mastered will not help his or her acquisition, nor will input that is too difficult for him or her. Instead, input should ideally be at the $i + 1$ level, where $i =$ the learner's current state of knowledge.

5.   The *affective filter hypothesis* states that "filters" exist that may prevent L2 learners from processing input and thus prevent acquisition. These affective filters include such factors as low motivation, negative attitude, poor self-confidence, and anxiety. The affective filters may account for individual variation in L2 acquisition, and Krashen (1985) contended that young children experience more success with L2 acquisition because they do not have affective filters to inhibit learning.

Implications for L2 Instruction.   The *natural approach* (Terrell, 1977, cited in Danesi, 2003) is an L2 teaching approach that stems from Krashen's (1985) monitor model. To use the natural approach, teachers must help ensure that students' affective filters are "down" and not "up." When students' affective filters are down, the students should have more success at acquiring the comprehensible input from their teacher because they are not thinking about the possibility of failure.

Teachers should also introduce grammar and other formal structures only so that students can use this information to "monitor" or make corrections to the output that results from their "acquired" system. Finally, and most important, teachers should ensure that the input they provide is comprehensible in order to push students to increasingly higher levels of competence in their L2.

Other Theories

Many other theories of L2 acquisition exist, and although we do not discuss them in this book, you should know that they have had considerable influence on L2 teaching approaches, methods, and techniques. For one example, see Theory to Practice: *Suggestopedia,* which describes a neurolinguistic method of L2 teaching: Suggestopedia. Danesi (2003) aptly summarized the dilemma of bridging the gap between theory and practice to ensure the effectiveness of L2 teaching:

DISCUSSION POINT

What purpose or purposes do you think an L2 teaching method such as Suggestopedia would best serve?

> Some teachers now reject the reformist theory-into-practice paradigm completely, since no scientifically-designed pedagogical method has ever proven itself to be universally effective. . . . Yet, despite the many successes that have been documented for contemporary immersion and languages-across-the-curriculum approaches, the search for appropriate classroom pedagogy goes on relentlessly. (p. 3)

THEORY TO PRACTICE

Suggestopedia

Suggestopedia is an L2 learning method that emerged during the 1970s (Lozanov, 1979, cited in H. D. Brown, 2001). It stems from learning theories that emphasize optimal conditions for the learner (i.e., relaxed state of consciousness), integration of the five senses in learning, and judicious integration of the right hemisphere of the brain through the use of visual images, color, music, and creativity. Language classes using Suggestopedia include four main stages:

Stage 1. Presentation: The teacher prepares the students to relax and to adopt a positive frame of mind for learning.

Stage 2. First Concert—"Active Concert": In this stage, the teacher presents language material for the students to learn. For example, the teacher may do a dramatic reading of text and accompany the reading with classical music.

Stage 3. Second Concert—"Passive Review": In this stage, the teacher invites the students to relax and listen to Baroque music. The teacher then reads the text quietly in the background as the music plays. This method is supposed to enable students to acquire new material effortlessly.

Stage 4. Practice: In the final stage, the students use games and puzzles to review what they learned. The teacher then requests that the students cursorily read the material from the lesson that day once before going to bed and once again first thing in the morning.

SUMMARY

This chapter begins with a discussion of the close connection between language and culture. We discuss infant-directed speech as an example of how adults socialize young children *through* the use of language and *to* the use of language. In the next section, we examine the process of language evolution and change. We discuss several American English dialects, including some regional and sociocultural dialects. We also discuss the process of language evolution through pidgins and creoles.

In the following section, we define bilingualism and describe two types: simultaneous and sequential. We examine the debate on whether bilingual individuals have two language systems or a single system and describe the process of code switching that bilingual people use. We also distinguish between bilingualism and second language acquisition, describe the second language process of interlanguage, and provide a historical account of attitudes and policies regarding dual language instruction. An examination of research on English as a second language and English as a foreign language completes this section.

Finally, we compare some prevailing nurture-inspired theories (the cognitive theory with attention-processing model and the interaction hypothesis) and nature-inspired theories (universal grammar and the monitor model) of L2 acquisition. To bridge theory with practice, we also provide some instructional implications for each of these theories.

KEY TERMS

accents, p. 289
communicative accommodation, p. 289
comprehensible input, p. 311
critical period hypothesis, p. 310
dual language learners, p. 297
dual language system hypothesis,
    p. 300
general all-purpose verbs, p. 307
home language stage, p. 305
interlanguage, p. 302
interutterance mixing, p. 301
intrautterance mixing, p. 301

language fossilization, p. 302
language productivity, p. 307
language stabilization, p. 302
majority ethnolinguistic community,
    p. 298
minority ethnolinguistic community,
    p. 299
nonverbal period, p. 306
second language acquisition, p. 302
telegraphic and formulaic use, p. 306
unitary language system hypothesis,
    p. 300

For online resources related to chapter content, including audio samples, valuable Web sites, suggested readings, and self-quizzes, please go to the Companion Website at http://www.prenhall.com/pence

10

Language Disorders in Children

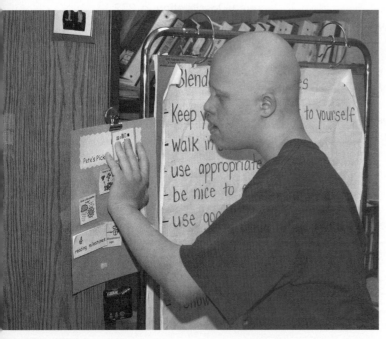

In many of the preceding chapters, we discuss major milestones that characterize how most children develop language from infancy into adolescence. You might assume that all children and adolescents meet these major milestones at about the same time and in about the same manner. Unfortunately, such an assumption would not be true, as we mentioned in Chapter 1 when discussing the concept of language disorders. As noted in Chapter 1, language is a complex human trait that can be affected by heritable weaknesses in the language mechanism as well as by certain developmental disabilities and brain injuries. Children with language disorders, whether present at birth or acquired later, face significant challenges in language development. Children who are born with a language disorder typically experience delays in obtaining critical language precursors, such as babbling and gesturing, in the first year of life. In the toddler and preschool years, they are slow to achieve important early language milestones, such as speaking the first word, combining words into sentences, and initiating conversation with adults or peers. During the school-age years, these children often struggle with academic skills that rely on language proficiency, such as reading and writing. These children are also likely to have problems with complex language tasks, such as using and understanding figurative language (e.g., idioms, proverbs) and abstract language. As adults, persons with language disorders face ongoing challenges to living and working in a culture that places enormous value on language proficiency. Although language disorders can affect persons at any age, from infancy to old age, in this chapter we focus our attention on language disorders affecting children from birth through adolescence.

WHAT IS A LANGUAGE DISORDER?

Practitioners and researchers use many terms to describe language disorders in children, including *language delay, language impairment, language disability,* and *language-learning disability*. The term **language delay** carries the connotation that children exhibiting problems with language development are experiencing a late start with language development and can be expected to catch up with their peers (Leonard, 2000). However, many children with language disorders do not eventually catch up with their peers; rather, the gap in language skills between children developing normally and those with language disorders often widens over time. Therefore, the term *language delay* is not an accurate characterization of language disorders in children. Instead, the terms *language impairment* and **language disorder** provide the

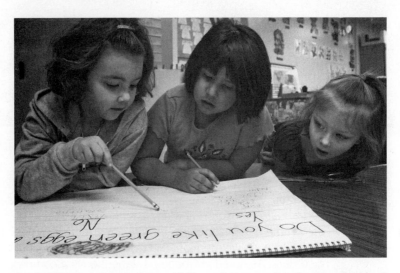

When professionals determine whether a child has a language disorder, they consider the extent to which language difficulties affect the child's social, psychological, and educational performance.
(*Photo Source:* Patrick White/Merrill.)

most accurate representation of the language difficulties a child exhibits; these terms are currently preferred for describing children experiencing significant challenges in language development relative to that of other children (Paul, 2001). The term *language disability* may also be used; it suggests that a child's language difficulties are exerting a significant, negative impact on activities or functions of daily living (Paul, 2001). The term **language-learning disability** is often used to describe language disorders in older children who experience difficulties with academic achievement in areas associated with language, such as reading, writing, and spelling (Heward, 2003).

According to the American Speech–Language–Hearing Association (ASHA; 1993), a *language disorder* is present when an individual exhibits the following:

> [I]mpaired comprehension and/or use of a spoken, written, and/or other symbol system. The disorder may involve (1) the form of language (phonology, morphology, and syntax), (2) the content of language (semantics), and/or (3) the function of language in communication (pragmatics) in any combination. (p. 40)

When professionals apply this theoretical definition to identifying whether a given child has a language disorder, they also consider the extent to which a child's language difficulties (a) have an adverse impact on social, psychological, and educational functioning; (b) may represent a language difference; and (c) are significant enough to be considered disordered.

Social, Psychological, and Educational Impact

If a child exhibits substantial difficulty with language but the difficulty has no adverse social, psychological, or educational impact, one question to ask is whether the child does, in fact, have a language disorder (Fey, 1986). This question relates to the importance of differentiating the concepts of *disease, activity,* and *participation in life*. These concepts require important consideration when practitioners determine whether a particular child exhibits a language disorder. The World Health Organization (2001) differentiates these concepts as follows:

- **Disease** refers to the underlying physiological condition that impedes performance. For language disorders, *disease* refers to an underlying neurological impairment (the *genotype* of the disease) that causes a person to have difficulties with comprehension and/or production of language form, content, or use.

- **Activity** refers to the behavioral or performance deficits that result from the disease. In language disorders, this term refers to the impact of the underlying neurological impairment on the child's comprehension and/or production of language form, content, and use in everyday circumstances—or the *phenotype* of the disease.

- **Participation in life** refers to how the disease affects the quality of life for the child and his or her family, including possible impacts on social, psychological, and educational functioning.

Next, we consider how these three constructs may be differentiated for two children—Shamika and Jorge—each of whom has a language disorder. Shamika and Jorge are 6-year-old children. The speech–language pathologist at their school diagnosed each child with *specific language impairment* (SLI), a developmental impairment of language presumed to occur because of a neurological weakness in basic language processing. Within the classroom, both children show moderate impairment of language comprehension and production, including difficulties in syntax, phonology, and semantic development. Thus, in terms of *disease* and *activity,* Shamika and Jorge are similar. However, the children differ with regard to the impact of SLI on their *participation in life.* Jorge has significant difficulty communicating effectively with his peers and teachers and performs poorly on language tasks within the classroom, including comprehending literature and developing reading skills. In contrast, Shamika seems to have no difficulty communicating with peers and adults in the classroom and is progressing well in all academic domains. These differences between the two children result from various developmental forces (e.g., temperament, intelligence, gender) and environmental forces (e.g., caregiver–child relationship, classroom quality, access to early intervention). For a given child, these forces interact to promote *risk* (vulnerability to the effects of a disease) or *resilience* (the ability to withstand the effects of a disease). Although Shamika and Jorge are similar with regard to the genotype and phenotype of language disorder, the effect of the underlying disorder varies considerably with respect to the two children's participation in life. Therefore, one argument could be that Shamika does not have a language disorder, whereas Jorge does—a distinction based on consideration of the impact of a disease on how well a child can function in social, psychological, and educational contexts.

Language Disorders and Language Differences

In Chapter 1, we discussed how a comparison of any two children of about the same age will reveal considerable differences in their language content, form, and use.

Numerous genetic, developmental, and environmental factors interact to affect a child's language development. We noted in Chapter 1 that *language difference* is a general term used to describe the normal variability seen among children in their language development. People who identify and treat language disorders in children recognize that sometimes a fine line exists between a language difference and a language disorder. These two concepts differentiate between normal variability in language development and variability that reflects an underlying neurological impairment affecting language development.

How do professionals differentiate language differences from language disorders? In large part, such differentiation requires a careful understanding of the **cultural context** in which a child is learning and applying his or her language abilities. A particular cultural community's approach to socializing children can influence the amount and quality of language that children experience in their home and community. In turn, children's exposure to language in the home and other caregiving contexts is a strong and unique contributor to children's language acquisition. In addition, professionals must be aware of how language acquisition may vary for children who are learning several languages at once (i.e., bilingualism) or who are speaking nonmainstream dialects. Children who are learning English as a second language may differ significantly from native English speakers in their attainment of English-language milestones.

Any two cultural communities can vary substantially in their approaches to child socialization. For instance, adult members of one cultural community may believe that children "should be seen but not heard"; therefore, in that community children rarely participate in conversations among adults. In another cultural community, adults may believe that children should be frequent and active participants in conversations among adults. These differences in socialization practices can affect children's language development. As another example, adults in one cultural community may socialize often with their infants through direct parent–infant talk, whereas in another community adults may rarely speak directly to infants. Again, such variability in the way adults socialize children in their cultural community directly affects the quantity and quality of language that children in the community experience. From a cultural perspective, no "right" or "wrong" way to socialize children in a cultural community exists, although variability in child socialization practices can readily influence children's rate of language development.

When professionals can attribute a given child's variability in language acquisition to a language difference (rather than a disorder), they can still provide suggestions to families and other caregivers on how to maximize the child's language development. For instance, a professional may provide the parents of a toddler who is a late talker, and is learning several languages simultaneously, with specific strategies for increasing the quantity and quality of language input to their child in both languages. As another example, for a child who is slow to meet major language milestones because of limited exposure to language in the home environment, the professional may provide parents with information on how language input facilitates young children's language growth. See Multicultural Focus: *Differentiating Language Differences from Language Disorders* for a discussion on the importance of distinguishing between language differences and language disorders.

MULTICULTURAL FOCUS

Differentiating Language Differences from Language Disorders

Diagnosis of language disorders in young children requires professionals to be able to distinguish language differences from language disorders. This fact is especially true for professionals who work with pupils who speak several languages (i.e., who are bilingual), who are learning English as a second language (ESL), or who speak an English dialect that differs from the mainstream dialect. Unfortunately, many of the tests and tasks professionals use to identify language disorders were developed for monolingual speakers of the Standard American English dialect. Therefore, they may be insufficiently sensitive for differentiating between children who are typically developing and those who have a language impairment.

Consider, for instance, the use of language sample analysis (LSA), one procedure discussed in this chapter that professionals use to study a child's language abilities. A common technique used in LSA is to analyze a child's grammatical morphology, including examining for the presence of specific bound morphemes that serve important grammatical roles (e.g., plural and past tense verb markers, auxiliary verbs, articles). The professional examines a child's use of grammatical morphology in spoken language, then compares it against developmental norms that indicate when specific morphemes emerge in typical language development. The results of a number of studies show that analysis of grammatical morphology is useful for identifying children with language impairment because children with such impairment show delays in their development of grammatical morphology and often omit grammatical morphemes in their spontaneous language use (Rice, Wexler, & Cleave, 1995; Rice & Wexler, 1996). LSA is a useful way for identifying such omissions, and it is often used as a companion to other standardized tests in language assessment.

Next, consider a scenario in which an experienced professional collects a language sample from a 5-year-old girl and analyzes it for the following grammatical morphemes (Paradis, 2005): third person singular *-s,* past tense *-ed,* irregular past tense, *be* and *do* as auxiliary and copula verbs, plural *-s,* and articles. The professional calculates how often the child omits each grammatical morpheme in her language sample, then compares her omission rates against normative references identifying when 5-year-old children typically use these morphemes. The professional finds that the child omits these morphemes at much higher rates than expected (e.g., 64% for third-person singular, 67% for past tense regular) and determines that a language disorder is present.

Unfortunately, this professional may have made an error because the child is a native Spanish speaker who is learning ESL. As recent studies have shown, the grammatical morphology of children who are learning ESL may look similar to that of children with language impairment, particularly their omission of grammatical morphemes (Paradis, 2005). In addition, children's mastery of grammatical

(continued)

morphology varies considerably in that some children acquire English grammatical morphology rapidly, whereas other children do so much more slowly (Paradis, 2005). Thus professionals must ensure that their analyses of children's spontaneous language samples are sensitive enough to differentiate between differences and disorders. Paradis (2005) identified four approaches to improving the sensitivity of such analyses:

1. Assess children in their native language whenever possible.
2. Know how language develops for bilingual children, children learning ESL, and nonmainstream dialect speakers and have expectations based on this knowledge.
3. Use a variety of tools for studying a child's language skills.
4. Whenever possible, compare a child's language skills to those of children who have a similar language background.

The Meaning of *Significant*

The definition of *language disorder* presented at the beginning of this chapter is somewhat vague in specifying the level of impairment that must be present to signal the presence of a language disorder. Often, experts use the term **significant** to specify the impairment level a child must exhibit to have a language disorder (Paul, 2001). However, what does *significant* mean in both relative and absolute terms? Currently, no gold standard is available by which to define the term *significant* as it applies to language disorders.

Typically, professionals who identify language disorders rely on the use of standardized tests that measure a child's language comprehension and expression in the form, content, and use areas. Professionals administer tests to children to identify whether their language abilities are sufficiently poorer than those of children of the same age and cultural background. The professional (or the organization in which he or she works, such as a public school system) sets a threshold to demarcate the line of significance, which is used to identify whether the child's test performance exceeds or does not meet this threshold. Children whose test scores do not meet the threshold are considered to have language skills that are significantly different from normal. For instance, an often-used threshold is a standard score of 85 on a valid and reliable standardized test of language. This standard score equates to one standard deviation below the mean (−1 SD), as shown in Figure 10.1. About 16% of all children who are given a particular test of language receive a score of 84 or less, and when tested by professionals who use the −1 SD threshold, these children will likely be identified as having a language disorder if their disorder concomitantly affects their participation in life. Conversely, children who receive a score of 86 or 87 will not be considered to have a language disorder. This demarcation raises the question as to whether children who receive a score of 84 on the test are functionally different in their language skills relative to the children receiving a score of 86 or 87. In all likelihood, they are not.

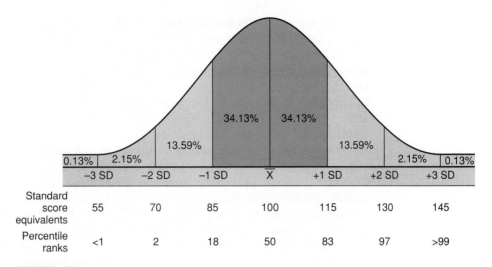

	−3 SD	−2 SD	−1 SD	X	+1 SD	+2 SD	+3 SD
Standard score equivalents	55	70	85	100	115	130	145
Percentile ranks	<1	2	18	50	83	97	>99

FIGURE 10.1

Normal curve for standardized test scores.

SD = standard deviation.

Source: Justice, Laura M., *Communication Sciences and Disorders: An Introduction,* 1st Edition, © 2006. Reprinted by permission of Pearson Education, Inc., Upper Saddle River, NJ.

To complicate matters further, not all professionals use the same threshold to identify significance and to demarcate normal language from disordered language. Some professionals use a lower standard score—81—as their threshold, which corresponds to approximately 10% of all children given the test. Professionals who work within public school systems typically use the threshold adopted by their system to determine whether a child is eligible for services for a language disorder. You should recognize that thresholds used to qualify children for language services can vary substantially among school districts; thus, eligibility for language services in one particular school district does not necessarily equate with exhibition of a language disorder.

Our point is that no clear-cut approach is currently available to identify when a child exhibits disordered language, given the ambiguity of the term *significant* and the lack of a gold standard method for differentiating normal language from disordered language. Thus, as an important supplement to administering standardized tests and analyzing children's scores on the tests, professionals must rely on their personal subjective impressions obtained from careful observation of children in different contexts to determine whether language difficulties are present and significant enough to warrant diagnosis of a disorder.

Prevalence and Incidence

Language disorders are the most common type of communication impairment affecting children. They are the most frequent cause for administering early intervention and special education services to children from toddler through elementary-school ages.

Primary language impairment, a significant language impairment in the absence of any other developmental difficulty (e.g., mental retardation, brain injury), affects about 7–10% of children older than 5 years (Beitchman et al., 1989; Tomblin et al., 1997). Because this disorder is specific to language, it is commonly called *specific language impairment,* or, as mentioned previously, SLI. Many children with SLI continue to experience significant problems with language skills into middle and later adolescence (Catts, Fey, Tomblin, & Zhang, 2002; Catts, Fey, Zhang, & Tomblin, 2001; C. J. Johnson et al., 1999).

The prevalence of **secondary language impairment,** language disorders resulting from (i.e., secondary to) other conditions, is more difficult to estimate. Common types of secondary language impairment include mental retardation, autism, and traumatic brain injury. About 1 in 1,000 children exhibit mild to severe mental retardation (Fujiura & Yamaki, 1997), and about 1 in 500 children exhibit autism or an autism spectrum disorder (Ehlers & Gillberg, 1993; Yeargin-Allsopp, 2003). Both developmental conditions typically result in a language disorder. Approximately 2% of all children sustain significant head injuries each year (U.S. Department of Health and Human Services, 1999), which can also result in a significant language disorder. In a given year, about 600,000 schoolchildren in public schools receive services for mental retardation, 65,000 children receive services for autism, and 14,000 children receive services for brain injuries (U.S. Department of Education, 2001).

WHO IDENTIFIES AND TREATS CHILDREN WITH LANGUAGE DISORDERS?

Various professionals are involved with identifying and treating language disorders in children. Some professionals provide direct services, whereas others provide indirect services. *Direct services* include diagnosing language disorders and treating children with disorders through clinical and educational interventions. *Indirect services* include screening children for the possibility of language disorders and referring them for direct services, as well as counseling parents on approaches to supporting language development in the home environment (see Theory to Practice: *Language Intervention in the Home Environment*).

The professionals most closely involved with direct and indirect services include speech–language pathologists, psychologists, general educators, special educators, early interventionists, audiologists, developmental pediatricians, and otorhinolaryngologists.

Speech–Language Pathologists

Speech–language pathologists, or SLPs, are frequently the lead direct service providers for children with language disorders. The scope of practice for SLPs is presented in Figure 10.2. As this figure shows, the SLP scope of practice related to language disorders includes a number of pertinent responsibilities, including prevention, screening, consultation, assessment and diagnosis, treatment delivery,

THEORY TO PRACTICE

Language Intervention in the Home Environment

A considerable body of research shows a strong, positive relationship between the quality of parent–child conversational interaction and children's early language accomplishments (e.g., Baumwell, Tamis-LeMonda, & Bornstein, 1997; Landry, Miller-Loncar, Smith, & Swank, 1997; Rush, 1999). This research lends support to social-interactionist accounts of language development that view language as a psychobiological process in which "frequent, relatively well-tuned affectively positive verbal interactions" are critical for supporting language growth in early childhood (R. Chapman, 2000, p. 43). Researchers have drawn on this theoretical perspective to design interventions that parents can use at home to accelerate language growth in their children with language disorders.

One example of this translation of theory to practice is an intervention approach called *interactive focused stimulation* (IFS; Girolametto et al., 1996). IFS is a parent-training program that teaches parents optimal ways to interact with their children during conversational exchanges. The basic premise of IFS is to teach parents to provide "frequent, highly concentrated presentations of preselected language targets" (Girolametto et al., 1996, p. 1275). For instance, when increasing vocabulary usage is a goal, parents learn ways to identify words to target during conversation with their children (e.g., words their children comprehend but do not yet use). They also learn how to incorporate these words often in their play with their children by using different conversational behaviors (e.g., modeling the words, expanding on their children's production of the words) and by setting up many routines in which the target words can be readily used. One study of an 11-week IFS training program for parents of toddlers with language impairment showed that when parents increased their use of IFS, their children made gains in their receptive vocabulary and use of different words during conversational interactions with their parents (Girolametto et al., 1996). Studies like these are important not only for improving professionals' access to evidence-based approaches for early language intervention, but also for confirming theoretical understanding of how children develop language.

and counseling. Therefore, typical services SLPs provide include screening children for possible language disorders, conducting evaluations of children suspected of having language disorders, diagnosing language disorders, and developing and administering treatments to remediate language disorders.

SLPs work in many settings, including public and private schools, hospitals, rehabilitation facilities, home health agencies, community and university clinics, private practices, group homes, state agencies, universities, and corporations (ASHA, 2001). Currently, more than 100,000 SLPs in the United States have been certified by the American Speech–Language–Hearing Association (ASHA);

The practice of speech–language pathology includes prevention, diagnosis, habilitation, and rehabilitation of communication, swallowing, or other upper aerodigestive disorders; elective modification of communication behaviors; and enhancement of communication. The practice involves the following 12 responsibilities:

1. Providing prevention, screening, consultation, assessment and diagnosis, treatment, intervention, management, counseling, and follow-up services for disorders of
   (a) Speech, including articulation, fluency, resonance, and voice
   (b) Language, including comprehension and expression in oral, written, graphic, and manual modalities; language-based processing; and preliteracy and language-based literacy skills
   (c) Swallowing or other upper aerodigestive functions
   (d) Cognitive aspects of communication
   (e) Sensory awareness related to communication, swallowing, or other upper aerodigestive functions

2. Establishing augmentative and alternative communication techniques and strategies

3. Providing services, such as speech–reading, to individuals with hearing loss and their families or caregivers, and providing hearing screening

4. Using instrumentation to observe, collect data, and measure parameters of communication and scaffolding

5. Selecting, fitting, and establishing the effective use of prosthetic or adaptive devices for communication and swallowing

6. Collaborating to assess central auditory-processing disorders and providing treatment when speech, language, and other cognitive abilities are affected

7. Educating and counseling individuals and families about communication and swallowing

8. Advocating for persons with communication disorders through community awareness, education, and training programs to promote and facilitate access to full participation in communication

9. Collaborating with other health professionals, including providing referrals as individual needs dictate

10. Addressing behaviors and environments that affect communication and swallowing functions

11. Providing services to modify or enhance communication performance, such as accent modification, or care and improvement of the professional voice or the transgendered voice

12. Recognizing the need to provide and appropriately accommodate services to individuals from diverse cultural backgrounds and adjust services appropriately

FIGURE 10.2

Scope of practice for speech–language pathologists.

Source: From *Scope of Practice in Speech–Language Pathology,* by the American Speech–Language–Hearing Association, 2001, Rockville, MD: Author. Copyright 2001 by the American Speech–Language–Hearing Association. Adapted with permission.

however, most regions of North America have a significant shortage of SLPs. This shortage is not likely to be resolved soon because the U.S. Department of Labor (Hecker, 2001) has named speech–language pathology as one of the top 30 fastest growing professions. In addition to the shortage of SLPs who can fill direct service positions in schools, clinics, and hospitals, doctoral-level SLPs, who can serve as academic faculty in university SLP training programs, are in short supply.

Psychologists

Psychologists also have important responsibilities with regard to identifying and treating child language disorders, including conducting research necessary for helping people understand how to identify and treat such disorders (American Psychological Association, 2003). *Cognitive and perceptual psychology* and *developmental psychology* are two branches of psychology in which research relevant to child language disorders is conducted. Researchers in these fields conduct basic and applied research on human perception, thinking, and memory; in particular, developmental psychologists emphasize growth in these capacities during the life span. These researchers helps answer such important questions as "What demographic factors predict whether a child will persist in or resolve his or her early language difficulties?" (e.g., Bishop, Price, Dale, & Plomin, 2003) and "How does teacher input in the classroom influence children's rate of language development?" (e.g., J. Huttenlocher, Vasilyeva, Cymerman, & Levine, 2002).

Clinical psychologists, clinical neuropsychologists, rehabilitation psychologists, and *school psychologists* often work more directly with children with language disorders. These professionals work in public and private schools, clinics, and hospitals, and many of them provide services through private practice. Typically, identification and treatment of language disorders is only a small part of what these professionals do.

Clinical psychologists screen for and diagnose language impairments, often as part of a larger psychoeducational assessment that examines a child's strengths and needs in many areas of development (e.g., nonverbal intelligence, perceptual skills, learning aptitude). Clinical psychologists may offer specialized treatments for various types of language disorders, such as those exhibited by children with autism or by children who have difficulty processing auditory information.

Clinical neuropsychologists and rehabilitation psychologists may oversee the diagnosis and treatment of childhood and adolescent language disorders resulting from traumatic injuries, such as acquired brain injuries. They may also work with individuals with developmental disabilities (e.g., cerebral palsy, autism) to promote these persons' community involvement and adjustment.

School psychologists typically work in private and public schools. They perform essential activities as part of school-based teams that identify children with language disorders and develop educational programs to remediate or compensate for these disorders.

General Educators

General educators include preschool, elementary, middle school, and high school teachers. General educators have the important role of identifying children in their classrooms who show signs of difficulty with language within the educational context. General educators must be knowledgeable about not only the course of typical language development but also signs of impaired development. Common signs of language difficulties from preschool into adolescence are listed in Table 10.1.

TABLE 10.1
Common Signs of Language Disorders: Preschool to Adolescence

Student's age or grade	Language difficulties
Preschool	• Omission of grammatical inflections, including present progressive (*-ing*), plural (*-s*), possessive (*'s*), past tense regular and irregular verbs, and auxiliary verbs • Slow development of and errors with pronouns • Shorter sentence length • Problems forming questions with inverted auxiliaries • Immature requests (resembling those of younger children) • Difficulty with group conversations (conversing with more than one child) • Difficulty with oral resolution of conflicts • Longer reliance on gesture for getting needs met • Difficulty initiating with peers • Difficulty sustaining turns in conversation • Difficulty comprehending complex directions and narratives
Elementary grades	• Word-finding problems accompanied by pauses and circumlocutions • Naming errors (e.g., "shoes" for *pants*) • Slower processing speed in language comprehension • Difficulty responding to indirect requests • Difficulty maintaining topics • Difficulty recognizing the need for conversational repair • Problems with figurative and nonliteral language • Problems with abstract language concepts • Problems providing sufficient information to listeners • Poor cohesion of narratives • Difficulty asking for help or clarification • Difficulty providing details
Adolescence	• Difficulty expressing ideas about language • Inappropriate responses to questions and comments • Poor social language • Problems providing sufficient information to listeners • Redundancy • Inadequate sense of limits or boundaries • Difficulty expressing needs and ideas • Difficulty initiating conversations with peers

(continued)

TABLE 10.1   (*continued*)

Student's age or grade	Language difficulties
	• Immature conversational participation • Difficulty asking for help or clarification • Difficulty providing details • Problems with organizing complex information in oral or written language • Word-finding difficulties • Socially inappropriate discourse with peers or adults • Frequent pauses, hesitations, or repetitions when speaking • Delays in responding during conversations or other language tasks

Source: Adapted from "Verb Use in Specific Language Impairment," by G. Conti-Ramsden and M. Jones, 1997, *Journal of Speech, Language, and Hearing Research, 40,* 1298–1313; *Children with Specific Language Impairment,* by L. B. Leonard, 2000, Cambridge: MIT Press; "Intervention for Word-Finding Deficits in Children," by K. K. McGregor and L. B. Leonard, in *Language Intervention: Preschool Through the Elementary Years* (pp. 85–105), edited by M. Fey, J. Windsor, and S. Warren, 1995, Baltimore: Brookes; *Understanding Language Disorders: The Impact on Learning,* by V. L. Ratner and L. R. Harris, 1994, Eau Claire, WI: Thinking; and "Verb Use by Language-Impaired and Normally Developing Children," by R. Watkins, M. Rice, and C. Molz, 1993, *First Language, 37,* pp. 133–143.

When a general educator suspects that a child in his or her classroom may have impaired language abilities, the educator must request the school's **child study team** (also called the *evaluation team*) to engage in a systematic process that typically involves **prereferral intervention,** or identification of approaches to support the child's language skills in the classroom environment (Heward, 2003). General educators are therefore one of the most important referral sources for children suspected of having language disorders. The child study team typically comprises the general educator, the child's parents, and other professionals (e.g., school psychologist, special educator, SLP). The child study team identifies approaches the general educator may use to support the child's language performance in the classroom. If these approaches do not alleviate the general educator's concerns about the child's language performance, the child study team then conducts a *multifactored evaluation* (MFE) to evaluate the child carefully and determine whether a language disorder is present. If the team identifies a language disorder, they also use the MFE to identify the types of special education services the child should receive to treat his or her language disorder and to support his or her academic development.

Whenever possible, children with language disorders receive special education services in the **least restrictive environment** (LRE). The LRE is a federal mandate of the Individuals with Disabilities Education Act (IDEA), which stipulates that children with disabilities should receive their education to the maximum extent possible in the same contexts as those of their peers without disabilities. Therefore, many children with language disorders receive their education in the regular classroom along with children who do not have language disorders. Consequently, general educators must be skilled at differentiating their instruction to support the academic growth of children with language disorders.

Special Educators

Special educators have a critical role to play in supporting the educational progress of children identified with language disorders. The field of special education has grown as a result of federal legislation mandating the free and appropriate education of children with disabilities in U.S. schools. Currently, more than 300,000 special educators teach the nearly 6 million children with disabilities in U.S. schools (Individuals with Disabilities Education Act [IDEA] Data, 2003; U.S. Department of Education, 1999). Nearly one fourth of these children have speech and language disabilities (IDEA Data, 2003).

To meet the needs of these pupils with disabilities, special educators work directly with students from preschool through the secondary grades to deliver general and specialized interventions geared toward helping them succeed academically. Special educators use a variety of approaches to do so: They may be lead teachers or coteachers in classrooms serving primarily children with disabilities; they may consult and collaborate with teachers who have one or more students with disabilities; or they may deliver specialized interventions outside the classroom in pullout programs. Some special educators serve as *itinerant teachers;* they do not have their own classroom but coteach or collaborate with a number of teachers. Many itinerant special educators have a special area of expertise, such as the education of children with autism or children who are Deaf, and thus go into classrooms in which these children are served to collaborate with teachers and provide services in the least restrictive classroom environment.

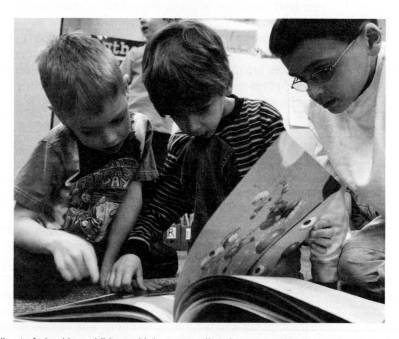

According to federal law, children with language disorders are entitled to receive their education in the least restrictive environment.

(*Photo Source:* Patrick White/Merrill.)

Although special educators may screen and test children for language disorders, their primary responsibility is to design, deliver, and monitor individualized education program (IEPs) and individualized family service plans (IFSPs), which specify educational interventions and annual goals for children identified with language disorders who receive special education services in public school programs. IEPs (for 3- to 21-year-olds with disabilities) and IFSPs (for infants to 2-year-olds with disabilities) are required by IDEA and its subsequent amendments. IDEA allocates federal funds to the 50 states to provide intervention services to children from infancy through age 21 years who have identified disabilities or delays in language and other areas of development (e.g., mental and motor development). Organizations may also use federal funds to provide interventions to newborns through 2-year-olds who exhibit significant medical, biological, and environmental risk conditions making them vulnerable for later disability.

Early Interventionists

Early interventionists (sometimes called *child development specialists*) are professionals who specialize in interventions for infants and toddlers. The field of early intervention is new, growing out of the 1986 reauthorization and amendment (P.L. 99-457) of the original 1975 Education for All Handicapped Children Act. The original act legislated special education services for children ages 6–21 years, with some support available for preschool programs serving children ages 3–5 years. In light of concerns raised about access to services for children who were even younger, the 1986 reauthorization provided federal support to states to implement early intervention services to children with identified or suspected disabilities from birth to age 2 years. The states needed well-trained professionals—early interventionists— to support the design and implementation of their early intervention systems. Public Law 99-457 provided states with considerable flexibility in determining the credentials needed by early intervention personnel, and the training provided to and required by these professionals still varies greatly across the United States.

Early interventionists undoubtedly have one of the most critical roles to play in serving the needs of children with language disorders. Given the importance of the first few years of life to language development, these professionals work with children with language disorders during the best "window of opportunity" for optimizing the children's developmental trajectory. In delivering their early intervention services, these professionals often work directly in families' homes, side by side with the parents of infants and toddlers to teach them ways to support their children's language learning in the home environment.

Typically, early interventionists work from a clinic, hospital, or community-based organization that has received a grant from the state to provide early intervention services in a particular region. The organization is responsible for serving infants to 2-year-olds in the region who have developmental delays (e.g., slow progress in language development), physical or medical conditions that often result in developmental delays (e.g., low birth weight, HIV), and environmental conditions linked to later developmental problems (e.g., extreme poverty, abuse). For children deemed eligible for early intervention services, an IFSP is developed to identify the specific early intervention services to be provided, including the intensity, type, and location of services. The IFSP also sets specific objectives for the child and family, and early interventionists oversee progress toward these objectives.

Audiologists

Audiologists are specialists in identifying, assessing, and managing disorders of the auditory, balance, and other neural systems (ASHA, 1996). Audiologists are often involved as collaborators in the treatment of language disorders when hearing loss is involved, and they work closely with SLPs and other professionals to design interventions. For instance, for a child born with profound hearing loss, they might deliver auditory–verbal therapies that simultaneously promote the child's use of residual hearing and his or her language production and comprehension. When an audiologist suspects that hearing loss may be affecting a child's language development, he or she also plays a critical role in referring the child to as SLP for language assessment.

Audiologists work in many settings, including schools, hospitals, rehabilitation facilities, community and university clinics, private practices, and universities. More than 12,000 audiologists currently work in the United States, and the field is expected to expand dramatically during the next decade because audiology is one of the top 30 fastest growing professions (Hecker, 2001).

Developmental Pediatricians

Developmental pediatricians play an important role in the early identification and ongoing treatment of language disorders in children of all ages. These specialized pediatricians have expertise in managing complex disorders that affect various aspects of development in young children. For instance, children with cerebral palsy often have a variety of developmental needs. This prenatal or perinatal developmental disturbance of the motor system can affect not only speech and language but also fine and gross motor skills, feeding and swallowing development, general height and weight growth, and, in some cases, intellectual functioning. The developmental pediatrician manages complex cases of developmental disability, such as those occurring with cerebral palsy. He or she evaluates the child regularly to monitor many developmental achievements and provides referrals for specialized assessments and interventions. Typically, developmental pediatricians work in clinics and hospitals and see primarily children with complex developmental disorders, including not only cerebral palsy but also autism, Down syndrome, and Rett syndrome, to name a few.

Otorhinolaryngologists

Otorhinolaryngologists, also known as *ear–nose–throat specialists,* or ENT specialists, are close collaborators in the diagnosis and management of language disorders resulting from injury to or illness of the ear, nose, or throat. They are particularly important team members for children who exhibit slow language development as a function of otitis media (OM) or other types of hearing loss. OM is one of the most common causes of hearing loss in children. It results from a viral or bacterial infection of the middle-ear space, and in some instances the middle-ear space is filled with fluid, which dampens the hearing ability. Some estimates indicate that at least 50% of all children experience at least one case of otitis media, which may be an underestimation because symptoms of the disease often are not obvious (ASHA, 2005). When OM persists either in a single case of the disease or through chronic infections (e.g., five or six in a given year), a child may exhibit delays in language acquisition. The ENT specialist has the key role of halting the progress of OM by administering antibiotics or inserting pressure-equalizing tubes (PE tubes) into the eardrum to equalize pressure between the middle ear and the outer ear and to release any fluids in the middle-ear space. ENT specialists often work closely with SLPs and audiologists to promote the language and hearing achievements of children with chronic hearing loss.

WHAT ARE THE MAJOR TYPES OF CHILD LANGUAGE DISORDERS?

In this section, we describe the defining characteristics of, causes of, and risk factors for five conditions typically associated with language disorders among children and adolescents: specific language impairment, autism spectrum disorder, mental retardation, traumatic brain injury, and hearing loss.

Specific Language Impairment

Defining Characteristics

As mentioned previously, *specific language impairment* (SLI; also called *primary language disorder*) is a developmental disability in which an individual shows a significant impairment of expressive or receptive language that cannot be attributed to any other causal condition (Tomblin, Zhang, Buckwalter, & O'Brien, 2003). Children with SLI have typical hearing skills (although they may have a history of middle-ear infections); normal intelligence; and no obvious neurological, motor, or sensory disturbances, such as seizures or brain injury.

Children are typically diagnosed with SLI after their third birthday (Rescorla & Schwartz, 1990). Although signs of language difficulty may be present as early as the first and second years of life, toddlers who are slow to talk are typically classified as "late talkers" rather than language impaired. Some estimates suggest that most late talkers (about 50–60%) outgrow their language problems by age 3 years (Paul, Spangle-Looney, & Dahm, 1991; Rescorla, Roberts, & Dahlsgaard, 1997; Thal & Tobias, 1992). Therefore, a formal diagnosis of SLI is usually not made until a child is 3 years old or more, when practitioners can more clearly determine whether the child is exhibiting a true language disorder rather than a late start.

Although children with SLI characteristically exhibit a late start in language, they differ from late talkers in that most of them have enduring difficulties with language. According to recent epidemiological research, about 50% of kindergartners with SLI continue to exhibit a significant language impairment in fourth grade (Tomblin et al., 2003). Children with SLI whose language impairment affects both expression and comprehension of language show lower remission rates between kindergarten and fourth grade than those of children with deficits in only language expression or comprehension (Tomblin et al., 2003).

Although children with SLI show considerable individual differences in the domains of language affected and the severity of the disorder, they often share five common traits:

1. Many children with SLI have strengths in some areas of language and weaknesses in others (Conti-Ramsden, Crutchley, & Botting, 1997). For instance, a child may have relatively intact grammatical skills but exhibit poor pragmatic and semantic performance. As another example, a child may have deficits in the expression of language but relatively good comprehension.

2. Many children with SLI have a history of slow vocabulary development. On average, children with SLI produce their first words at about age 2 years (compared with about 1 year for nonimpaired children), and they continue to struggle with learning new words through the elementary years (see Leonard, 2000). When provided the opportunity to learn a new word, children with SLI learn the word more slowly than their nonimpaired same-age peers do (Nash & Donaldson, 2005). Experts attribute these delays in vocabulary learning to a generalized deficit in processing linguistic stimuli (Kail, 1994).

3. Many children with SLI show considerable difficulties with grammatical production and comprehension that begin during toddlerhood and continue through school age (Conti-Ramsden & Jones, 1997). During toddlerhood and the preschool years, children with SLI are likely to omit key grammatical morphemes, such as articles and auxiliary verbs; they produce shorter utterances; and they may have problems with pronoun usage (e.g., substituting possessive pronouns for subjective pronouns, such as "Her did it"). One area of particular weakness is verb development (Leonard, 2000). Children with SLI use verbs less frequently than same-age peers do, use fewer types of verbs, and show delayed development of verb morphology, particularly the use of auxiliary verbs (Conti-Ramsden & Jones, 1997; Rice, 1996; Watkins & Rice, 1994).

4. Children with SLI also tend to have difficulty adjusting academically; for example, they may have problems with social skills, behavior, and attention (Fujiki, Brinton, Morgan, & Hart, 1999; Fujiki, Brinton, & Todd, 1996; Redmond & Rice, 1998) as well as with more academically oriented skills, such as literacy and mathematics (Pence, Skibbe, Justice, Bowles, & Beckman, 2006). Difficulties with reading development—such as timely development of the alphabetic principle and application of reading comprehension strategies—are common sources of academic difficulty for children with SLI (Catts et al., 2002; see Research Paradigms: *Prospective and Retrospective Longitudinal Studies*).

5. Most children diagnosed with SLI have long-term difficulties with language achievement. As many as 60% of children who exhibit SLI at kindergarten age continue to show language weaknesses in adolescence and adulthood, and resolution is most unlikely for children who exhibit impairment of both language expression and language comprehension (in contrast, resolution is most likely for children with expressive-only impairment; C. J. Johnson et al., 1999; Stothard, Snowling, Bishop, Chipchase, & Kaplan, 1998; Tomblin et al., 2003).

RESEARCH PARADIGMS

Prospective and Retrospective Longitudinal Studies

The results of a number of studies have revealed that young children with language impairment face significant challenges in the later development of their reading ability (e.g., Catts et al., 2002; Gallagher, Frith, & Snowling, 2000). For instance, Catts and colleagues found that about 50% of kindergartners later exhibit poor reading skills in second grade. Some experts contend that preschool language impairment and school-age reading disability are two manifestations of a single underlying developmental language disorder (Scarborough, 2001). Next, we consider two approaches researchers use to study the co-occurrence of early language impairment and later reading disability: prospective and retrospective longitudinal studies.

A *prospective longitudinal study* is a research design in which researchers follow children forward in time as they develop. Researchers test children intermittently (e.g., every 6 months) to track their development. In longitudinal studies, researchers may follow children for several months or for many years. An example of a prospective longitudinal study of reading outcomes for children with language impairment is that of Catts and colleagues (2002). In this study, an initial sample of 7,218 kindergartners were tested by using a comprehensive battery of language and cognitive measures. From these children, a subset of children with language impairment (LI; $n = 328$) were identified and tested again in second and fourth grade. The second- and fourth-grade test battery included measures of language, cognition, and reading ability. The researchers used data from the test battery to identify the percentage of children with LI who exhibited reading disability in second and fourth grade, finding that 53% and 48% of kindergartners with LI had reading disability in second and fourth grade, respectively. (In contrast, about 8% of children with no history of LI had reading disability in second and fourth grade.) This prospective study quantified the increased risk for reading problems among children with LI.

Another way to study the relationship between language impairment and reading disability is a *retrospective longitudinal study*. In such studies, researchers follow children across time to identify those who exhibit a reading disability in the elementary grades, then look backward to determine whether language difficulties were present earlier. An example of this type of research design is Scarborough's (1990) longitudinal study of 78 children who were tracked from toddlerhood to second grade; she recruited children from families "in which someone has experienced a severe childhood reading problem" (p. 1729) because reading problems often "run in" families. She used this strategy to increase the likelihood that a large percentage of children being followed would have a reading disability by second grade; of the children followed, 36% had a reading disability in second grade, with a high incidence (65%) for the children with family members

(continued)

who were reading disabled. An important feature of this study was Scarborough's retrospective analysis of the early language skills of children who later developed a reading disability. Scarborough had tested the children at ages 30, 36, and 60 months using a battery of language measures, including standardized tests and spontaneous language samples. Scarborough found that children who exhibited a reading disability in second grade had language problems in the toddler and preschool years. For instance, at age 30 months, children with a reading disability had poorer grammatical and phonological skills than those of children who did not have a reading disability. On the basis of her retrospective analyses, Scarborough contended that "potentially important differences between children who do and do not become disabled readers are evidenced by the third year of life" (p. 1740), a finding that converges with the results of prospective studies (such as that by Catts and colleagues [2002] discussed previously) showing the increased risk for reading disability for children with LI.

SLI Subgroups

Children with SLI comprise a heterogeneous group. Some children with SLI have problems in both language expression and language comprehension, whereas other children have difficulties with only expression. Likewise, some children with SLI have deficits in all the language domains, whereas other children have a more focal impairment that affects only one area of language functioning (e.g., grammar). Researchers have long been interested in determining whether children with SLI can be classified into specific subgroups, or typologies (e.g., Aram & Nation, 1975; Fletcher, 1992).

One tool for identifying subgroups from among a larger population is *cluster analysis,* a statistical approach in which data are organized into meaningful clusters of scores. Researchers can use cluster analysis to identify subgroups of children with SLI by statistically analyzing their scores for a range of language tasks, including phonological, syntactic, morphological, semantic, and pragmatic measures (Conti-Ramsden et al., 1997; Rapin & Allen, 1987). Such research reveals six major subgroups of SLI (Conti-Ramsden et al., 1997; Rapin & Allen, 1987), as shown in Table 10.2.

Causes and Risk Factors

No known cause for SLI has been identified, although advances in brain-imaging and epidemiological research suggest a strong biological and genetic component to this disorder (Gauger, Lombardino, & Leonard, 1997). Children who have immediate family members with language impairment are more likely than other children to develop SLI, and 20–40% of children with SLI have a sibling or parent with a language disorder (Ellis Weismer, Murray-Branch, & Miller, 1994; Rice, Haney, & Wexler, 1998; Tomblin, 1989; van der Lely & Stollwerck, 1996). Current theories on the cause of SLI

TABLE 10.2

Subtypes of Specific Language Impairment

LI subtype	Expressive or receptive LI	Characteristics
Verbal dyspraxia	Expressive	• Severe problems with articulation of speech sounds and expressive phonology • Intact pragmatics, syntax, and morphology, although production of syntax and morphology is difficult to assess because of the child's unintelligible speech
Phonological programming deficit syndrome	Expressive	• Moderate problems with phonology and poor reading ability • Relatively intact pragmatics, syntax, and morphology
Phonological–syntactic deficit syndrome	Expressive and receptive	• Moderate-to-severe problems with phonology, syntax, and morphology • Relatively intact semantic and pragmatic skills • Most common of all six subtypes: present in about one third of all children with specific language impairment
Lexical–syntactic deficit syndrome	Expressive or expressive and receptive	• Moderate-to-severe problems with syntax, morphology, and vocabulary, particularly word-finding and naming abilities • Relatively intact phonology and pragmatics
Semantic–pragmatic deficit syndrome	Receptive	• Mild-to-moderate problems with semantics and pragmatics, particularly the comprehension of oral information • Relatively intact phonology, syntax, and morphology, which results in other people's viewing children with this syndrome as not having specific language impairment but as having "bizarre" language
Verbal auditory agnosia	Receptive and expressive	• Significant difficulties across all language domains • Least common of all six subtypes

LI = language impairment.
Source: Adapted from "The Extent to Which Psychometric Tests Differentiate Subgroups of Children with Specific Language Impairment," by G. Conti-Ramsden, A. Crutchley, and N. Botting, 1997, *Journal of Speech, Language, and Hearing Research, 40,* pp. 765–777; and "Developmental Dysphasia and Autism in Preschool Children: Characteristics and Subtypes," by I. Rapin and D. A. Allen, in *Proceedings of the First International Symposium on Specific Speech and Language Disorders in Children* (pp. 20–35), edited by J. Martin, P. Fletcher, P. Grunwell, and D. Hall, 1987, London: Association for All Speech-Impaired Children (AFASIC).

suggest that biological or genetic factors predispose a child to SLI, which can then interact unfavorably with additional risk factors present in the child's developmental environment. Risk factors that may increase a child's vulnerability to SLI include both environmental (e.g., child neglect and abuse) and physical (e.g., exposure to toxins, undernutrition, chronic middle-ear infections) health factors.

Autism Spectrum Disorder

Defining Characteristics

Autism spectrum disorder (ASD) is an umbrella term that includes four conditions: autism, childhood disintegrative disorder, Asperger's syndrome, and pervasive developmental disorder—not otherwise specified (PDD–NOS). Together, these conditions affect about 1 in 500 children, with a higher prevalence among boys and among children with family members who are affected (American Psychiatric Association, [APA], 1994).

Autism. **Autism** is a severe developmental disability with symptoms that emerge before a child's third birthday. Diagnosis of autism requires three conditions to be met, as shown in Table 10.3 (APA, 1994). The first is impaired social interactions with other people. Children with autism characteristically display an inability or a lack of interest in developing relationships with peers and in participating in social games or routines as well as little awareness of others' feelings or needs (APA, 1994).

The second condition is moderate to severe impairment of communication skills. Some children with autism never develop any functional spoken language skills, and the speech of children who do develop spoken language is often characterized by idiosyncratic, repetitive language, such as *echolalia*. **Echolalia** refers to stereotypical repetitions of specific words or phrases, such as when a 4-year-old repeatedly says "Ticket, please. Thank you." Many children with autism also have difficulty initiating or reciprocating in communicative interactions with other people, and they seldom engage in periods of sustained joint attention with adults.

The third condition is restrictive, repetitive, and stereotypical behaviors and interests. Children with autism may have few interests and be overly preoccupied with certain objects or activities. For instance, a child may be preoccupied with a particular puzzle and spend hours each day putting the puzzle together and then taking it apart. Stereotypical behaviors are also common, such as rocking back and forth, humming, or flapping the arms.

Childhood Disintegrative Disorder. Under the ASD umbrella, **childhood disintegrative disorder** describes children younger than 10 years who appear to be developing normally until at least their second birthday but then display a significant loss or regression of skills in two or more of the following areas: language, social skills, bowel and bladder control, play, or motor skills (APA, 1994). Like children with autism, children with disintegrative disorder display significant problems in their social interactions and communication skills and show restricted and repetitive behaviors and interests.

Asperger's Syndrome. Children with **Asperger's syndrome** are often referred to as "higher functioning" children with autism. Children and adolescents with Asperger's often have substantial problems with social interaction and show restricted and

TABLE 10.3
Diagnostic Criteria for Autism Spectrum Disorder

Disorder	Onset	Hallmark criteria

Autism	Before age 3 years	Abnormal functioning in social interaction, communication, and behavior, with at least six specific areas of deficit (at least two must be from Social Interaction and at least one in the other two categories):
		
		A. Social Interaction
		  1. Marked impairment in using multiple nonverbal behaviors (eye-to-eye gaze, facial expression, body posture, gestures)
		  2. Failure to develop peer relationships appropriately
		  3. Lack of spontaneous seeking to share enjoyment, interests, or achievements with other people
		  4. Lack of social or emotional reciprocity
		B. Communication
		  1. Delay in or total lack of development of spoken language
		  2. Marked impairment in the ability to sustain conversation with other people
		  3. Stereotyped and repetitive use of language or idiosyncratic language
		  4. Lack of varied, spontaneous, or make-believe play or social imitative play
		C. Behavior
		  1. Preoccupation with one or more stereotyped patterns of interest that is abnormal in intensity or focus
		  2. Inflexible adherence to specific nonfunctional routines or rituals
		  3. Repetitive motor movements
		  4. Persistent preoccupation with parts of objects

Childhood disintegrative disorder	Between ages 2 and 10 years	Normal development for at least the first 2 years; significant loss of skills in two or more of the following areas: language, social skills or adaptive behavior, bowel or bladder control, play, and motor skills. Significant impairment must also be observed in at least two of the following areas: A. Social Interaction: Including impaired nonverbal behaviors, failure to develop peer relationships, and lack of emotional reciprocity B. Communication: Including lack of spoken language, inability to sustain or initiate conversation, and repetitive use of language C. Behavior: Including restrictive, repetitive, or stereotyped patterns of behavior and interests

Asperger's syndrome	Before or after age 3 years	No clinically significant delay in language, cognitive, self-help, and adaptive behavioral skills, but significant impairment in two or more of the following areas:
		
		A. Social Interaction
		
		  1. Impairment in the use of nonverbal behaviors
		  2. Failure to develop peer relationships

(continued)

TABLE 10.3   (*continued*)

Disorder	Onset	Hallmark criteria
		3. Lack of spontaneous seeking to share enjoyment, interests, or achievements with other people
		4. Lack of social or emotional reciprocity
		B. Behavior
		1. Preoccupation with one or more stereotyped patterns of interest that is abnormal in intensity or focus
		2. Inflexible adherence to specific nonfunctional routines or rituals
		3. Repetitive motor movements
		4. Persistent preoccupations with parts of objects
Pervasive developmental disorder—not otherwise specified	Before or after age 3 years	Severe and pervasive impairment of social interaction, communication, or behavior, but the criteria are not met for diagnosis of autistic disorder, childhood disintegrative disorder, or Asperger's syndrome

Source: Adapted with permission from the *Diagnostic and Statistical Manual of Mental Disorders,* Fourth Edition, Text Revision (Copyright 2000). American Psychiatric Association.

idiosyncratic behavioral patterns and interests. The language skills of children with Asperger's are generally well developed and are not viewed as clinically disordered. However, these children may use language in idiosyncratic and unconventional ways and have difficulty using language in social situations and comprehending abstract or figurative language. For instance, they may understand only the literal meaning of idiomatic phrases (e.g., "We really need to *hit the books* to prepare for this test" and "She really is *out of her mind*"). Children with Asperger's may also have considerable difficulty using language as a social tool and for developing and maintaining social relationships. They may have difficulty initiating conversations with peers and use situationally inappropriate language.

Pervasive Developmental Disorder—Not Otherwise Specified. **Pervasive developmental disorder—not otherwise specified** (PDD–NOS) describes severe problems with social interactions and communication and repetitive behaviors and overly restricted interests, but do not otherwise meet the specific diagnostic criteria for autism, childhood disintegrative disorder, or Asperger's syndrome.

Causes and Risk Factors

Autism spectrum disorders are neurobiological disorders that result from an organic brain abnormality (Lord & Risi, 2000). Some factors may increase a child's risk for developing autism. Certain prenatal and perinatal complications, particularly maternal rubella and anoxia (lack of oxygen to the brain), are associated with an increased risk for autism (APA, 1994), as is the presence of some developmental or physical disabilities, such as encephalitis (an inflammation of the brain) and

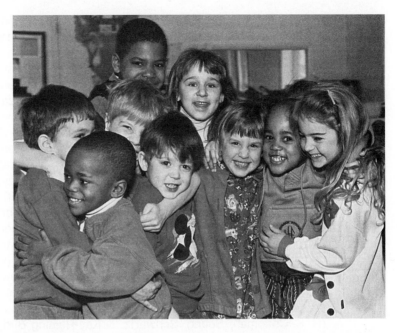

Children with autism display an inability to develop, or a lack of interest in developing, relationships with peers and instead participate in social games or routines with other people.
(*Photo Source:* Barbara Schwartz/Merrill.)

fragile X syndrome (a genetic disorder that results in mental retardation). Seizure disorder is seen in 25% of children with autism, which suggests a commonality in the brain structures affected by ASD and seizures (APA, 1994). Also, extreme sensory deprivation can have a profound impact on communication and social development and in severe cases may result in patterns of development consistent with those of ASD (Kenneally, Bruck, Frank, & Nalty, 1998).

Mental Retardation

Defining Characteristics

Mental retardation (MR) is a "condition of arrested or incomplete development of the mind, which is especially characterized by impairment of skills manifested during the developmental period" (American Association on Mental Retardation [AAMR], 2002, p. 103). MR is diagnosed in children younger than age 18 years who meet two criteria: (a) significant limitations in intellectual functioning and (b) significant limitations in adaptive behavior (AAMR, 2002). Thus, children with MR exhibit limitations in intelligence such as difficulty reasoning, planning, solving problems, thinking in abstract terms, comprehending abstract and complex concepts, and learning skills. These children also experience limitations in adaptive behavior and the activities of daily living, including difficulties with conceptual skills (communication, functional academics, self-direction, health and safety), social skills (social relationships, leisure), and practical skills (self-care, home living, community participation, work).

MR ranges from mild to profound, and because of the interrelationships among intellectual functioning and language ability, most children with MR have at least mild language impairment (see Table 10.4). In mild cases, the most common type, MR may affect an individual only minimally, such that the individual exhibits mild language difficulties yet is able to participate fully in society and to develop strong social relationships with few adaptive limitations. In profound cases, which occur far less frequently, an individual's intellectual and adaptive functioning is severely affected. A person with profound MR may be unable to care for him- or herself, to communicate with other people, or to participate in any community or employment activities.

The language skills of a person with MR usually parallel the degree of intellectual impairment. In general, children with MR show delays in early communicative behaviors (e.g., pointing to request, commenting vocally) and are slow to use their first words and to produce multiword combinations (Rosenberg & Abbeduto, 1993). Children with mild MR may have well-developed oral language skills with only minor difficulties with abstract concepts, figurative language, complex syntax, conversational participation, and communicative repairs (Ezell & Goldstein, 1991; Kuder, 1997). Children and adolescents who have Down syndrome, a relatively common cause of MR, typically produce short sentences (about three words long), use a fairly small expressive vocabulary, and exhibit a slowed rate of speech (R. S. Chapman, Seung, Schwartz, & Kay-Raining Bird, 1998). Function words, such as copula and auxiliary verbs (*is, were, does*), are frequently omitted as well as pronouns, conjunctions, and articles. Language comprehension tends to be better than language expression for these children. Despite these difficulties, many children with mild levels of MR exhibit language skills that allow them to participate fully in the academic curricula of their schools, to communicate competently with peers and adults, and to relay their needs and interests to other people.

Comparatively, children with more severe forms of MR display more significant deficits in language expression and comprehension. Some individuals with MR never learn to express themselves orally. They may produce only a few words or sounds and few gestures. In addition, they may be able to comprehend only single, simple words representing concrete actions or objects (e.g., *sit, cup*). For some individuals with more severe forms of MR, an augmentative and alternative communicative (AAC) system can facilitate their ability to express themselves. For instance, an individual with profound MR who cannot produce any words may learn to point to pictures representing common actions (e.g., *eat, drink, walk, toilet*) as a means of representing his or her needs and wants.

Causes and Risk Factors

MR can occur for many reasons, although in about 30–40% of all cases the cause cannot be identified (APA, 1994). For the other 60–70% of cases, prenatal damage to the developing fetus due to chromosomal abnormalities or maternal ingestion of toxins accounts for the majority of cases (about 30%). Environmental influences and other mental conditions, such as sensory deprivation (e.g., neglect) or the presence of autism, account for about 15–20% of all cases. Pregnancy and perinatal problems—such as fetal malnutrition, prematurity, anoxia (lack of oxygen to the child's brain before, during, or following birth), and viral infections—account for an additional

TABLE 10.4

Categories of Mental Retardation

Type	Cases (%)	IQ range	Adaptive skills
Mild	85	50–69	• Has mild learning difficulties but can work, maintain good social relationships, and contribute to society • Can acquire academic skills to about a sixth-grade level • By adulthood can usually achieve social and vocabulary skills adequate for minimal self-support; supervision and assistance likely needed • Can usually live successfully in community, either independently or in supervised settings
Moderate	10	35–49	• Has marked developmental delays in childhood but can develop some degree of independence in self-care and acquire adequate communication and academic skills • May have difficulties with peers in adolescence because of problems with social conventions • Can benefit from vocational training • In adulthood needs varying degrees of support to live and work in community but can perform unskilled and semiskilled work with supervision • Adapts well to community life, usually in supervised settings
Severe	3–4	20–34	• Has significant developmental delays; acquires few or no speech or language skills in preschool years but may later develop minimal communication skills • Can master some preacademic skills (sight reading of important words) • Needs continuous levels of support to care for self and participate in community activities but can adapt well to community life with close supervision
Profound	1–2	<20	• Is severely limited in self-care, contingence, and communication abilities and in mobility; such limitations are usually identified with a neurological condition that accounts for the mental retardation • Needs constant aid and supervision, but some individuals can perform simple tasks with much support

Source: Adapted with permission from the *Diagnostic and Statistical Manual of Mental Disorders,* Fourth Edition, Text Revision (Copyright 2000). American Psychiatric Association.

10% of cases. Medical conditions such as trauma, infection, and poisoning cause about 5% of all cases of MR, and heredity alone accounts for 5% of the cases.

Traumatic Brain Injury

Defining Characteristics

Traumatic brain injury (TBI) refers to damage or insult to an individual's brain tissue sometime after birth. Young children, adolescent males, and older persons have the highest risk, and males are affected twice as often as females (U.S. Department of Health and Human Services, 1999). Mild injuries, characterized by a concussion and loss of consciousness for 30 min or less, are the most common type of brain injury and usually have few lasting repercussions. In contrast, a severe injury is accompanied by a coma of 6 hours or more (Russell, 1993). Such injuries can result from infection (e.g., meningitis), disease (e.g., brain tumor), and physical trauma (e.g., gunshot wound). Some of the more common causes of TBI in children include abuse (e.g., shaken baby syndrome), intentional harm (e.g., being hit on the head), accidental poisoning through ingestion of toxic substances (e.g., prescription medications, pesticides), car accidents, and falling.

The most common type of TBI is a **closed-head injury** (CHI), in which brain matter is not exposed or penetrated. CHI may occur in a car accident, in which a child in the rear seat is thrown forward and then backward with sudden deceleration. Another example of CHI is the brain injury resulting from shaken baby syndrome, in which an infant or a toddler is so rigorously shaken that the child's brain sustains diffuse injury. In contrast, with **open-head injuries** (OHI), the brain matter is exposed through penetration, as would occur with a gunshot wound. OHI tends to cause a more focal brain injury than that resulting from CHI. However, in both CHI and OHI, the immediate injury to the brain—whether diffuse or focal—is often accompanied by secondary brain injuries that result from the primary trauma. For instance, an individual who sustains a CHI may then experience anoxia (a lack of oxygen to brain tissue) or edema (swelling of the brain tissue), both of which can cause additional brain damage (Brooke, Uomoto, McLean, & Fraser, 1991).

Most children with an acquired brain injury have a history of normal language skills. Injury to the brain typically damages the frontal and temporal lobes of the brain, which house the centers for many of the executive (e.g., reasoning, planning, hypothesizing) and language functions. Language disorders resulting from brain injury are influenced by the *severity* of the injury, the *site* of damage, and the *characteristics of the child* before the injury occurred (S. B. Chapman, 1997). Children with more severe injuries have less chance of a full language recovery than do children with more mild injuries. However, even children with more mild cases of TBI may show long-lasting cognitive and language impairments, even though the effects may not be immediately apparent until years later when damaged areas of the brain are applied to certain skills and activities (Goodman & Yude, 1996).

The aspect of language most commonly impaired with TBI is language use, or pragmatics. About 75% of all children with severe CHI have problems with discourse; for example, they may produce language that is fragmented and difficult to follow and have difficulty with word retrieval (S. B. Chapman, 1997; Russell, 1993). Brain injury may also affect a child's cognitive, executive, and behavioral skills (Russell, 1993; Taylor, 2001). Such effects include difficulties with sustained and selective attention (maintaining attention during an ongoing activity, including when distractions are present), storing new information, retrieving known information, planning and setting goals, organizing, reasoning and solving problems, being self-aware, and monitoring behavior (Taylor, 2001). Children and adolescents with brain injury may be more likely to exhibit aggression, irritability, depression, and anxiety. Because the prevalent long-term repercussions of brain injury are more subtle than obvious physical manifestations are, brain injury is often referred to as an *invisible epidemic* (U.S. Department of Health and Human Services, 1999).

Causes and Risk Factors

The most common causes of brain injuries are automobile accidents, falls, and sports injuries (Beukelman & Yorkston, 1991). For children, recreational and sports injuries, such those sustained from bicycling, playing football, and riding horses, are common causes of brain injury. Risk factors for incurring brain injury include (a) participating in contact sports or other recreational activities that may result in a fall or collision and (b) using drugs or alcohol during these activities or when driving or riding in vehicles.

Hearing Loss

Defining Characteristics

A *hearing loss* is a physical condition in which an individual cannot detect or distinguish the full range of sounds normally available to the human ear. It can result from prenatal, perinatal, or postnatal damage to any of the structures that carry auditory information from the external world to the brain centers that process auditory information. As shown in Figure 10.3, hearing loss resulting from damage to the outer or middle ear is termed **conductive loss,** whereas hearing loss resulting from damage to the inner ear or auditory nerve is termed **sensorineural loss.** Conductive and sensorineural loss may occur *bilaterally* (both ears are affected) or *unilaterally* (only one ear is affected and the other is intact). Hearing loss that results from damage to the centers of the brain that process auditory information is called **auditory-processing disorder,** or APD.

Individuals with hearing loss compose a heterogeneous group based on not only the type of loss (conductive, sensorineural, APD) but also the timing and severity of the loss. A hearing loss present at birth is termed a **congenital hearing loss.** About 50% of all cases of congenital hearing loss occur for unknown reasons (Gallaudet Research Institute, 2001). Several of the more prevalent causes include genetic transmission (i.e., one or both of the child's parents carry a gene for hearing loss), in utero infections (e.g., herpes, rubella), prematurity, pregnancy complications, and trauma during the birth process. A hearing loss that occurs after birth is termed an **acquired hearing loss,** and prominent causes include noise exposure, infection, use of ototoxic medications (i.e., medications that damage the hearing structures), and chronic middle-ear infections (Martin & Greer Clark, 2002). Acquired hearing loss is often differentiated into that acquired after birth but before the child has developed language, termed a **prelingual hearing loss,** and that acquired sometime after the child has developed language, termed a

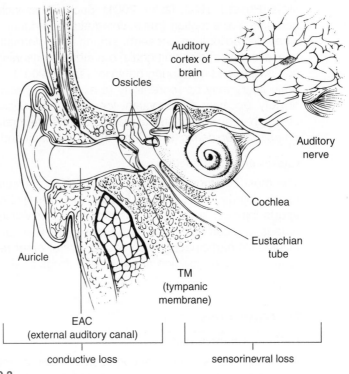

Auditory
cortex of
brain

Ossicles

Auditory
nerve

Cochlea

Eustachian
tube

Auricle

TM
(tympanic
membrane)

EAC
(external auditory canal)

conductive loss   sensorinevral loss

FIGURE 10.3

Types of hearing loss based on location of auditory damage.

Source: Justice, Laura M., *Communication Sciences and Disorders: An Introduction,* 1st Edition, © 2006.
Adapted by permission of Pearson Education, Inc., Upper Saddle River, NJ.

postlingual hearing loss. Postlingual hearing loss has less of an impact on a
child's language development than does prelingual loss.

Whether prelingual or postlingual, hearing loss ranges in severity from mild to
profound (see Table 10.5). Professionals typically determine the severity of loss using
the *decibel (dB) scale,* which is the standard unit of sound intensity, or loudness.
The range of human hearing is from 0 dB (the threshold of sound) to 140 dB, which
corresponds to a continuum from the drop of a pin (0 dB) to a fire alarm close to
your ear (140 dB). Experts use the decibel scale to identify the threshold at which
an individual with hearing loss can hear sound (Pakulski, 2006):

> 16–25 dB: Minimal loss
>
> 26–40 dB: Mild loss
>
> 41–55 dB: Moderate loss
>
> 56–70 dB: Moderately severe loss
>
> 71–90 dB: Severe loss
>
> 91 dB or higher: Profound loss

Because audition is the primary way in which children experience language, the
impact of any hearing loss can profoundly influence a child's language acquisition.

TABLE 10.5
Severity of Hearing Loss and Possible Effects

Degree of hearing impairment (dB HL)	Potential speech and language effects	Potential educational effects
Normal hearing (−10 to +15)	May have difficulty discriminating speech in the presence of background noise	• None
Minimal loss (16–25)	May have difficulty detecting faint and distant speech, listening in a noisy room, and detecting word–sound distinctions (e.g., verb tenses, plural forms, possessives)	• May miss 10% of classroom instruction • May appear inattentive or uninterested • May be more fatigued because of increased listening effort
Mild loss (26–40)	Depending on degree of loss, may miss 25–50% of speech signals, including many consonants necessary for intelligibility, which will affect language development and articulation	• May appear to daydream or listen only when interested • Likely to be more fatigued or irritable
Moderate loss (41–55)	Without sound amplification, will miss 75% or more of speech signals; thus, will likely have delayed syntax, limited vocabulary, imperfect speech production, and voice-quality issues	• Will have difficulty with receptive and expressive language, reading, spelling, and other school concepts • Will miss most classroom instruction presented orally
Moderately severe loss (56–70)	Will miss as much as 100% of all speech signals, so will have marked difficulty in both one-on-one and group conversations, will have delayed language and syntax and reduced voice quality and speech intelligibility, and will produce unintelligible speech 75% of the time	• Will not be able to keep up with oral instruction and will fall behind academically • All subjects likely to be affected
Severe loss (71–90) *and* *profound loss* (91+)	Without sound amplification, may not develop speech or language, or preexisting skills will deteriorate for acquired conditions	• Without intervention, will not be able to participate in a typical academic setting
Unilateral loss (mild or worse)	May have difficulty hearing faint or distant speech, localizing sounds, and understanding speech in poor listening conditions	• May miss important oral instructions or descriptions (particularly in a noisy room), which will lead to incomplete concept development or misunderstanding

dB HL = decibels hearing level.
Source: Justice, Laura M., *Communication Sciences and Disorders: An Introduction,* 1st Edition, © 2006. Reprinted by permission of Pearson Education, Inc., Upper Saddle River, NJ. (Adapted from *Facilitating Hearing and Listening in Young Children,* by C. Flexer, 1994, San Diego, CA: Singular.)

This fact is particularly true for children whose hearing loss occurs prelingually. However, the extent to which hearing loss affects a child's language development depends on a number of factors, including the following four:

1. *Timing of the loss:* At what age did the loss occur?
2. *Severity of the loss:* How severe is the loss? Is it unilateral or bilateral?
3. *Age of identification:* At what age was the loss identified?
4. *Exposure to language input:* How much language exposure does the child receive?

Of these factors, the third and fourth are unequivocally the most important because they are most strongly related to whether the child with hearing loss acquires typical or atypical language. A child with even a profound hearing loss but whose loss is identified early and whose exposure to language input is not compromised can develop language at virtually the same rate as that of a child without hearing loss. For instance, a child with profound hearing loss who experiences sign language in the home environment because his or her parents are native users of sign will likely progress at a normal language development rate. Likewise, a child with profound hearing loss whose loss is identified early and soon after undergoes cochlear implantation that makes spoken language audible may also progress typically in speech and language acquisition (Dawson, Blamey, Dettman, Barker, & Clark, 1995; T. A. Meyer, Svirsky, Kirk, & Miyamoto, 1998). Cochlear implants are a relatively new intervention for children age 12 months and older with severe to profound hearing loss. This intervention is a desirable approach for parents who want their child who is Deaf to develop as an oral language user. In the year 2000, more than 7,000 children had undergone cochlear implantation in the United States (Ertmer, 2002). A cochlear implant requires surgical implantation of a receiver–stimulator (implanted in a hollowed-out portion of the mastoid bone) and an electrode array (implanted in the cochlea), which accompany external hardware worn by the user (microphone, speech processor, transmitter, and power supply; for a comprehensive discussion, see Moore & Teagle, 2002). Although children with implants have variable language outcomes (Pisoni, Cleary, Geers, & Tobey, 2000), for many children with profound hearing loss, cochlear implants provide a promising option for accelerating their language growth to approximate that of normal development (e.g., Ertmer, Strong, & Sadagopan, 2003).

For children whose hearing loss is not identified early and for whom no consistent avenue to experiencing language input (whether sign or spoken) is ensured, the loss can severely compromise their language acquisition. This outcome is true even for relatively mild loss, such as might occur for the child who experiences chronic middle-ear infections accompanied by fluid in the middle ear. For children with mild to more severe hearing loss that is not identified or acted on consistently and proactively, language acquisition is often significantly delayed. These children often show language impairment that transcends all five domains of language. With regard to morphology and syntax, children with hearing loss will show delays in their acquisition of simple and more complex syntax and their production of grammatical morphemes (Tye-Murray, 2000). In the area of semantics, children

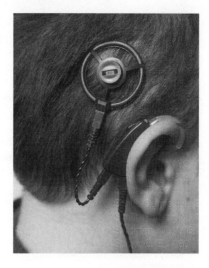

A cochlear implant involves surgical implantation of a receiver–stimulator and an electrode array. These components process auditory information in the surrounding environment, which makes hearing possible for persons with profound hearing loss.

(*Photo Source:* James King-Holmes/Photo Researchers Inc.)

with hearing loss show delayed growth in vocabulary and use fewer different words during communication (Nicholas & Geers, 1997). With regard to phonology, children with hearing loss show delays in their acquisition of expressive phonology, including distortions of consonants (Shriberg, Friel-Patti, Flipsen, & Brown, 2000). Finally, in the area of pragmatics, children with hearing loss may communicate less frequently with their peers and show delays in their production of different communicative intentions (e.g., questioning, responding; Nicholas & Geers, 1997).

Causes and Risk Factors

Hearing loss is a relatively common condition among children. As many of 50% of young children experience fluctuating hearing loss as a result of chronic otitis media (ASHA, 2005). Although relatively few children exhibit severe or profound permanent hearing loss (about 1–2%), as many as 8% exhibit hearing loss serious enough to affect their language and educational achievement (ASHA, 2005). The causes of hearing loss are numerous; several of the more prevalent causes are listed in Figure 10.4.

HOW ARE CHILD LANGUAGE DISORDERS IDENTIFIED AND TREATED?

Identification of Language Disorders

Identifying children who exhibit language disorders requires administration of a *comprehensive language evaluation*, most often conducted by a certified SLP. The goal of the evaluation is to determine whether a language disorder is present and, if so, to develop a profile of the child's linguistic strengths and weaknesses and a plan for intervention. The comprehensive language evaluation typically includes a case history and an interview, followed by a comprehensive assessment of language skills.

- Family history of congenital hearing loss
- Congenital infection linked to hearing loss (e.g., herpes, rubella)
- Craniofacial anomaly affecting the ear
- Low birth weight
- Ototoxic medications
- Bacterial meningitis and other infectious diseases associated with hearing loss (e.g., measles)
- Low Apgar scores at birth
- Mechanical ventilation for 10 days or longer
- Presence of a syndrome associated with hearing loss (e.g., Down syndrome)
- Head trauma during or soon after birth

FIGURE 10.4

Prevalent causes of hearing loss.

Source: Adapted from "1990 Position Statement," by Joint Committee on Infant Hearing, 1991, *ASHA, 33* (Suppl. 5), pp. 3–6; and *Introduction to Audiology* (5th ed.), by F. Martin, 1994, Upper Saddle River, NJ: Prentice Hall.

Case History and Interview

The case history involves administering a questionnaire and interviewing the child's parents; examples of questions are provided in Figure 10.5. The case history documents a child's developmental history, general health, medical conditions and allergies, family size and resources, language and communicative history, current skills, interests, and behaviors as well as the parents' and child's perception of suspected

1. What age was your child when he or she started to babble?
2. When did your child say his or her first word?
3. What are some examples of words your child used when he or she started talking?
4. When did your child start to produce short sentences?
5. Have you ever noticed occasions when your child had difficulty expressing him- or herself? Can you give me an example of one of those times and what you did in response?
6. How would you describe your child's conversational style? Does he or she often start conversations with you? When you ask him or her questions, does your child usually respond?
7. Give me an example of a question you often ask your child. How does he or she typically respond?
8. How well does your child communicate with peers who are the same age? How long does a typical conversation last?
9. When eating dinner at your home with your child, what are some typical things he or she might say?
10. Share with me some specific concerns you have about your child's communication, speech, and language. How long have you had these concerns?

FIGURE 10.5

Example of a case history questionnaire.

problems. Typically, after a parent completes a case history questionnaire, the professional interviews him or her to focus on certain areas, particularly language and communication. For instance, the professional is likely to ask pointed questions about how a child gets his or her needs met in the home environment, which words he or she uses often, and when he or she met specific language milestones (e.g., putting two words together).

Comprehensive Language Assessment

The SLP designs and administers a comprehensive assessment of a child's language abilities. This assessment is often completed during several hours in a private, quiet location. For young children, the assessment may be broken into several test sessions to prevent fatigue in or frustration of the child. It also often involves observation of the child in different contexts, including the classroom for school-age children. The assessment is designed to analyze both comprehension and production in all language domains. For younger children who are not yet talking, the analysis covers the development of critical language precursors, including babbling, gesturing, affect and expression, participation in early communicative routines, and periods of joint attention. For older children, the analysis covers not only oral and written language skills, including reading, writing, and spelling, but also children's performance on classroom and curriculum-based tasks.

One important characteristic of the comprehensive language assessment is that it focuses on functional aspects of language so that the professional can study the extent to which a child's language skills affect his or her ability to function at home and in school. For young children, the assessment examines children's ability to use language skills in their daily lives to get their needs met through various communicative functions. Such functions include requesting objects and actions; expressing feelings of interest, pleasure, and excitement; responding to other people's questions, requests, and comments; and using social behaviors such as greeting other people (Halliday, 1975). For older children, the analysis examines the extent to which children's language skills affect their ability to participate in the school curriculum and to interact with friends, teachers, and parents effectively.

The professional uses many tests and tasks to conduct the comprehensive language assessment, including criterion-referenced tasks, norm-referenced tests, dynamic assessment, and observational measures. **Criterion-referenced tasks** are used to examine a child's performance level for a particular type of language task, such as the percentage of one-step directions (e.g., "Give me the cup") the child can perform correctly. For instance, a professional might use a criterion-referenced task to study a child's understanding of various locational and spatial terms, such as *in, on, under, below, next to, beside, above,* and *behind.* By providing the child a ball and a box, the professional could assess the child's performance by using a series of directives, such as "Put the ball *under* the box" and "Put the ball *next to* the box." The child's performance on the criterion-referenced task is calculated by dividing the number of items responded to correctly by the number of tasks administered. Criterion-referenced tasks can be used both to provide a baseline examination of a child's skills in a given area and to monitor children's performance gains with time.

Norm-referenced tests are used to examine children's level of language performance against that of a national sample of same-age peers. This type of testing often requires the use of commercially available tests, such as the Clinical Evaluation of Language Fundamentals (CELF)—Preschool (CELF–Preschool; Wiig, Secord, & Semel, 1992) and the CELF–Preschool–2 (Semel, Wiig, & Secord, 2004). This norm-referenced test is used with children ages 3–7 years and includes six subtests that cover expressive and receptive language skills in the areas of morphology, syntax, and vocabulary.

Dynamic assessment is used to examine how children's performance on a particular language task is advanced by giving different types of assistance. With dynamic assessment, the professional engages a child in a learning trial to determine exactly how much and what kind of support is needed to improve the child's language performance. For instance, noting that the child uses only one type of communicative intention (commenting), the professional would use dynamic assessment to determine how much and what kind of support is needed for the child to use a new communicative intention (e.g., requesting). The professional might design a "communicative temptation" in which he or she places a desired object in a box and models a request for the child ("Tell me . . . 'Want box'") to identify how much support is needed to entice the child to request. Unlike criterion-referenced and norm-referenced tasks, which reveal what a child can do independently, dynamic assessment addresses how support and interaction can help the child attain more advanced language forms and functions.

Observational measures are used to examine children's language form, content, and use in naturalistic activities with peers or parents. Two types of observational measures are commonly used in language assessment. The first is *conversational analysis.* In conversational analysis, the professional observes a child during interactions with other people to study his or her ability to initiate conversation, to use different communicative intentions, to take turns, to maintain topics, to identify breakdowns in conversation, and to attend to listener needs. The second type is *language sample analysis* (LSA). With LSA, the professional collects a sample of spontaneous language from the child, typically comprising at least 50 utterances, then analyzes the sample for all aspects of language. Some common measures used in LSA are listed in Table 10.6. Various computer programs, such as the Systematic Analysis of Language Transcripts (SALT; J. Miller & Iglesias, 2006), are available for use with LSA. For instance, after inputting a language sample into the SALT computer program, the professional can run standard statistics on the sample, including calculating the mean length of utterance, the total number of words, the total number of different words, and the use of conjunctions.

Diagnosis

Once the professional completes the comprehensive language evaluation, he or she assesses the findings to determine whether a language disorder is present and, if so, to make a diagnosis. The diagnosis usually involves designating the type of impairment (primary, secondary), affected domains (form, content, use), and severity (mild, moderate, severe, profound). In addition, the diagnosis may include a *prognosis statement.* An excellent or good prognosis means that a disorder is likely to resolve, whereas a poor prognosis means that a disorder is unlikely to resolve. In some cases, professionals do not write a prognosis statement until further

TABLE 10.6
Examples of Various Measures Used in Language Sample Analysis

Language area	Measure
Semantics	• Total number of words • Number of different words • Use of rare words • Lexical ties across utterances • Naming errors • Word-finding problems (e.g., hesitations, circumlocutions)
Phonology	• Percentage of consonants produced correctly • Inventory of different consonants used • Types of consonant errors (omissions, substitutions, distortions) • Consonant use patterns across different syllable structures
Syntax and morphology	• Mean length of utterance • Grammatical morpheme use • Percentage of grammatically correct utterances • Percentage of complex utterances • Conjunction use • Elaborated noun phrase use • Verb phrase use • Variety of sentence types
Pragmatics	• Length of conversational turns • Number of initiations • Contingency of responses • Responses to conversational breakdowns • Variety of communicative intentions

information from other specialists is obtained or an observation period to see how the child responds to treatment has passed.

Treatment of Language Disorders

The nature of a child's language disorder drives the course of treatment. For instance, if a child has a severe language disorder, his or her treatment approach will be more intensive than that for a child with mild problems. Likewise, a child whose language disorder is secondary to autism will receive a treatment approach distinct from that of a child whose language disorder is secondary to traumatic brain injury. The professional develops a **treatment plan** that is unique to the child's needs and strengths. The plan specifies (a) treatment targets, (b) treatment strategies, and (c) treatment contexts.

Treatment Targets

Treatment targets, also called *treatment objectives,* are the aspects of language addressed during treatment. For instance, a treatment target for a 2-year-old might be to produce two-word utterances to communicate needs, whereas a treatment target for an adolescent might be to comprehend figurative language (e.g., jokes heard on the playground). A treatment target for a young child with autism might be to communicate nonverbally for various purposes (request, reject, comment), whereas a treatment target for a first grader with traumatic brain injury might be to answer questions with appropriate, on-topic responses. Some professionals may emphasize only one or two objectives at a time, whereas others may target many objectives simultaneously.

In developing treatment targets, professionals set both long-term and short-term objectives. Long-term objectives specify the long-term goal of treatment, such as "Juan will achieve receptive vocabulary skills commensurate with those of his same-age peers" or "when interacting with other people, Anika will use a full range of communicative intentions to meet her needs." Short-term objectives specify a series of intermediate goals that, when achieved, ultimately lead to the desired long-term objective. For instance, to achieve Anika's long-term objective, a treatment plan for a therapy session might include these two short-term objectives:

1. Anika will use five requests for actions (through gesture, vocalizations, or words) from her peers, given a model by the therapist, during each of three consecutive sessions.

2. Anika will spontaneously use words to pose three requests for actions or objects from her peers during each of three consecutive sessions.

Treatment Strategies

Treatment strategies are the ways in which treatment targets are addressed. **Child-centered approaches** are those in which the child is "in the driver's seat" (Paul, 1995, p. 68). The child sets the pace and chooses the materials, and the professional seeks ways to facilitate language form, content, or use in the context of child-selected activities. One example of a child-centered treatment approach is *focused stimulation* (Cleave & Fey, 1997; Fey, Cleave, Long, & Hughes, 1993; Girolametto, Pearce, & Weitzman, 1996). With focused stimulation, the adult provides multiple and highly salient models of language targets that are goals for the child. For instance, if a child cannot request using the word *want,* the clinician would set up communicative temptations in the context of play-based interactions to entice the child to use the word *want.* The clinician would also repeatedly model use of this word ("I *want* the cookie," "The boy *wants* candy," "The dog *wants* the bone"). To make the word stand out, he or she might say it loudly, slowly, or with dramatic pitch changes (Fey, Long, & Finestack, 2003). During focused stimulation, the child is not required to respond; however, the parent or professional arranges the environment and uses oral techniques to *entice* the child's oral participation and use of language targets. Focused stimulation and other child-centered strategies are often used with young children (infants and preschoolers) and can be implemented by parents in the home following training by a professional (Girolametto et al., 1996).

Clinician-directed approaches are those in which the adult (therapist, teacher, parent) is in the driver's seat. The adult selects the activities and materials and sets the pace of instruction. Rather than waiting for opportunities to occur that address a particular treatment target, the clinician deliberately structures a therapy session with frequent, ongoing opportunities for the child to experience and practice a form, content, or use target. Clinician-directed approaches are especially useful for older children and can be used to target skills that arise infrequently in naturalistic communications. These approaches are also used to teach children with language disorders how to apply specific strategies to compensate for underlying challenges with language comprehension and production. For instance, the professional (therapist) might use a barrier game in which he or she places a barrier between him- or herself and the child. The therapist then gives the child an illustration featuring a complex event and asks the child to describe the picture sufficiently so that the therapist can reproduce it. During the barrier task, the therapist coaches the child to use a **comprehension monitoring** strategy in which the child pauses periodically to check whether the listener is following his or her instructions.

Comprehension monitoring is one strategy children with language disorders can be trained to use to promote more effective communication with other people. A *strategy* is the way an individual approaches a task; it includes both cognitive and behavioral components (i.e., how a person thinks and acts when doing something). **Strategy training** can be an effective way to improve children's abilities to complete diverse language tasks, such as understanding jokes, initiating conversation with friends or adults, or deciphering unknown words when reading. Strategy instruction focuses on teaching students specific ways to approach a linguistic task. The steps in strategy instruction include the following six (Mercer, 1997):

1. Pretest the child on strategy knowledge.
2. Describe the strategy.
3. Model the strategy.
4. Have the child discuss and rehearse the strategy.
5. Have the child practice the strategy, providing feedback until acquisition occurs.
6. Have the child use the strategy in other settings.

Treatment Contexts

Treatment contexts are the settings in which treatment targets and strategies are used. Treatment contexts should include as many settings as possible to promote generalization of skills learned in treatment (i.e., the application of skills to many diverse settings). For instance, children may experience treatment targets and strategies at home with their parents, in the classroom with their teachers, and in the clinic with their SLPs. Clearly, collaboration among parents, teachers, SLPs, and other professionals is critical for ensuring that treatment occurs in many contexts.

For many young children receiving language intervention, treatment is often provided in the home environment. This approach allows parents to observe treatment targets and strategies directly. Home-based interventions are particularly prevalent for children younger than age 3 years who receive language therapy through early intervention services. For older children, treatment is usually provided in the school setting (preschool; elementary, middle, or high school), although parental involvement remains important and should occur at every opportunity. Some children receive language treatment in outpatient hospital clinics or private centers.

In the school setting, treatment contexts can vary. Although historically children received language intervention in a *pullout model,* in which language therapy was provided in a "speech room," this model is becoming less common. Frequently, children receive language intervention through collaborative classroom-based models, in which teachers and SLPs work together to target language goals within the classroom environment (Farber & Klein, 1999). SLPs may work individually with children in classrooms during small-group or center times, may coteach or collaborate to develop particular lessons with teachers, or may train teachers to integrate language enhancement techniques into their classroom instruction.

SUMMARY

A *language disorder* is present when an individual exhibits impaired comprehension or expression of a spoken, written, or other symbol system. Language disorders are the most prevalent type of communication impairment affecting children. When professionals identify a language disorder, they do so by considering the extent to which a child's language difficulties (a) have an adverse impact on social, psychological, and educational functioning; (b) may represent a *language difference* (rather than a disorder); and (c) are significant enough to be considered disordered.

Various professionals are involved with identifying and treating language disorders in children. *Speech–language pathologists* (SLPs) are frequently the lead service providers for children with language disorders. Their responsibilities include prevention, screening, consultation, assessment and diagnosis, and treatment delivery. *Cognitive* and *developmental psychologists* conduct important basic and applied research relevant to theoretical understanding of language disorders. *Clinical, rehabilitation,* and *school psychologists,* as well as *clinical neuropsychologists,* may work directly with children with language disorders, screening for and identifying the disorders. *General educators* and *special educators* have the important role of supporting the educational achievement of children with language disorders in the school setting. *Early interventionists* specialize in assessment and treatment of developmental disabilities in infants and toddlers; thus, they play a critical role in early identification and intervention for young children with suspected or diagnosed language disorders. *Audiologists* are specialists in auditory system disorders and are involved with assessing and treating language disorders when the auditory system is involved. *Developmental pediatricians* often manage the referral process for children whose language disorders are accompanied by more complex health or developmental challenges. *Otorhinolaryngologists* work with children whose language disorders result from disease or infection of the ear, nose, or throat.

Five prevalent developmental conditions associated with language disorder are *specific language impairment* (SLI), *autism spectrum disorder* (ASD), *mental retardation* (MR), *traumatic brain injury* (TBI), and *hearing loss.* SLI is a primary language impairment in which children show significant challenges with language development in the absence of any other known developmental difficulty. *ASD* is an umbrella term that encompasses four neurologically based developmental disorders characterized by disordered communication, repetitive behaviors, difficulties with social relationships, and restricted interests. MR is a developmental disability associated with language disorders ranging from mild to profound. Language disorders resulting from TBI are typically characterized by discourse problems and additional executive difficulties. Hearing loss may be accompanied by a language disorder if it is not detected and early intervention is not instituted.

Identification of a language disorder requires administration of a *comprehensive language evaluation.* It typically includes a case history, an interview, and completion of a comprehensive language assessment using standardized norm-referenced tasks, criterion-referenced tasks, dynamic assessment, and observational measures. The treatment of language disorders typically follows a treatment plan that specifies language targets, treatment strategies, and treatment contexts. It may use a child-directed approach or a clinician-directed approach.

KEY TERMS

acquired hearing loss, p. 343
activity, p. 317
Asperger's syndrome, p. 336
auditory-processing disorder, p. 343
autism, p.336
child-centered approaches, p. 352
childhood disintegrative disorder, p. 336
child study team, p. 327
clinician-directed approaches, p. 352
closed-head injury, p. 342
comprehension monitoring, p. 353
conductive loss, p. 343
congenital hearing loss, p. 343
criterion-referenced tasks, p. 349
cultural context, p. 318
disease, p. 317
dynamic assessment, p. 350
echolalia, p. 336
language delay, p. 315

language disorder, p. 315
language-learning disability, p. 316
least restrictive environment, p. 327
mental retardation, p. 339
norm-referenced tests, p. 349
observational measures, p. 350
open-head injuries, p. 342
participation in life, p. 317
pervasive developmental disorder—
    not otherwise specified, p. 338
postlingual hearing loss, p. 344
prelingual hearing loss, p. 343
prereferral intervention, p. 327
primary language impairment, p. 322
secondary language impairment, p. 322
sensorineural loss, p. 343
significant, p. 320
strategy training, p. 353
treatment plan, p. 351

For online resources related to chapter content, including audio samples, valuable Web sites, suggested readings, and self-quizzes, please go to the Companion Website at http://www.prenhall.com/pence

GLOSSARY

accents (p. 289)   Varieties of language that vary only in pronunciation, not in vocabulary or grammar. Contrast *dialects.*

acoustics (p. 13)   The study of sound.

acquired brain injuries (p. 36)   Damage to the brain occurring in utero (before birth) and perinatally (during the birth process), as well as after birth. See also *closed-head injury; open-head injury; traumatic brain injury.*

acquired hearing loss (p. 343)   Hearing loss that occurs after birth as a result of such factors as noise exposure, infection, use of ototoxic medications, and chronic middle-ear infections. Contrast *congenital hearing loss.* See also *postlingual hearing loss; prelingual hearing loss.*

acquisition rate (p. 24)   How fast language is learned.

activity (p. 317)   The behavioral or performance deficits that result from a disease. With regard to language disorders, the impact of an underlying neurological impairment on a person's comprehension or production of language form, content, and use in everyday circumstances. See also *disease; participation in life.*

afferent (p. 116)   Used to describe the pathway of information as it moves *toward* the brain. Afferent pathways carry sensory information from the distal body structures to the brain; such pathways are also called *ascending pathways.* Contrast *efferent.*

age of mastery (p. 197)   The age by which most children produce a sound in an adultlike manner. See also *customary age of production.*

agent (p. 196)   In an event, the entity that performs the action. See also *goal; location; source; theme.*

agrammaticism (p. 7)   Omission of grammatical markers. In speech, agrammaticism is characterized by a "telegraphic" quality (e.g., "Tommy go store now"). Can occur with damage to certain areas of the left frontal lobe of the brain.

allocortex (p. 122)   In evolutionary terms, the original and older human brain. It and the neocortex compose the cerebrum.

allophones (p. 22)   The subtle variations of phonemes that occur as a result of contextual influence on how phonemes are produced in different words. Example: The two /p/

phonemes in *pop* are produced differently and are thus allophones. See also *phonology.*

alphabetic principle (p. 236)   The relationship between letters or combinations of letters (graphemes) and sounds (phonemes).

alphabet knowledge (p. 223)   Knowledge about the letters of the alphabet. A type of metalinguistic ability important to emergent literacy development.

applied research (p. 43)   Studying language development to test different approaches and practices that pertain to real-world settings, or to address specific problems in society and to inform practices relevant to language development. Contrast *basic research.*

arachnoid mater (p. 120)   The second layer of the meninges. A delicate membrane separated from the pia mater by the subarachnoid space. See also *dura mater; pia mater.*

articulation (p. 8)   Manipulation of a breath of air by the oral articulators—including tongue, teeth, and jaw—so that it comes out as a series of speech sounds that are combined into words, phrases, and sentences. One of four systems involved in speech. See also *phonation; resonation; respiration.*

Asperger's syndrome (p. 336)   A type of autism in which the person is considered "higher functioning." Persons with Asperger's have problems with social interaction; difficulty understanding figurative or abstract language; and restricted, idiosyncratic behavioral patterns and interests. Their language skills are well developed and not considered clinically disordered, but their language may be used in idiosyncratic and unconventional ways. See also *autism; childhood disintegrative disorder; pervasive developmental disorder.*

assessment (p. 213)   Ongoing procedures used to identify a child's needs, family concerns, and resources. Less formal than an evaluation and often encourages more parent and caregiver participation than do evaluations.

assimilation (p. 197)   The process by which children change one sound in a syllable so that it takes on the features of another sound in the same syllable. A context-dependent change. Includes velar assimilation.

audition (p. 13) The perception of sound, including general auditory perception and speech perception. See *hearing.*

auditory perception (p. 14) How the brain processes any type of auditory information (e.g., a clap of the hands), not just speech. Contrast *speech perception.*

auditory-processing disorder (p. 343) Abbreviated APD. Hearing loss that results from damage to the centers of the brain that process auditory information. Contrast *conductive loss; sensorineural loss.*

autism (p. 336) A severe developmental disability with symptoms that emerge before a child's third birthday. Diagnostic criteria are impaired social interaction with other people; moderately to severely impaired communication skills; and restrictive, repetitive, and stereotypical behaviors and interests. See also *Asperger's syndrome; childhood disintegrative disorder; pervasive developmental disorder.*

axon (p. 117) The single efferent nerve extension from the cell body of a neuron. Extends from the cell body for a distance of 1 mm to 1 m, at which point it arborizes into a number of terminal branches. It, along with the dendrites, serves as a vehicle for the cell body to receive and transmit information from other neurons. One of four parts of a neuron. See also *cell body; dendrites; presynaptic terminal.*

babbling (p. 156) A young child's production of syllables that contain pairs of consonants and vowels (*C–V sequences* when the consonant precedes the vowel). Usually begins between ages 6 and 10 months. See also *jargon; marginal babbling; nonreduplicated babbling; reduplicated babbling.*

basic research (p. 43) Also called *theoretical research.* Studying language development primarily to generate and refine the existing knowledge base. See also *use-inspired basic research.* Contrast *applied research.*

bilingualism (p. 29) Technically, a process by which people acquire *two* first languages. In this text, for the sake of simplicity, a process by which people acquire *two or more* first languages. The two languages can be learned simultaneously or sequentially. A type of language difference (rather than disorder). Contrast *monolingualism; second language acquisition.*

bound morphemes (p. 83) Grammatical morphemes that cannot be freestanding; they must be attached to other morphemes: prefixes and suffixes. Contrast *free morphemes.*

brainstem (p. 128) One of the three divisions of the brain. Sits directly on top of the spinal cord and serves as a conduit between the rest of the brain and the spinal cord. Comprises the midbrain, the pons, and the medulla oblongata. It has three primary roles: (a) a key transmitter of sensory information to the brain and of motor information away from the brain; (b) a major relay station for the cranial nerves supplying the head and face and for controlling the visual and auditory areas; and (c) a center for metabolic control and arousal. See also *cerebellum; cerebrum.*

Broca's area (p. 124) Named after the French physician Paul Broca. A region of the left frontal lobe of the cerebrum, important for the fine coordination of speech output. See also *premotor cortex; primary motor cortex.*

categorical scope (p. 193) A principle that builds on the principle of extendibility by limiting the basis for extension to words that are taxonomically similar.

caudal (p. 115) A positional term that describes the specific nervous system structures along the horizontal and vertical axes of the neuraxis. With regard to the horizontal axis, it means "toward the back of the brain." With regard to the vertical axis, it means "toward the bottom of the spinal cord (near the coccyx, or tailbone)." Contrast *dorsal; rostral; ventral.*

cell body (p. 117) The center of a neuron, containing its nucleus. One of four parts of a neuron. See also *axon; dendrites; presynaptic terminal.*

central nervous system (p. 111) Abbreviated CNS. The brain and the spinal cord. Contrast *peripheral nervous system.*

cerebellum (p. 128) One of three major divisions of the brain. Oval-shaped "little brain" that resides posterior to the brainstem. It is primarily responsible for regulating motor and muscular activity and has little to do with the "rational" part of the brain that involves conscious planning responses. It coordinates motor movements, maintains muscle tone, monitors movement range and strength, and maintains posture and equilibrium. See also *brainstem; cerebrum.*

cerebrospinal fluid (p. 120) Abbreviated CSF. Along with bone and the meninges, it shields the central nervous system by circulating between the two innermost layers of the meninges: the pia mater and the arachnoid mater.

cerebrum (p. 122) Also known as the *cerebral cortex.* The largest of the three major divisions of the brain. Plays roles in language, conceptual thinking, creativity, planning, and the form and substances of human thoughts. Consists of right and left hemispheres and is organized into six lobes of four types: one frontal, one occipital, two temporal, and two parietal lobes. Comprises the allocortex and the neocortex. See also *brainstem; cerebellum.*

child-centered approaches (p. 352) Treatment plan strategies in which the child sets the pace and chooses the materials, and the clinician seeks ways to facilitate language form, content, or use in the context of the child-selected activities. One example is focused stimulation. Contrast *clinician-directed approaches.*

childhood disintegrative disorder (p. 336) A disorder in children younger than age 10 years, who appear to be developing normally until at least their second birthday but then display a significant loss or regression of skills in two or more of the following areas: language, social skills, bowel or bladder control, play or motor skills. See also *Asperger's syndrome; autism; pervasive developmental disorder.*

child study team (p. 327) Also called the *evaluation team.* Group of people—including the general educator, a child's parents, and other professionals (e.g., school psychologist, special educator, speech–language pathologist)—who engage in the systematic process of identifying approaches for the general educator to use to support the child's language skills in the classroom. This team also conducts multifactored evaluation to determine whether the child has a language disorder. See also *prereferral intervention.*

clinician-directed approaches (p. 352) Treatment plan strategies in which the adult (therapist, teacher, parent) selects the activities and materials and sets the pace of instruction. One example is comprehension monitoring. Contrast *child-centered approaches.*

closed-head injury (p. 342) Abbreviated CHI. The most common type of traumatic brain injury (TBI), in which brain matter is not exposed or penetrated. One cause in infants is shaken baby syndrome. Usually results in a more diffuse brain injury. Contrast *open-head injuries.*

coarticulation (p. 15) The overlapping of phonemes during human speech.

code switching (p. 29) When speakers who have more than one language in common alternate between the languages. Bilingual children may code switch to fill in lexical or grammatical gaps, for pragmatic effect, or to follow the social norms of their community. Example: A child who is bilingual in Spanish and English may produce an English sentence with Spanish syntax. See also *interutterance mixing; intrautterance mixing.*

communication (p. 8) The process of sharing information among individuals. Communication can involve only language (e.g., communication in an Internet chat room), or language, hearing, and speech (e.g., a spoken conversation).

communication breakdowns (p. 18) Communication problems that occur when receivers do not provide appropriate types or amounts of feedback or when senders do not attend to the feedback. See also *conversational repair.*

communication function (p. 102) The intention of a communication used in a social context, such as instrumental, regulatory, interactional, personal, heuristic, or imaginative.

communication units (C units; p. 281) Each C unit consists of an independent clause and any of its modifiers, such as a dependent clause. Can include incomplete sentences and sentence fragments. C units are coded in transcripts of language samples to assess a student's language form. Contrast *terminable units (T units).*

communicative accommodation (p. 289) The way in which a culture deals with infant-directed speech. It can range from highly child centered to highly situation centered.

complex syntax (p. 92) Grammatically well-formed sentences containing phrases, clauses, and conjunctions, which are used to organize the internal structures of the sentences. Contrast *simple syntax.*

comprehensible input (p. 311) Language input that is just slightly ahead of the learner's current state of grammatical knowledge. Also known as the *i + 1 level,* where *i* is the learner's current state of knowledge. Part of Krashen's (1985) theory that language that contains structures a second language (L2) learner has already mastered will not help his or her acquisition of the L2, nor will input that is too difficult.

comprehension monitoring (p. 353) A strategy used during a barrier task, in which the child must pause periodically to check whether the listener is following his or her instructions. Part of a clinician-directed approach to training children with language disorders to communicate more effectively with other people. See also *strategy training.*

conductive loss (p. 343) Hearing loss resulting from damage to the outer or middle ear. Contrast *auditory-processing disorder; sensorineural loss.*

congenital hearing loss (p. 343) A hearing loss present at birth. About 50% of all cases occur for unknown reasons. Causes include genetic transmission, in utero infections, prematurity, pregnancy complications, and trauma during the birth process. Contrast *acquired hearing loss.*

connectionist models (p. 128) Models that attempt to represent the computational architecture of the brain as it processes various types of information, particularly that which is specific to higher order cognition, such as reasoning and problem solving. According to such models, information processing within the brain involves a network of distributed processors that interact with one another by means of excitatory and inhibitory connections.

content (p. 20) Synonymous with *semantics.* The meaning of language. The words used and the meaning behind them. One of the three language domains. See also *contextualized; decontextualized; form; lexicon; use.*

contextualized (p. 20) Relying on the immediate context, or setting, to convey content. Contrast *decontextualized.*

contextualized language (p. 222) The language used, beginning in infancy, that is grounded in the immediate context, or the here and now. Contrast *decontextualized language.*

conventionality (p. 193) A principle stating that for children to communicate successfully, they must adopt the terms people in their language community understand.

conversational repair (p. 19) When a communication breakdown occurs and the sender or receiver adjusts the exchange to mend the breakdown. It requires the receiver to provide ongoing feedback and the sender to monitor the receiver's feedback closely.

conversational schema (p. 103)   Also called a *conversational framework*. Framework of a conversation, including initiating and establishing a topic, engaging in a series of turns that maintain the topic, and resolving and closing the topic.

conversations (p. 103)   Exchanges with other people.

corpus callosum (p. 122)   The band of fibers that connects the two hemispheres of the cerebrum. Serves as a conduit for communication between them. See also *longitudinal fissure*.

cranial nerves (p. 119)   The 12 pairs of nerves that emerge from the brain.

criterion-referenced tasks (p. 349)   Tasks used to examine a child's performance level for a particular type of language task, such as understanding locational and spatial terms. Typically used as part of a comprehensive language assessment. See also *dynamic assessment; norm-referenced tests; observational measures*.

critical period (p. 25)   Also called *sensitive period*. The window of opportunity during which children develop language most rapidly and with the most ease.

critical period hypothesis (p. 310)   The theory that the time between birth and puberty is crucial for language acquisition and that adolescents and adults may experience difficulty acquiring a second language.

cultural context (p. 318)   The cultural setting in which a child learns and applies language. Practitioners must take it into account when differentiating between a language difference and a language disorder.

C units (p. 281)   See *communication units*.

customary age of production (p. 197)   The age by which 50% of all children can produce a given sound in multiple positions in words in an adultlike way. Contrast *age of mastery*.

declarative pointing (p. 164)   Pointing by an infant to call an adult's attention to objects and to comment on objects. Involves a social process between an infant and an adult. Occurs after age 10 months. Contrast *imperative pointing*.

declarative sentences (p. 89)   Sentences that make a statement. Contrast *interrogative sentences; negative sentences*.

decontextualized (p. 20)   Not relying on the immediate context, or setting, to convey content. Contrast *contextualized*.

decontextualized language (p. 222)   Language that relies heavily on itself in the construction of meaning. Begins to emerge during the preschool period. Contrast *contextualized language*.

deep-structure ambiguity (p. 268)   A form of sentential ambiguity in which a noun serves as an agent in one interpretation and as an object in another. Example: *The duck is ready to eat* can mean "The duck is ready to be eaten" or "The duck is hungry." Contrast *surface-structure ambiguity*.

deictic terms (p. 232)   Words whose use and interpretation depend on the location of a speaker and listener within a particular setting. To use such terms correctly, children must be able to adopt their conversational partner's perspective. Examples: The terms *here* and *this,* used to indicate proximity to the speaker, and the terms *there* and *that,* used to indicate proximity to the listener.

dendrites (p. 117)   The afferent extensions from the single cell body of a neuron. They bring nerve impulses into the cell body from the axonal projections of other neurons. One of four parts of a neuron. See also *axon; cell body; presynaptic terminal*.

dendritic sprouting (p. 138)   The formation of new synaptic connections among neurons. Is necessary for experience-dependent plasticity.

derivational morphemes (p. 82)   Prefixes and suffixes added to root words to create derived words. See also *derivational relations*. Contrast *grammatical morphemes*.

derivational relations (p. 84)   The relationship among a corpus of words that share a common root word. Example: *friend, friendless, befriend*. See also *derivational morphemes*.

diagnostic assessments (p. 278)   Evaluations performed anytime during the school year to obtain an in-depth look at a specific child's instructional needs.

dialects (p. 29)   Regional or social variations of a language that differ from one another in terms of their pronunciation, vocabulary, and grammar. Dialects can evolve within specific geographic regions or sociocultural communities. A type of language difference (rather than disorder). Example: African American Vernacular English. Contrast *accents*.

disease (p. 317)   An underlying physiological condition that impedes performance. With regard to language disorders, an underlying neurological impairment that causes a person to have difficulties with comprehension or production of language form, content, or use. See also *activity; participation in life*.

dishabituation (p. 174)   Describes a phase in a task used to renew an infant's interest in a stimulus according to a predetermined threshold. Contrast *habituation*.

domain general (p. 55)   The same as in other situations. In the context of language development, domain-general language processes are the same as the processes used in other situations such as solving problems and perceiving objects and events in the environment. Contrast *domain specific*.

domain specific (p. 7)   Dedicated solely to a certain task. In the context of language development, domain-specific language processes are dedicated solely to the tasks of comprehending and producing language. Contrast *domain general*.

dorsal (p. 115) A positional term experts use when describing the specific nervous system structures along the horizontal and vertical axes of the neuraxis. With regard to the horizontal axis, it means "toward the top of the brain." With regard to the vertical axis, it means "toward the back of the spinal cord (the side nearest the back)." Contrast *caudal; rostral; ventral.*

dual language learners (p. 297) People who learn two or more languages simultaneously, sequentially, as a second language in school in the United States, or as a foreign language in another country.

dual language system hypothesis (p. 300) The idea that bilingual children have two separate language systems from the start. According to this theory, bilingual children do not move through stages whereby they eventually differentiate between the two languages. Contrast *unitary language system hypothesis.*

dura mater (p. 120) Literal meaning is "hard mother." The third and outermost layer of the meninges. Consists of thick, fibrous tissue that completely encases the brain and the spinal cord. See also *arachnoid mater; pia mater.*

duration (p. 148) In terms of speech, the length of sounds. One of three prosodic characteristics of speech. Contrast *frequency; intensity.*

dynamic assessment (p. 350) An examination of how a child's performance on a particular language task improves by giving the child different types of assistance. Typically used as part of a comprehensive language assessment. See also *criterion-referenced tasks; norm-referenced tests; observational measures.*

early consonants (p. 99) Consonants that emerge early in speech sound development. Contrast *late consonants.*

echolalia (p. 336) Stereotypical repetitions of specific words or phrases. Commonly seen in association with autism spectrum disorder, which includes Asperger's syndrome, autism, childhood disintegrative disorder, and pervasive developmental disorder.

ecological validity (p. 214) The extent to which the data resulting from an assessment or an evaluation can be extended to multiple contexts, including the child's home and day care settings.

efferent (p. 116) Used to describe the pathway of information as it moves *away* from the brain. Efferent pathways carry motor impulses from the central nervous system to more distal body structures; such pathways are also called *descending pathways.* Contrast *afferent.*

egocentric speech (p. 61) Speech that describes the worldview from only the speaker's perspective. Self-centered speech. One of the earliest forms of speech; a precursor to true dialogue.

emergent literacy (p. 222) The earliest period of learning about reading and writing. Children in this stage of literacy are not yet reading and writing in a conventional sense, but their emerging knowledge about print and sounds forms an important foundation for the reading instruction that begins in formal schooling.

enrichment (p. 68) The process through which teachers, clinicians, and other adults provide children, adolescents, and adults with an enhanced language-learning environment that builds on existing skills and promotes the development of new and more advanced language skills. One of three direct applications of language theory and research to practice. See also *intervention and remediation; prevention.*

evaluation (p. 213) A method used to determine a child's initial and continuing eligibility for services under the Individuals with Disabilities Education Act. Includes a determination of the child's status across developmental areas. Contrast *assessment.*

event-related potentials (p. 194) Abbreviated ERPs. The electrical responses of the brain to particular stimuli, including linguistic stimuli. Used in neuroimaging.

executive functions (p. 123) Functions that govern the organized, goal-directed, and controlled execution of critical human behaviors, such as monitoring and controlling purposeful behaviors, overriding impulses, and controlling information processing. The frontal lobe of the cerebrum controls these functions.

experience-dependent plasticity (p. 138) Brain modification that results from highly specific types of experiences. Contrast *experience-expectant plasticity.*

experience-expectant plasticity (p. 138) Changes in the brain structure that occur as a result of normal experiences. Contrast *experience-dependent plasticity.*

expressive elaboration (p. 274) When the components of story grammar are combined in an expressive or artful manner of storytelling.

expressive language (p. 170) The language a person produces spontaneously, without imitating another person's verbalizations. Includes content, form, and use. Contrast *receptive language.*

expressive lexicon (p. 74) The volume of words a person uses; a "mental dictionary." Contrast *receptive lexicon.*

extended mapping (p. 229) A full and complete understanding of the meaning of a word.

extendibility (p. 192) The notion that words label categories of objects, not just the original exemplar.

extralinguistic feedback (p. 17) See *nonlinguistic feedback.*

fast mapping (p. 86) A type of task in which the rate at which children map a new word to its referent is determined. Contrast *slow mapping.*

feedback (p. 12) (a) In models of speech production, information about the timing, delivery, and precision of speech output that is relayed back to the origination of the perceptual target and motor schema. It provides information about what is to come next at the perceptual and motor levels. Speakers are seldom aware of feedback on a conscious level. (b) In models of communication, information provided by the receiver to the sender. The sender responds to this feedback to modulate the flow of communication. See also *linguistic feedback; nonlinguistic feedback.*

fictional narrative (p. 238) A child's spoken or written description of an imaginary event. Contrast *personal narrative.*

figurative language (p. 258) Language used in nonliteral and often abstract ways. Used to evoke mental images and sense impressions in other people. See also *hyperboles; idioms; irony; metaphors; proverbs; similes.*

form (p. 20) How words, sentences, and sounds are organized and arranged to convey content. One of the three language domains. See also *content; use.*

formative evaluations (p. 278) Assessment of the language process (rather than the products) of language learning and development. Practitioners use these assessments to determine the types of language-learning activities to implement. Contrast *summative evaluations.*

free morphemes (p. 83) Grammatical morphemes that can stand alone; they include not only words with clear semantic referents (e.g., *dream, dog*) but also words that serve primarily grammatical purposes (e.g., *his, the*). Contrast *bound morphemes.*

frequency (p. 13) How fast air particles move back and forth during the creation of sound. Pitch. One of three prosodic characteristics of speech. Contrast *duration; intensity.*

frontal lobe (p. 123) The largest of six lobes in the cerebrum. Resides in the most anterior part of the brain, behind the forehead. Activates and controls both fine and complex motor activities and controls executive functions. Includes the prefrontal cortex, primary motor cortex, and premotor cortex. See also *Broca's area; occipital lobe; parietal lobes; temporal lobes.*

fronting (p. 198) Replacement of sounds normally produced farther back in the mouth (e.g., /k/) with sounds produced father forward in the mouth (e.g., /t/). A place-of-articulation change that is not context dependent. Example: *Cake* becomes "take."

functional flexibility (p. 271) The ability to use language for various communicative purposes (e.g., requesting, stating, persuading).

functional magnetic resonance imaging (p. 113) Abbreviated fMRI. A type of brain imaging that allows researchers and physicians to identify the brain structures involved in specific mental functions. Noninvasive procedure that maps neural activities to specific neural regions according to change in blood oxygen levels that correspond to changes in neural activity.

gender differences (p. 31) Language differences relating to gender. Example: Girls usually begin talking before boys do. Usually minor, particularly as children move into the preschool years.

general all-purpose verbs (p. 307) Also called *GAP verbs.* The verbs *make, do,* and *go.* Children rely on these verbs heavily during the fourth stage of L2 development, or the period of language productivity.

General American English (p. 22) Abbreviated GAE. Also called *Standard American English.* Dialect used most commonly in the United States (i.e., assigned the highest social status). Includes about 39 phonemes.

genetic epistemology (p. 61) The study of the development of knowledge. French psychologist Jean Piaget is know for his theories on genetic epistemology.

goal (p. 196) In an event, the ending point for movement. See also *agent; location; source; theme.*

grammatical morphemes (p. 82) Also called *inflectional morphemes.* Small units of language added to words to allow grammatical inflection of the words. Examples: the plural *-s,* the possessive *'s,* the past tense *-ed,* and the present progressive *-ing.* See also *bound morphemes; free morphemes.* Contrast *derivational morphemes.*

gray matter (p. 118) Nervous tissue consisting of the cell bodies of neurons and the dendrites. Where information is generated and processed. Contrast *white matter.*

habituation (p. 174) Describes a task involving presenting an infant with the same stimulus repeatedly until his or her attention to the stimulus decreases by a predetermined amount. Contrast *dishabituation.*

hearing (p. 8) The sensory system that allows speech to enter into and be processed by the human brain. See also *communication; speech.*

heritable language impairment (p. 34) See *primary language impairment.*

Heschl's gyrus (p. 126) Named after the Austrian anatomist Richard L. Heschl. A small left temporal lobe region that appears to be specialized for processing speech, particularly its temporal aspects.

home language stage (p. 305) First stage of learning English as a second language. During this stage, children use their home language in the classroom with other children and adults. They usually cease to do so upon realizing that it does not promote successful communication with other people. See also *language productivity; nonverbal period; telegraphic and formulaic use.*

homographs (p. 268) Words that are spelled the same and may sound alike (e.g., *row a boat* vs. *row of homes*) or may sound different from each other (e.g., *record player* vs. *record a movie*). A type of lexical ambiguity at the level of the word. See also *homonyms; homophones.*

homonyms (p. 268) Words that are alike in spelling and pronunciation but differ in meaning (e.g., *brown bear* vs. *bear weight*). A specific type of homophone.

homophones (p. 267) Words that sound alike and may be spelled alike (*brown bear* vs. *bear weight*) or may be spelled differently (e.g., *brown bear* vs. *bare hands*). A type of lexical ambiguity at the word level. See also *homographs; homonyms.*

horizontal axis (p. 114) The part of the neuraxis that runs from the anterior (frontal) pole of the brain to the posterior (occipital) pole. See also *vertical axis.*

hyperbole (p. 260) A type of figurative language that uses exaggeration for emphasis or effect. Example: *I nearly died laughing.*

iconic communication (p. 16) See *intentional communication.*

idioms (p. 260) Expressions that contain both literal and figurative language. Two types of idioms are opaque and transparent. Example: *He got out of the wrong side of bed.*

imperative pointing (p. 164) Pointing by an infant to request an adult to retrieve an object for him or her. Occurs around age 10 months. Contrast *declarative pointing.*

inflection point (p. 75) The point in a vocabulary spurt that differentiates between the slow and the rapid stages of vocabulary development.

inner language (p. 8) Thoughts and ideas that an individual keeps to him- or herself after they are formulated. Contrast *written language.*

innervate (p. 119) To supply nerves to a particular region or part of the body.

intensity (p. 13) How far apart air particles move when they are going back and forth during the creation of sound. Loudness. One of three prosodic characteristics of speech. Contrast *duration; frequency.*

intentional communication (p. 16) Also called *iconic communication.* Communication that is relatively more precise in intent than symbolic communication, but unlike symbolic communication, the relationship between the communicative behavior and its referent is not arbitrary. Rather, it relies on the shared spatial position among the sender, the recipient, and the referent. The relationship between the message and its referent is transparent. Example: When a chimpanzee points to a banana. See also *preintentional communication.* Contrast *symbolic communication.*

intentionality hypothesis (p. 103) The theory that children's development of language form and content is fostered in part by their experience with other people as they use language to engage with these people.

interlanguage (p. 302) The language system speakers create during second language (L2) acquisition. It includes elements of the first language (L1) and the L2 as well as elements found in neither of the two languages. Example: L1 phonology combined with L2 syntax, such as "I bring not the children" by a speaker with German as the L1 and English as the L2.

interrogative sentences (p. 90) Sentences that ask a question. Contrast *declarative sentences; negative sentences.*

intersubjective awareness (p. 163) Recognition of when one person shares a mental focus on some external object or action with another person.

interutterance mixing (p. 301) When code switching occurs between utterances. Contrast *intrautterance mixing.*

intervention and remediation (p. 68) Programs or strategies used to help children, adolescents, and adults who exhibit difficulties with some aspect of language development. One of three direct applications of language theory and research to practice. See also *enrichment; prevention.*

intonation (p. 148) The prominence placed on various parts of sentences. Contrast *stress.*

intrautterance mixing (p. 301) When code switching occurs within a single utterance. Contrast *interutterance mixing.*

irony (p. 550) A type of figurative language that involves incongruity between what a speaker or writer says and what actually happens. Puns and sarcasm make use of irony. Two types of irony are verbal and dramatic.

jargon (p. 157) A special type of babbling that contains the true melodic patterns of an infant's native language. Such babbling resembles questions, exclamations, and commands, even in the absence of recognizable words. See also *marginal babbling; nonreduplicated babbling; reduplicated babbling.*

joint attention (p. 104) Attention focused on a mutual object. For infants, maintaining joint attention requires them to coordinate their attention between the social partner and the object. Prerequisite to development of a conversational schema.

language (p. 4) A rule-governed, code-based tool shared by the members of a community. Used to represent thoughts and ideas to other people who know the code.

language acquisition device (p. 63) Professor of linguistics Noam Chomsky's innate, species-specific module dedicated to language and not other forms of learning.

language comprehension (p. 53) The ability to understand language. Contrast *language production.*

language delay (p. 315) A late start to language development that is expected to resolve at some point.

language difference (p. 28) The variability among language users. Example: Girls speak earlier than boys do. See also *bilingualism; dialects; gender differences.* Contrast *language disorder.*

language disorder (p. 315)   Significant language development difficulties relative to those experienced by children developing normally. See also *primary language impairment; secondary language impairment.* Contrast *language difference.*

language fossilization (p. 302)   When the speech of a second language speaker becomes permanently established in the interlanguage.

language impairment (p. 31)   See *language disorder.*

language-learning disability (p. 316)   A language disorder in an older child that results in difficulties with academic achievement in areas associated with language, such as reading, writing, and spelling.

language production (p. 48)   The ability to use language expressively. Contrast *language comprehension.*

language productivity (p. 307)   The fourth stage of second language development, in which children are not yet proficient speakers of their second language but their communicative repertoire continues to expand. See also *home language stage; nonverbal period; telegraphic and formulaic use.*

language stabilization (p. 302)   In second language (L2) acquisition, when the interlanguage stops evolving and L2 learners reach a plateau in their language development.

late consonants (p. 99)   Consonants emerging later in speech sound development. Contrast *early consonants.*

least restrictive environment (p. 327)   Abbreviated LRE. The environment in which a child with disabilities should receive education. It should, to the maximum extent, be the same as that of the child's peers without disabilities. Part of the Individuals with Disabilities Education Act (IDEA) mandate.

left hemisphere (p. 122)   One of two mirror-image halves of the cerebrum. See also *corpus callosum; longitudinal fissure.* Contrast *right hemisphere.*

lexical ambiguity (p. 267)   When words or phrases have multiple meanings. Provides the humor in jokes, riddles, comics, and so forth. Example: *That was a real bear* (*bear* has several meanings). See also *sentential ambiguity.*

lexicon (p. 20)   A vocabulary system, or "mental dictionary." Used to convey content. For each word a child learns, he or she creates an entry in the lexicon. The entry contains a series of symbols that compose the word, the sound of the word, the meaning of the word, and its part of speech.

linguistic feedback (p. 17)   The use of speech or vocalizations (e.g., "mm-hmm") to relay information to the sender about his or her message. See also *nonlinguistic feedback; paralinguistic feedback.*

liquid gliding (p. 236)   When a glide consonant, such as /w/, replaces a liquid consonant, such as /r/, so that, for example, *rabbit* is pronounced "wabbit." This phonological process may persist past a child's fifth birthday.

literate language (p. 268)   Language used without the aid of context cues to support meaning: highly decontextualized language.

location (p. 196)   In an event, the place where an action occurs. See also *agent; goal; source; theme.*

longitudinal fissure (p. 122)   The long cerebral crevice that separates the two hemispheres of the cerebrum. See also *corpus callosum.*

magnetic resonance imaging (p. 112)   A technology that allows scientists to obtain detailed images of both the anatomy and the physiology of the nervous system.

majority ethnolinguistic community (p. 298)   A group of people who speak a language that the majority of people in an area (e.g., country, state, province) value and assign high social status. Example: Standard American English (SAE) speakers in the United States. Contrast *minority ethnolinguistic community.*

marginal babbling (p. 156)   An early type of babbling containing short strings of consonant-like and vowel-like sounds. Usually emerges as infants gain control of their articulation, at around age 5–8 months. See also *jargon; nonreduplicated babbling; reduplicated babbling.*

meninges (p. 120)   One shield of the central nervous system, comprising three layers that completely encase the CNS. Comprises the pia mater, arachnoid mater, and dura mater.

mental lexicon (p. 74)   The volume of words a person understands and uses. See also *expressive lexicon; receptive lexicon.*

mental retardation (p. 339)   Abbreviated MR. A condition of arrested development of the mind. Diagnostic criteria are significant limitations in both intellectual functioning and adaptive behavior. May range from mild to severe. Down syndrome is a common cause of MR.

metalinguistic ability (p. 222)   The ability to view language as an object of attention (e.g., preschoolers exhibit metalinguistic ability when they pretend to write or make up rhyming patterns). See also *alphabet knowledge; phonological awareness; print awareness.*

metalinguistic competence (p. 257)   The ability to think about and analyze language as an object of attention. Acquired mainly in the school-age years.

metaphor (p. 258)   A type of figurative language that conveys similarity through an expression that refers to something it does not denote literally. Components of metaphors are the topic and the vehicle. Two types of metaphors are predictive and proportional.

minority ethnolinguistic community (p. 299)   A group of people who speak a language that few people in the community speak or value. Example: Japanese speakers in the United States. Contrast *majority ethnolinguistic community.*

model (p. 9) A representation of an unknown event on the basis of the best current evidence governing the event.

modularity (p. 7) A cognitive science theory about how the human mind is organized within the brain structures. It contends that the human brain contains a set of highly specific modules—or regions developed to process specific types of information.

monolinguism (p. 29) Acquisition of only one language. Contrast *bilingualism*.

morphemes (p. 5) The smallest units of language that carry meaning. They are combined to create words. Example: *pre + school + s = preschools*.

morphology (p. 22) The rules of language governing the internal organization of words. One of the components of the language domain of form. See also *phonology; pragmatics; semantics; syntax*.

morphophonemic development (p. 271) When an individual attains the ability to make sound modifications by joining certain morphemes (/əz/ in *matches*), to use vowel shifting (/aɪ/ to /ɪ/ in *decide–decision*), and to use stress and emphasis to distinguish phrases from compound words (*green house* vs. *greenhouse*).

myelin (p. 118) The coating sheathing each neuron. The myelin sheath contributes to the rapid relay of nerve impulses, particularly within white matter, and protects the neuron.

myelinization (p. 118) The growth of the myelin sheath, a slow process that is not complete until late childhood.

narrative (p. 238) A child's spoken or written description of a real or a fictional event from the past, the present, or the future. See also *fictional narrative; personal narrative*.

negative sentences (p. 90) Sentences that express negation and rely on such words as *no, not, can't, don't*, and *won't*. Contrast *declarative sentences; interrogative sentences*.

neocortex (p. 121) Means "new cortex" or "new rind." The enlarged outer layers of the brain that, during evolution, grew over the older human brain, or allocortex. The neocortex and the allocortex compose the cerebrum. Controls most of the functions that exemplify human thought and language, including speech, language, reasoning, planning, and problem solving.

neural plasticity (p. 137) The malleability of the central nervous system, or the ability of the sensory and motor systems to organize and reorganize by generating new synaptic connections or by using existing synapses for alternative means. See also *experience-dependent plasticity; experience-expectant plasticity*.

neuraxis (p. 114) The horizontal and vertical axes along which the human nervous system is organized. See also *horizontal axis; vertical axis*.

neuroanatomy (p. 111) The anatomical structures of the nervous system. See also *neurophysiology; neuroscience*.

neurolinguists (p. 112) Experts who study the structures and functions of the nervous system that relate to language.

neurons (p. 117) The billions of highly specialized cells that compose the nervous system.

neurophysiology (p. 111) The way the anatomical structures of the nervous system work together as a complex unit and as separate, distinct biological units. See also *neuroanatomy; neuroscience*.

neuroscience (p. 111) The branch of science involving the study of the anatomy and physiology of the nervous system. See also *neuroanatomy; neurophysiology*.

neurotransmitters (p. 118) Chemical agents that help transmit information across the synaptic cleft between two neurons.

nonlinguistic feedback (p. 17) The use of eye contact, facial expression, posture, and proximity to relay information to the sender about his or her message. It may supplement linguistic feedback or stand alone. See also *paralinguistic feedback*.

nonostentive word-learning contexts (p. 77) Also called *inferential contexts*. Situations in which little contextual information is provided about a novel word. Contrast *ostentive word-learning contexts*.

nonreduplicated babbling (p. 157) Also known as *variegated babbling*. Babbling consisting of nonrepeating consonant–vowel combinations, such as "da ma goo ga." Occurs around age 6–10 months. See also *jargon; marginal babbling*. Contrast *reduplicated babbling*.

nonverbal period (p. 306) Second stage of learning English as a second language (ESL). During this period, children learn little to no language, instead beginning to acquire their second language receptively. Some children in this stage use gestures to communicate until they acquire a sufficient number of words in their second language. See also *home language stage; language productivity; telegraphic and formulaic use*.

normative research (p. 48) Studies in which experts compile data from individuals on a certain aspect of language development and from these data determine and chart the ages (or grades) by which children typically meet certain milestones.

norm-referenced tests (p. 349) Tests used to examine children's level of language performance against that of a national sample of same-age peers. Typically used as part of a comprehensive language assessment. See also *criterion-referenced tasks; dynamic assessment; observational measures*.

novel name–nameless category (N3C) (p. 193) A principle stating that a nameless object included in a group of known objects should be the recipient of a novel label. Supporting the principle of object scope, the principle of N3C is based on the principle of mutual exclusivity but does not presuppose that children avoid attaching more than one label to an object.

object scope (p. 193)   A principle stating that words map to whole objects. See also *whole object assumption.*

obligatory contexts (p. 84)   Situations in which a mature grammar specifies use of a grammatical marker. Example: In the sentence *The girl's hat is lost,* the possessive *'s* is considered obligatory. Used by researchers studying children's achievement of grammatical morphology.

observational measures (p. 350)   Analyses used to examine children's language form, content, and use in naturalistic activities with peers or parents. Two types are conversational analysis and language sample analysis (LSA). Typically used as part of a comprehensive language assessment. See also *criterion-referenced tasks; dynamic assessment; norm-referenced tests.*

occipital lobe (p. 124)   One of the six lobes of the cerebrum composing the posterior portion of the brain. It is functionally specialized for visual reception and processing. See also *frontal lobe; parietal lobes; temporal lobes.*

open-head injuries (p. 342)   Abbreviated OHIs. Traumatic brain injuries (TBIs) in which the brain matter is exposed through penetration. One cause is gunshot wounds. Usually result in a more focal brain injury. Contrast *closed-head injury.*

operant conditioning (p. 59)   A concept in B. F. Skinner's behaviorist theory that describes how behaviors are shaped by responses to the behaviors. The result is that behaviors that are reinforced become stronger and those that are punished become suppressed.

oral communication (p. 16)   The combination of speaking and listening.

oral language (p. 222)   Language that is spoken. Comprises three domains: content, form, and use.

ostentive word-learning contexts (p. 77)   Situations in which a lot of contextual information is provided about a novel word, either linguistically or extralinguistically. Contrast *nonostentive word-learning contexts.*

outcome assessments (p. 278)   Evaluations conducted to help determine the discrepancy between expected and observed outcomes in a particular area.

overextension (p. 189)   Three types of overgeneralizations children make: categorical, analogical, and relational (e.g., calling all four-legged animals "dog" after learning the word *dog,* calling the moon "ball," and calling a watering can "flower," respectively). See also *overlap.* Contrast *underextension.*

overgeneralization (p. 62)   A concept in the competition model that describes when children who are learning language make an irregular past tense verb regular by adding a /d/, /t/, or /ɪd/ sound.

overlap (p. 190)   Overextension of a word in certain circumstances and underextension of the same word in other circumstances. Example: Using the word *candy* to refer to jelly beans and grandmother's pills (overextension) but not to chocolate bars (underextension).

paralinguistic (p. 160)   Aspects of communication outside the linguistic information, such as pitch, loudness, posture, and eye contact. With infant-directed speech, paralinguistic features include a high overall pitch, exaggerated pitch contours, and slower tempos than those of adult-directed speech.

paralinguistic feedback (p. 18)   The use of pitch, loudness, and pauses, all of which are superimposed over linguistic feedback, to relay information to a sender about his or her message. See also *nonlinguistic feedback.*

parietal lobes (p. 125)   Two of the six lobes of the cerebrum. They reside posterior to the frontal lobe on the left and right sides (above the ears). Their key functions include perceiving incoming sensory and perceptual information and integrating it with the executive functions of the frontal lobe, comprehending oral and written language, and calculating mathematics. Include the primary somatosensory cortex and the sensory association cortex. See also *frontal lobe; occipital lobe; temporal lobes.*

participation in life (p. 319)   How a disease affects the quality of life of a child and his or her family, including possible impacts on social, psychological, and educational functioning. See also *activity; disease.*

peripheral nervous system (p. 112)   Abbreviated PNS. The cranial and spinal nerves, which carry information inward to and outward from the brain and spinal cord. Contrast *central nervous system.*

personal narrative (p. 238)   A child's spoken or written description of a factual event. Contrast *fictional narrative.*

pervasive developmental disorder—not otherwise specified (p. 338)   Abbreviated PDD–NOS. A disorder in which a person has severe problems with social interactions and communication and displays repetitive behaviors and overly restricted interests but does not otherwise meet the specific diagnostic criteria for autism, childhood disintegrative disorder, or Asperger's syndrome.

phonation (p. 8)   When a breath of air that has been respirated travels over the vocal cords. One of four systems involved in speech. See also *articulation; resonation; respiration.*

phoneme (p. 10)   The smallest unit of sound that can signal a difference in meaning. In the production of syllables and words, a series of phonemes are strung together. Examples: /m/ + /a/ = "ma."

phonemic awareness (p. 99)   The ability to attend to the phonemic units of words.

phonetic (p. 148)   Referring to phonemes (speech sounds) and combinations of phonemes. Infants pay close attention to the phonetic details of speech to learn words. Contrast *prosodic*.

phonetically consistent forms (p. 184)   Abbreviated PCFs. The idiosyncratic wordlike productions that children use consistently and meaningfully but that do not approximate adult forms. PCFs have a consistent sound structure, but children may use them to refer to more than a single referent. Example: "aaah" to refer to both water and the desire to be picked up.

phonetic module (p. 132)   According to some experts, a specialized processor that is designed specifically for processing the phonetic segments of speech.

phonological ambiguity (p. 267)   A type of sentential ambiguity in which varying pronunciations of a word change the meaning of a sentence. Example: *She needs to visit her psychotherapist* vs. *She needs to visit her psycho therapist*.

phonological awareness (p. 69)   The ability to focus on the sounds that make up syllables and words, through implicit or explicit analysis. A type of metalinguistic ability important to emergent literacy. See also *phonemic awareness*.

phonological knowledge (p. 98)   Knowledge of internal representations of the phonemes composing a native language. See also *phonological production*.

phonological processes (p. 197)   The systematic and rule-governed speech patterns that characterize speech, including syllable structure changes, assimilation, place-of-articulation changes, and manner-of-articulation changes.

phonological production (p. 98)   Using the phonemes composing a native language to produce syllables and words. See also *phonological knowledge*.

phonology (p. 22)   The rules of language governing the sounds used to make syllables and words. One of the components of the language domain of form. See also *allophones; morphology; pragmatics; semantics; syntax*.

phonotactic cues (p. 98)   Sounds following the phonotactic rules of a native language that allow infants to parse the speech stream. Example: In English, the phoneme sequence /g/ + /z/ does not usually start a word but can end it (*dogs*). Contrast *prosodic cues*.

phonotactic rules (p. 97)   The rules of a person's native language that specify "legal" orders of sounds in syllables and words and the places where specific phonemes can and cannot occur.

phonotactics (p. 24)   How sounds are organized in words. See also *phonology*.

phrasal coordination (p. 91)   The ability to connect phrases, such as with conjunctions. Example: *I'm putting on my coat and my hat*.

pia mater (p. 120)   The inner layer of the meninges. Wraps tightly around the brain and spinal cord. See also *arachnoid mater; dura mater*.

polysemous (p. 267)   Having more than one meaning.

postlingual hearing loss (p. 344)   A type of acquired hearing loss that occurs after birth and after a child has developed language. Contrast *prelingual hearing loss*.

pragmatics (p. 24)   Synonymous with *use*. The rules of language governing how language is used for social purposes. See also *morphology; phonology; semantics; syntax*.

prefrontal cortex (p. 123)   The most anterior portion of the frontal lobe of the cerebrum. The part of the brain that evolved most recently, is most developed, and is connected with all other sensory and motor systems of the brain. It regulates the depth of feelings—such as gloom, elation, calmness, and friendliness—and is involved with executive functions.

preintentional communication (p. 15)   Communication in which other people assume the relationship between a communicative behavior and its referent. Example: When an infant cries, the communicative partner must infer the referent or goal of the communication. See also *intentional communication*. Contrast *symbolic communication*.

prelingual hearing loss (p. 343)   A type of acquired hearing loss that occurs after birth but before a child has developed language. Contrast *postlingual hearing loss*.

premotor cortex (p. 123)   One component of the frontal lobe of the cerebrum. Important for speech and other motor functions. Controls musculature and programming patterns and sequences of movements. See also *primary motor cortex*.

prereading stage (p. 255)   Period from birth till the beginning of formal education. Some of children's most critical developments—oral language, print awareness, and phonological awareness—occur during this period.

prereferral intervention (p. 329)   Identification of approaches to use to support a child's language skills in the classroom when the child is suspected of having impaired language abilities. The child study team, or evaluation team, implements such intervention.

presynaptic terminal (p. 117)   The distal end of each terminal branch of an axon. A site at which the axonal connection of one neuron corresponds with the dendritic extension of another neuron.

prevention (p. 68)   To inhibit language difficulties from emerging and thus reduce the need to resolve such difficulties later in life. One of three direct applications of language theory and research to practice. See also *enrichment; intervention and remediation*.

primary language impairment (p. 322)   Also known as *heritable language impairment* or *specific language* impairment (SLI). A significant language impairment in the absence of any other developmental difficulty (e.g., mental retardation, brain injury). Affects approximately 7–10% of children older than age 5 years. The most common reason for administering early intervention and special education services to toddlers through fourth graders. Contrast *secondary language impairment*.

primary motor cortex (p. 123) One component of the frontal lobe of the cerebrum. Important for speech and other motor functions. Controls the initiation of skilled, delicate voluntary movements of the extremities and speech. See also *premotor cortex*.

primary somatosensory cortex (p. 125) Also called the *sensory strip* or *primary sensory cortex*. The region of the parietal lobes that, along with the sensory association cortex, resides just posterior to the primary motor cortex in the frontal lobe. Receives and processes sensory experiences of pain, temperature, touch, pressure, and movement from receptors throughout the body.

print awareness (p. 223) Understanding of the forms and functions of written language. A type of metalinguistic ability important to emergent literacy.

productivity (p. 27) The principle of combination whereby small numbers of discrete units are combined into seemingly infinite novel creations. This principle also applies to human activities other than language—such as mathematics and music.

progress-monitoring assessments (p. 278) Evaluations conducted routinely (at least three times a year) to document a child's rate of improvement in an area and to compare the efficacy of curricula and interventions.

prosodic (p. 148) Referring to the frequency (pitch), duration (length), and intensity (loudness) of sounds. Combinations of prosodic characteristics produce distinguishable stress and intonation patterns that infants can detect to parse the speech stream. Contrast *phonetic*.

prosodic cues (p. 98) Word and syllable intonation and stress patterns in a language that allow infants to break into the speech stream. Contrast *phonotactic cues*.

proverbs (p. 261) Statements that express the conventional values, beliefs, and wisdom of a society. A type of figurative language.

receiver (p. 15) The listener during communication. The person who takes in and then comprehends the information. Contrast *sender*.

receptive language (p. 170) The language people comprehend. Contrast *expressive language*.

receptive lexicon (p. 74) The volume of words a person understands. Contrast *expressive lexicon*.

receptive speech area (p. 126) See *Wernicke's area*.

reduplicated babbling (p. 157) Babbling that consists of repeating consonant–vowel pairs, such as "da da da." See also *jargon; marginal babbling*. Contrast *nonreduplicated babbling*.

reference (p. 192) A principle stating that words symbolize objects, actions, events, and concepts. Example: The word *Daddy* stands for or symbolizes someone's father.

referent (p. 5) The aspect of the world to which a word refers. Example: In English, the specific feeling to which the word *happy* refers.

referential communication (p. 15) See *symbolic communication*.

referential gestures (p. 185) Gestures such as holding a fist to an ear to indicate *telephone* or waving a hand to indicate *bye-bye*. Used by children beginning to transition from the prelinguistic stage to the one-word stage.

register (p. 105) Stylistic variations in language that are used in different situations. Example: How you vary your language form, content, and use when making a request of your best friend versus when making a request of your professor.

resonation (p. 8) The phase of speech that occurs after a breath of air has been respirated and phonated, when the air travels into and vibrates within the oral and nasal cavities. One of four systems involved in speech. See also *articulation; phonation; respiration*.

respiration (p. 8) The act of inspiring a breath of air into the lungs, expiring it from the lungs, and allowing it to travel up through the trachea, or windpipe, before it is phonated. One of four systems involved in speech. See also *articulation; phonation; resonation*.

responsiveness (p. 33) How prompt and appropriate a response is. With regard to language development, the promptness, contingency, and appropriateness of caregiver responses to children's bids for communication through words or other means.

right hemisphere (p. 122) One of two mirror-image halves of the cerebrum. See also *corpus callosum; longitudinal fissure*. Contrast *left hemisphere*.

rostral (p. 115) A positional term used to describe the specific nervous system structures along the horizontal and vertical axes of the neuraxis. With regard to the horizontal axis, it means "toward the front of the brain." With regard to the vertical axis, it means "toward the top of the spinal cord (near the brain)." Contrast *caudal; dorsal; ventral*.

screenings (p. 278) Brief assessments used to identify possible areas of difficulty that may signal a need for more in-depth evaluation.

secondary language impairment (p. 322) A language impairment resulting from, or secondary to, conditions such as mental retardation, autism, and traumatic brain injury. Contrast *primary language impairment*.

second language acquisition (p. 302) Also called *L2 acquisition* or *SLA*. The process by which children who have already established a solid foundation in their first language (L1) learn an additional language. Contrast *bilingualism*.

semantic bootstrapping (p. 64) The process by which children deduce grammatical structures by using word meanings they acquire by observing events around them. Contrast *syntactic bootstrapping*.

semanticity (p. 26) The species-specific aspect of language that allows people to represent the world. In particular, it allows people to represent decontextualized events.

semantic network (p. 78) A network in which the entries in a person's mental lexicon are stored according to their connective ties. See also *spreading activation*.

semantics (p. 21) Synonymous with *content*. The rules of language governing the meaning of individual words and word combinations. See also *morphology; phonology; pragmatics; syntax*.

sender (p. 15) The speaker during communication. The person who formulates and then transmits the information her or she wants to convey. Contrast *receiver*.

sensitive period (p. 136) With regard to the human brain, a time frame of development during which a particular aspect of neuroanatomy or neurophysiology that underlies a given sensory or motoric capacity undergoes growth or change. A critical window of opportunity for development. Example: Deprivation of visual input during the first 6 weeks of the life of a kitten (the critical window) results in permanent blindness.

sensorineural loss (p. 343) Hearing loss that results from damage to the inner ear or auditory nerve. Contrast *auditory-processing disorder; conductive loss*.

sensory association cortex (p. 125) The region in the parietal lobes that, along with the primary somatosensory cortex, resides just posterior to the primary motor cortex of the frontal lobe and is involved with processing sensory information.

sentential ambiguity (p. 262) When different components of a sentence have several meanings. See also *deep-structure ambiguity; phonological ambiguity; surface-structure ambiguity*.

significant (p. 320) A term often used to specify the impairment level a child must exhibit before he or she is considered to have a language disorder. Currently, no gold standard is available to use to define this term as it applies to language disorders.

similes (p. 259) A type of figurative language, similar to predictive metaphors, in which the comparison between the topic and the vehicle is made explicit by the word *like* or *as*. Examples: *sitting like a bump on a log; flat as a pancake*.

simple syntax (p. 94) Grammatically well-formed sentences containing simple noun phrases and verb structures. Contrast *complex syntax*.

slow mapping (p. 229) Gradually refining representations of a word with time and multiple exposures to the word in varying contexts. Occurs after fast mapping. Contrast *fast mapping*.

source (p. 196) In an event, the starting point for movement. See also *agent; goal; location; theme*.

species specificity (p. 26) When something pertains to only one species. Language is strictly a human capacity and thus species specific.

specific language impairment (p. 34) Abbreviated SLI. See *primary language impairment*.

speech (p. 8) The neuromuscular process by which humans turn language into a sound signal that is transmitted through the air (or another medium such as a telephone line) to a receiver. See also *articulation; communication; hearing; phonation; resonation; respiration*.

speech perception (p. 14) How the brain processes speech and language. The ability to understand the sounds and words of a native language. Studies of speech perception help researchers learn about the kinds of language abilities infants have when they are born and how children use their speech perception to learn language. Contrast *auditory perception*.

spinal nerves (p. 119) The 31 pairs of nerves that emerge from the spinal cord.

spreading activation (p. 79) A process in which activation of specific mental lexicon entries spreads across the semantic network according to the strength of connections among the entries.

stopping (p.) When a fricative consonant (e.g., /f/, /v/, /s/, /z/, /h/) or an affricate consonant (e.g., /dʒ/, /ts/) is replaced by a stop consonant (/p/, /b/, /t/, /d/, /k/, or /g/). Examples: *funny* becomes "punny"; *jump* becomes "dump."

strategy training (p. 353) A way to improve children's abilities to complete diverse language tasks, such as understanding jokes, initiating conversations with friends or adults, or deciphering unknown words when reading. Focuses on teaching students specific ways to approach a linguistic task. One example is comprehension monitoring.

stress (p. 148) In terms of speech, the prominence placed on certain syllables of multisyllabic words. Contrast *intonation*.

summative evaluations (p. 278) Assessments focused on the products (rather than the process) and final outcomes of language learning and development. Contrast *formative evaluations*.

supported joint engagement (p. 163) Joint attention in which adults use such techniques as speaking with an animated voice or showing an infant novel objects.

surface-structure ambiguity (p. 267) A type of sentential ambiguity in which varying stress and intonation in a sentence changes its meaning. Example: *I fed her bird seed* vs. *I fed her bird seed.* Contrast *deep-structure ambiguity.*

symbolic communication (p. 15) Also called *referential communication.* When an individual communicates about a specific entity (an object or event), and the relationship between the entity and its referent (e.g., a word) is arbitrary. This type of communication is not limited by space or time. Example: When an infant says "bottle" to request something to drink, the relationship between the word *bottle* and its referent is arbitrary. Contrast *intentional communication; preintentional communication.*

synapse (p. 118) The site where two neurons meet. For the two neurons to communicate, the nerve impulse must cross the synapse. See also *neurotransmitters; synaptic cleft.*

synaptic cleft (p. 118) The space between the axon of the transmitting neuron and the dendrite of the receiving neuron. See also *synapses; neurotransmitters.*

synaptic pruning (p. 137) When excess synapses are pruned after synaptogenesis. Occurs from the end of the first year of life into adolescence.

synaptogenesis (p. 137) The formation of synaptic connections. Occurs most rapidly during the first year of life, after which excess synapses are pruned (synaptic pruning).

syntactic bootstrapping (p. 64) The process by which children use the syntactic frames surrounding unknown verbs to successfully constrain the possible interpretations of the verbs. Contrast *semantic bootstrappping.*

syntax (p. 22) The rules of language governing the internal organization of sentences. One component of the language domain of form. See also *morphology; phonology; pragmatics; semantics.*

telegraphic and formulaic use (p. 306) The third stage of second language development. In this stage, children begin to imitate other people, to use single words to label items, and to use simple phrases that they memorize. The variety of communicative functions they can express is limited. See also *home language system; language productivity; nonverbal period.*

temperament (p. 106) A person's predominant behavioral style or personality type. Example: bold versus shy.

temporal lobes (p. 126) Two of the six lobes of the cerebrum. They sit posterior to the frontal lobe but inferior to the parietal lobes (behind the ears). They contain the functions for processing auditory information and language comprehension. Include Heschl's gyrus and Wernicke's area. See also *frontal lobe; occipital lobe; parietal lobes.*

terminable units (T units; p. 281) Each T unit consists of an independent clause and any of its modifiers, such as a dependent clause. T units are coded in transcripts of

language samples to assess a student's language form. Contrast *communication units (C units).*

theme (p. 196) In an event, the entity undergoing an action or a movement. See also *agent; goal; location; source.*

theory (p. 41) Descriptive statements that provide stable explanations for a given phenomenon.

traumatic brain injury (p. 36) Abbreviated TBI. Damage or insult to an individual's brain tissue sometime after birth. Ranges from mild (concussion with loss of consciousness for 30 min or less) to severe (accompanied by a coma of 6 hr or more). Causes include infection, disease, and physical trauma. See also *acquired brain injury; closed-head injury; open-head injuries.*

treatment plan (p. 351) An approach to helping a child with a language disorder develop language skills. The plan specifies treatment targets, treatment strategies, and treatment contexts. See also *child-centered approaches; clinician-directed approaches.*

T units (p. 281) See *terminable units.*

twin studies (p. 31) Research on identical and monozygotic twins used to estimate the contribution of genetics to language development, as well as the heritability of language disorders.

underextension (p. 190) Using words to refer to only a subset of possible referents. Example: Using the word *bottle* only in reference to baby bottles (and not glass bottles or plastic water bottles). See also *overlap.* Contrast *overextension.*

unitary language system hypothesis (p. 300) The idea that bilingual children have a single language system that eventually splits into two. According to this theory, children are not bilingual until they successfully differentiate between the two languages. Contrast *dual language system hypothesis.*

universal grammar (p. 63) Abbreviated UG. The system of grammatical rules and constraints that are consistent among all world languages. UG, proposed by the linguist Noam Chomsky, is a nature-inspired theory of second language acquisition because it rests on an innate, species-specific module dedicated solely to language acquisition. See also *critical period hypothesis; language acquisition device.*

universality (p. 25) The idea that all persons around the world have a cognitive infrastructure that they apply to the task of learning language.

use (p. 21) Synonymous with *pragmatics.* How language is used in interactions with other people to express personal and social needs. One of the three domains of language. See also *content; form.*

use-inspired basic research (p. 43) A type of basic research that concentrates on building connections between theory and practice.

variegated babbling (p. 157) See *nonreduplicated babbling.*

ventral (p. 115)   A positional term used to describe the specific nervous system structures along the horizontal and vertical axes of the neuraxis. With regard to the horizontal axis, it means "toward the bottom of the brain." With regard to the vertical axis, it means "toward the front of the spinal cord (the side nearest the belly)." Contrast *caudal; dorsal; rostral.*

vertical axis (p. 114)   The part of the neuraxis that extends from the superior portion of the brain downward along the entire spinal cord. See also *horizontal axis.*

vocabulary spurt (p. 74)   Near the end of the second year of a child's life, when he or she transitions from a slow stage of vocabulary development to a rapid stage of development. See also *inflection point.*

voice onset time (p. 150)   The interval between the release of a stop consonant such as *p, b, t, or d* and the onset of vocal cord vibrations.

Wernicke's area (p. 126)   Named after the German neurologist and psychiatrist Karl Wernicke. Also called the *receptive speech area.* Resides in the superior portion of the left temporal lobe near the intersection of the parietal, occipital, and temporal lobes—or parieto-occipitotemporal junction. Critical for language comprehension.

white matter (p. 118)   Nervous tissue consisting primarily of axonal fibers that carry information among gray matter tissues. An information conduit. Contrast *gray matter.*

whole object assumption (p. 193)   The assumption that words label whole objects and not object parts. See also *object scope.*

wh- questions (p. 90)   Interrogative sentences that use the *wh-* words, such as *who, what, where, when,* and *why.* Contrast *yes–no questions.*

written language (p. 8)   Thoughts and ideas that an individual writes down after they are formulated. Contrast *inner language.*

Wug Test (p. 210)   Elicited production task used to investigate children's acquisition of English morphemes, including the plural marker. Developed by Jean Berko (now Berko Gleason).

yes–no questions (p. 90)   Interrogative sentences that require a yes or no response. Contrast *wh- questions.*

zone of proximal development (p. 60)   Abbreviated ZPD. A concept in Vygotskian theory that describes the difference between a child's actual developmental level (determined through independent problem solving) and his or her potential developmental level (determined through problem solving in collaboration with a more competent adult or peer).

REFERENCES

Aboitiz, F., & Ricardo, G. V. (1997). The evolutionary origin of the language areas in the brain: A neuroanatomical perspective. *Brain Research Reviews, 25*, 381–396.

Adams, S., Kuebli, J., Boyle, P. A., & Fivush, R. (1995). Gender differences in parent–child conversations about past emotions: A longitudinal investigation. *Sex Roles, 33*, 309–323.

Adamson, L. B., & Chance, S. E. (1998). Coordinating attention to people, objects, and language. In A. M. Wetherby, S. F. Warren, & J. Reichle (Eds.), *Transitions in prelinguistic communication: Preintentional to intentional and presymbolic to symbolic* (pp. 15–37). Baltimore: Brookes.

Aitchinson, J. (1994). *Words in the mind: An introduction to the mental lexicon* (2nd ed.). Oxford, England: Blackwell.

Akhtar, N. (2005). The robustness of learning through overhearing. *Developmental Science, 8*, 199–209.

Akhtar, N., Jipson, J., & Callanan, M. A. (2001). Learning words through overhearing. *Child Development, 72*, 416–430.

Akhtar, N., & Tomasello, M. (1996). Twenty-four-month-old children learn words for absent objects and actions. *British Journal of Developmental Psychology, 14*, 79–93.

Amayreh, M. M. (2003). Completion of the consonant inventory of Arabic. *Journal of Speech, Language, and Hearing Research, 46*, 517–529.

American Association on Mental Retardation. (2002). *Mental retardation: Definition, classification, and systems of supports* (10th ed.). Washington, DC: Author.

American Psychiatric Association. (1994). *Diagnostic and statistical manual of mental disorders* (4th ed.). Washington, DC: Author.

American Psychiatric Association. (2000). *Diagnostic and statistical manual of mental disorders* (4th ed., Text Revision). Washington, DC: Author.

American Psychological Association. (2003). *Psychology: Scientific problem solvers*. Washington, DC: Author.

American Speech–Language–Hearing Association. (1993). Definitions of communication disorders and variations. *ASHA, 35*(Suppl. 10), 40–41.

American Speech–Language–Hearing Association. (1996). Central auditory processing: Current status of research and implications for clinical practice. *American Journal of Audiology, 5*(2), 41–54.

American Speech–Language–Hearing Association. (2001). *Scope of practice in speech–language pathology*. Rockville, MD: Author.

American Speech–Language–Hearing Association. (2005). Causes of hearing loss in children. Rockville, MD: Author. Retrieved January 5, 2005, from http://www.asha.org/public/hearing/disorders/causes.htm

Ammer, J., & Bangs, T. (2000). *Birth to three assessment and intervention system* (2nd ed.). Austin, TX: PRO-ED.

Anderson, E. (1992). *Speaking with style: The sociolinguistic skills of children*. Exeter, NJ: Heinemann.

Anderson, E. (2000). Exploring register knowledge: The value of "controlled improvisation." In L. Menn & N. R. Ratner (Eds.), *Methods for studying language production* (pp. 225–248). Mahwah, NJ: Erlbaum.

Anderson, K. J., & Leaper, C. (1998). Meta-analyses of gender effects on conversational interruption: Who, what, where, when, and how. *Sex Roles, 39*, 225–252.

Anderson, V., & Roit, M. (1996). Linking reading comprehension instruction to language development for language-minority students. *Elementary School Journal, 96*, 295–309.

Apel, K., & Masterson, J. J. (2001). *Beyond baby talk: From sounds to sentences—A parent's complete guide to language development*. Roseville, CA: Prima.

Aram, D. M. (1988). Language sequelae of unilateral brain lesions in children. In F. Plum (Ed.), *Language communication and the brain* (pp. 171–198). New York: Raven Press.

Aram, D., & Nation, J. E. (1975). Patterns of language behavior in children with developmental language disorders. *Journal of Speech and Hearing Research, 8*, 229–241.

Arlt, P. B., & Goodban, M. T. (1976). A comparative study of articulation acquisition as based on a study of 240 normals, aged three to six. *Language, Speech, and Hearing Services in Schools, 7*, 173–180.

Arnold, D. H., Lonigan, C. J., Whitehurst, G. J., & Epstein, J. N. (1994). Accelerating language development through picture-book reading: Replication and extension to a videotape training format. *Journal of Educational Psychology, 86*, 235–243.

Badian, N. A. (2000). Do preschool orthographic skills contribute to prediction of reading? In N. Badian (Ed.), *Prediction and prevention of reading failure* (pp. 31–56). Timonium, MD: York Press.

Bagby, J. H., Rudd, L. C., & Woods, M. (2005). The effects of socioeconomic diversity on the language, cognitive, and social-emotional development of children from low-income backgrounds. *Early Child Development and Care, 175*, 395–405.

Bailey, G., & Tillery, J. (2006). Sounds of the South. In W. Wolfram & B. Ward (Eds.), *American voices: How dialects differ from coast to coast* (pp. 11–16). Malden, MA: Blackwell.

Bakeman, R., & Adamson, L. B. (1984). Coordinating attention to people and objects in mother–infant and peer–infant interaction. *Child Development, 55*, 1278–1289.

Baker, C. (2000). *A parents' and teachers' guide to bilingualism* (2nd ed.). Tonawanda, NY: Multilingual Matters.

Baker, S. A., Golinkoff, R. M., & Petitto, L.-A. (2006). New insights into old puzzles from infants' categorical discrimination of soundless phonetic units. *Language Learning and Development, 2*, 147–162.

Baker, S. A., Idsardi, W. J., Golinkoff, R. M., & Petitto, L.-A. (2005). The perception of handshapes in American Sign Language. *Memory & Cognition, 33*(5), 887–904.

Baldwin, D. (1991). Infants' contribution to the achievement of joint reference. *Child Development, 62*, 875–890.

Baldwin, D. A. (1995). Understanding the link between joint attention and language. In C. Moore & P. J. Dunham (Eds.), *Joint attention: Its origins and role in development* (pp. 131–158). Hillsdale, NJ: Erlbaum.

Baldwin, D. A., & Baird, J. A. (1999). Action analysis: A gateway to intentional inference. In P. Rochat (Ed.), *Early social cognition: Understanding others in the first months of life* (pp. 215–240). Mahwah, NJ: Erlbaum.

Bangs, T., & Dodson, S. (1986). *Birth to three developmental scales.* Allen, TX: DLM Teaching Resources.

Bates, E., Camaioni, L., & Volterra, V. (1975). The acquisition of performatives prior to speech. *Merrill–Palmer Quarterly, 21*, 205–226.

Bates, E., Dale, P. S., & Thal, D. (1995). Individual differences and their implications for theories of language development. In P. Fletcher & B. MacWhinney (Eds.), *Handbook of child language* (pp. 96–151). Oxford, England: Basil Blackwell.

Bauer, D. J., Goldfield, B. A., & Reznick, J. S. (2002). Alternative approaches to analyzing individual differences in the rate of early vocabulary development. *Applied Psycholinguistics, 23*, 313–335.

Baugh, J. (2006). Bridging the great divide (African American English). In W. Wolfram & B. Ward (Eds.), *American voices: How dialects differ from coast to coast* (pp. 217–224). Malden, MA: Blackwell.

Baumwell, L., Tamis-LeMonda, C. S., & Bornstein, M. H. (1997). Maternal verbal sensitivity and child language comprehension. *Infant Behavior and Development, 20*, 247–258.

Bear, D. R., Invernizzi, M., Templeton, S., & Johnston, F. (2004). *Word study for phonics, vocabulary, and spelling instruction.* Upper Saddle River, NJ: Merrill Prentice Hall.

Becker Bryant, J. (2005). Language in social contexts: Communication competence in preschool years. In J. Berko Gleason (Ed.), *The development of language* (6th ed., pp. 191–229). New York: Allyn & Bacon.

Bedore, L. M., & Leonard, L. B. (2000). The effects of inflectional variations on fast mapping of verbs in English and Spanish. *Journal of Speech, Language, and Hearing Research, 43*, 21–33.

Behl-Chadha, G. (1996). Basic-level and superordinate-like categorical representations early in infancy. *Cognition, 60*, 105–141.

Beitchman, J., Hood, J., Rochon, J., Peterson, M., Mantini, T., & Majumdar, S. (1989). Empirical classification of speech/language impairment in children: I. Identification of speech/language categories. *Journal of the American Academy of Child & Adolescent Psychiatry, 28*(1), 112–117.

Bellugi, U. (1967). *The acquisition of negation.* Unpublished doctoral dissertation, Harvard University, Cambridge, MA.

Bereiter, C. (1966). *Teaching disadvantaged children to read.* Upper Saddle River, NJ: Prentice Hall.

Bereiter, C., & Engelmann, S. (1966). *Teaching disadvantaged children in the preschool.* Upper Saddle River, NJ: Prentice Hall.

Berko, J. (1958). The child's learning of English morphology. *Word, 14*, 150–177.

Bernstein, C. (2006). More than just yada yada yada (Jewish English). In W. Wolfram & B. Ward (Eds.), *American voices: How dialects differ from coast to coast* (pp. 251–257). Malden, MA: Blackwell.

Bernstein Ratner, N. (1986). Durational cues which mark clause boundaries in mother–child speech. *Journal of Phonetics, 14*, 303–309.

Bernstein Ratner, N., Berko Gleason, J., & Narasimhan, B. (1997). An introduction to psycholinguistics: What do language users know? In J. Berko Gleason & N. Bernstein Ratner (Eds.), *Psycholinguistics* (2nd ed., pp. 3–4). Fort Worth, TX: Harcourt Brace College.

Bernstein Ratner, N., & Pye, C. (1984). Higher pitch in BR is not universal: Acoustic evidence from Quiche Mayan. *Journal of Child Language, 11*, 515–522.

Beukelman, D. R., & Yorkston, K. M. (1991). Traumatic brain injury changes the way we live. In D. R. Beukelman & K. M. Yorkston (Eds.), *Communication disorders following traumatic brain injury: Management of cognitive, language, and motor impairments* (pp. 1–14). Austin, TX: PRO-ED.

Bhatnagar, S. C., & Andy, O. J. (1995). *Neuroscience for the study of communicative disorders.* Baltimore: Williams & Wilkins.

Bialystok, E., & Hakuta, K. (1994). *In other words: The science and psychology of second language acquisition.* New York: Basic Books.

Bialystok, E., & Miller, B. (1999). The problem of age in second-language acquisition: Influences from language, structure, and task. *Bilingualism: Language and Cognition, 2*, 127–145.

Bickerton, D. (1995). *Language and human behavior.* Seattle: University of Washington Press.

Biemiller, A. (1970). The development of the use of graphic and contextual information as children learn to read. *Reading Research Quarterly, 6*, 75–96.

Biemiller, A. (2005). Size and sequence in vocabulary development: Implications for choosing words for primary grade vocabulary instruction. In E. H. Hiebert & M. Kamil (Eds.), *Teaching and learning vocabulary: Bringing research to practice* (pp. 223–245). Mahwah, NJ: Erlbaum.

Bishop, D. V. M., Price, T. S., Dale, P. S., & Plomin, R. (2003). Outcomes of early language delay: II. Etiology of transient and persistent language difficulties. *Journal of Speech, Language, and Hearing Research, 46*, 561–575.

Bloom, A. (1979). *Emile: Or, On Education.* New York: Basic Books.

Bloom, L. (2000). The intentionality model of word learning: How to learn a word, any word. In R. M. Golinkoff, K. Hirsh-Pasek, N. Akhtar, L. Bloom, G. Hollich, L. Smith, et al. (Eds.), *Becoming a word learner: A debate on lexical acquisition* (pp. 19–50). New York: Oxford University Press.

Bloom, L., & Tinker, E. (2001a). V. General discussion. *Monographs of the Society for Research in Child Development, 66*(4), 73–82.

Bloom, L., & Tinker, E. (2001b). The intentionality model and language acquisition. *Monographs of the Society for Research in Child Development, 66*(4), vii–104.

Bloom, P. (2000). *How children learn the meanings of words.* Cambridge: MIT Press.

Bloom, P., & Markson, L. (2001). Are there principles that apply only to the acquisition of words? A reply to Waxman and Booth. *Cognition, 78*, 89–90.

Bono, M. A., & Stifter, C. A. (2003). Maternal attention-directing strategies and infant focused attention during problem solving. *Infancy, 4*, 235–250.

Bookheimer, S. (2002). Functional MRI of language: New approaches to understanding the cortical organization of semantic processing. *Annual Reviews of Neuroscience, 25*, 151–188.

Borden, G. J., Harris, K. S., & Raphael, L. J. (1994). *Speech science primer: Physiology, acoustics, and perception of speech* (3rd ed.). Baltimore: Williams & Wilkins.

Bornstein, M. H., Hahn, C.-S., & Haynes, O. M. (2004). Specific and general language performance across early childhood: Stability and gender considerations. *First Language, 24*, 267–304.

Bortfeld, H., & Whitehurst, G. J. (2001). Sensitive periods in first language acquisition. In D. Bailey, J. T. Bauer, F. J. Symons, & J. W. Lichtman (Eds.), *Critical thinking about critical periods* (pp. 173–192). Baltimore: Brookes.

Bowerman, M., & Choi, S. (2003). Space under construction: Language-specific spatial categorization in first language acquisition. In D. Gentner & S. Goldin-Meadow (Eds.), *Language in mind: Advances in the study of language and thought* (pp. 387–428). Cambridge: MIT Press.

Brackenbury, T., & Fey, M. E. (2003). Quick incidental verb learning in 4-year-olds: Identification and generalization. *Journal of Speech, Language, and Hearing Research, 46*, 313–327.

Bradley, R. H., & Corwyn, R. F. (2002). Socioeconomic status and child development. *Annual Review of Psychology, 53*, 371–399.

Brady, N. C., Marquis, J., Fleming, K., & McLean, L. (2004). Prelinguistic predictors of language growth in children with developmental disabilities. *Jsournal of Speech, Language, and Hearing Research, 47*, 663–677.

Brenowitz, E. A., & Beecher, M. D. (2005). Song learning in birds: Diversity and plasticity, opportunities and challenges. *Trends in Neuroscience, 28*, 127–132.

Brooke, M., Uomoto, J. M., McLean, A., & Fraser, R. T. (1991). Rehabilitation of persons with traumatic brain injury: A continuum of care. In D. R. Beukelman & K. M. Yorkston (Eds.), *Communication disorders following traumatic brain injury: Management of cognitive, language, and motor impairments* (pp. 15–46). Austin, TX: PRO-ED.

Brooks, P. J. (2004). Grammatical competence is not a psychologically valid construct. *Journal of Child Language, 31*, 467–470.

Brown, H. D. (2001). *Teaching by principles: An interactive approach to language pedagogy* (2nd ed.). White Plains, NY: Addison Wesley Longman.

Brown, R. (1973). *A first language: The early stages.* Cambridge, MA: Harvard University Press.

Brownell, R. (2000a). *Expressive One-Word Picture Vocabulary Test* (2000 ed.). Novato, CA: Academic Therapy.

Brownell, R. (2000b). *Receptive One-Word Picture Vocabulary Test.* Novato, CA: Academic Therapy.

Bruer, J. T. (2001). A critical and sensitive period primer. In D. Bailey, J. T. Bauer, F. J. Symons, & J. W. Lichtman (Eds.), *Critical thinking about critical periods* (pp. 3–26). Baltimore: Brookes.

Bruer, J. T., & Greenough, W. T. (2001). The subtle science of how experience affects the brain. In D. Bailey, J. T. Bauer, F. J. Symons, & J. W. Lichtman (Eds.), *Critical thinking about critical periods* (pp. 209–232). Baltimore: Brookes.

Bryant, G. A., & Tree, J. E. F. (2002). Recognizing verbal irony in spontaneous speech. *Metaphor and Symbol, 17*, 99–119.

Budwig, N. (1995). *A developmental-functionalist approach to child language.* Mahwah, NJ: Erlbaum.

Burgess, S. R., Hecht, S. A., & Lonigan, C. J. (2002). Relations of the home literacy environment (HLE) to the development of reading related abilities: A one-year longitudinal study. *Reading Research Quarterly, 37*, 408–426.

Burnham, D., Kitamura, C., & Vollmer-Conna, U. (2002). What's new pussycat? On talking to babies and animals. *Science, 296*, 1435.

Bus, A. G., van Ijzendoorn, M. H., & Pellegrini, A. D. (1995). Joint book reading makes for success in learning to read: A meta-analysis on intergenerational transmission of literacy. *Review of Educational Research, 65*, 1–21.

Butler, Y. G. (2004). What level of English proficiency do elementary school teachers need to attain to teach EFL? Case studies from Korea, Taiwan, and Japan. *TESOL Quarterly, 38*, 245–278.

Byrne, B., & Fielding-Barnsley, R. (1995). Evaluation of a program to teach phonemic awareness to young children: A 2- and 3-year follow-up and a new preschool trial. *Journal of Educational Psychology, 87*, 488–503.

Bzoch, K., & League, R. (1991). *Receptive–Expressive Emergent Language Test—Second edition (REEL–2).* Los Angeles, CA: Western Psychological Services.

Bzoch, K. R., League, R., & Brown, V. L. (2003). *Receptive–Expressive Emergent Language Test—Third edition (REEL–3).* Austin, TX: PRO-ED.

Caldera, Y. M., Huston, A. C., & O'Brien, M. (1989). Social interactions and play patterns of parents and toddlers with feminine, masculine, and neutral toys. *Child Development, 60*, 70–76.

Callanan, M., Akhtar, N., Sussman, L., & Sabbagh, M. (2003). *Learning words in directive and ostensive contexts.* Unpublished manuscript, University of California, Santa Cruz.

Camaioni, L., Perucchini, P., Bellagamba, F., & Colonnesi, C. (2004). The role of declarative pointing in developing a theory of mind. *Infancy, 5*, 291–308.

Campbell, M. T., & Plumb, G. (n.d.). Generic names for soft drinks by county [Map]. In A. McConchie (Ed.), *The great pop vs. soda controversy.* Retrieved September 26, 2006, from http://www.popvssoda.com/countystats/totalcounty.html

Capirci, O., Iverson, J. M., Pizzuto, E., & Volterra, V. (1996). Communicative gestures during the transition to two-word speech. *Journal of Child Language, 23*, 645–673.

Carey, S. (1978). The child as word learner. In M. Halle, J. Bresnan, & A. Miller (Eds.), *Linguistic theory and psychological reality* (pp. 264–293). Cambridge: MIT Press.

Carey, S., & Bartlett, E. (1978). Acquiring a single new word. *Papers and Reports on Child Language Development, 15*, 17–29.

Cartwright, J. (2000). *Evolution and human behavior.* Cambridge: MIT Press.

Caselli, M. C. (1983). Communication to language: Deaf children's and hearing children's development compared. *Sign Language Studies, 39*, 113–144.

Caselli, M. C., Volterra, V., & Pizzuto, E. (1984, April). *The relationship between vocal and gestural communication from the one-word to the two-word stage.* Paper presented at the International Conference on Infant Studies, New York, NY.

Catts, H. W., Fey, M. E., Tomblin, J. B., & Zhang, X. (2002). Longitudinal investigation of reading outcomes in children with language impairment. *Journal of Speech, Language, and Hearing Research, 45*, 1142–1157.

Catts, H. W., Fey, M. E., Zhang, X., & Tomblin, J. (2001). Estimating the risk of future reading difficulties in kindergarten children: A research-based model and its clinical implications. *Language, Speech, and Hearing Services in Schools, 32*, 38–50.

Chall, J. S. (1996). *Stages of reading development.* Fort Worth, TX: Harcourt Brace.

Champlin, C. A. (2000). Hearing science. In R. B. Gillam, T. P. Marquardt, & F. N. Martin (Eds.), *Communication sciences and disorders: From science to clinical practice* (Chap. 5). San Diego, CA: Singular.

Chaney, C. (1998). Preschool language and metalinguistic skills are links to reading success. *Applied Psycholinguistics, 19*, 433–466.

Chaney, C. (1994). Language development, metalinguistic awareness, and emergent literacy skills of 3-year-old children in relation to social class. *Applied Psycholinguistics, 15*, 371–394.

Chapman, R. (2000). Children's language learning: An interactionist perspective. *Journal of Child Psychology and Psychiatry, 41*, 33–54.

Chapman, R. S., Seung, H. K., Schwartz, S. E., & Kay–Raining Bird, E. (1998). Language skills of children and adolescents with Down syndrome: II. Production deficits. *Journal of Speech, Language, and Hearing Research, 41*, 861–873.

Chapman, S. B. (1997). Cognitive–communicative abilities in children with closed head injury. *American Journal of Speech–Language Pathology, 6*, 50–58.

Charity, A. H., Scarborough, H. S., & Griffin, D. M. (2004). Familiarity with School English in African American children and its relation to early reading achievement. *Child Development, 75*, 1340–1356.

Charles-Luce, J., & Luce, P. A. (1990). Similarity neighbourhoods of words in young children's lexicons. *Journal of Child Language, 17*, 205–215.

Charles-Luce, J., & Luce, P. A. (1996). An examination of similarity neighbourhoods in young children's receptive vocabularies. *Journal of Child Language, 22*, 727–735.

Choi, S., & Gopnik, A. (1995). Early acquisition of verbs in Korean: A cross-linguistic study. *Journal of Child Language, 22*, 497–530.

Choi, S., McDonough, L., Bowerman, M., & Mandler, J. M. (1999). Early sensitivity to language-specific spatial categories in English and Korean. *Cognitive Development, 14*, 241–268.

Chomsky, N. (1965). *Aspects of the theory of syntax.* Cambridge: MIT Press.

Chomsky, N. (1978). *Syntactic structures.* The Hague, The Netherlands: Mouton. (Original work published 1957)

Clark, E. V. (1993). *The lexicon in acquisition.* New York: Cambridge University Press.

Clark, E. V., & Sengul, C. J. (1978). Strategies in the acquisition of deixis. *Journal of Child Language, 5*, 457–475.

Cleave, P. L., & Fey, M. E. (1997). Two approaches to the facilitation of grammar in children with language impairments:

Rationale and description. *American Journal of Speech–Language Pathology, 6*, 22–32.

Colombo, J., Shaddy, D. J., Richman, W. A., Maikranz, J. M., & Blaga, O. M. (2004). The developmental course of habituation in infancy and preschool outcome. *Infancy, 5*, 1–38.

Conn, J. (2006). Dialects in the mist (Portland, OR). In W. Wolfram & B. Ward (Eds.), *American voices: How dialects differ from coast to coast* (pp. 149–155). Malden, MA: Blackwell.

Conti-Ramsden, G., Crutchley, A., & Botting, N. (1997). The extent to which psychometric tests differentiate subgroups of children with specific language impairment. *Journal of Speech, Language, and Hearing Research, 40*, 765–777.

Conti-Ramsden, G., & Jones, M. (1997). Verb use in specific language impairment. *Journal of Speech, Language, and Hearing Research, 40*, 1298–1313.

Cooper, R. P., & Aslin, R. N. (1990). Preference for infant-directed speech in the first month after birth. *Child Development, 61*, 1584–1595.

Coplan, J. (1993). *Early Language Milestone Scale* (2nd ed.). Austin, TX: PRO-ED.

Craig, H. K., Washington, J. A., & Thompson-Porter, C. (1998). Average C-unit lengths in the discourse of African American children from low-income, urban homes. *Journal of Speech, Language, and Hearing Research, 41*, 433–444.

Crais, E. R. (1995). Expanding the repertoire of tools and techniques for assessing the communication skills of infants and toddlers. *American Journal of Speech–Language Pathology, 4*, 47–59.

Creusere, M. A. (1999). Theories of adults' understanding and use of irony and sarcasm: Applications to and evidence from research with children. *Developmental Review, 19*, 213–262.

Csibra, G., Bíró, S., Koós, O., & Gergely, G. (2003). One-year-old infants use teleological representations of actions productively. *Cognitive Science, 27*, 111–133.

Curenton, S., & Justice, L. M. (2004). Low-income preschoolers' use of decontextualized discourse: Literate language features in spoken narratives. *Language, Speech, and Hearing Services in Schools, 35*, 240–253.

Dale, E. (1965). Vocabulary measurement: Techniques and major findings. *Elementary English, 42*, 895–901.

Dale, P. (1991). The validity of a parent report measure of vocabulary and syntax at 24 months. *Journal of Speech and Hearing Research, 34*, 565–571.

Dale, P. (1996). Parent report assessment of language and communication. In K. Cole, P. Dale, & D. Thal (Eds.), *Assessment of communication and language* (Vol. 6, pp. 161–182). Baltimore: Brookes.

Dale, P. S., & Fenson, L. (1996). Lexical development norms for young children. *Behavior Research Methods, Instruments, & Computers, 28*, 125–127.

Dale, P. S., Price, T. S., Bishop, D. V. M., & Plomin, P. (2003). Outcomes of early language delay: I. Predicting persistent and transient language difficulties at 3 and 4 years.

Journal of Speech, Language, and Hearing Research, 46, 544–560.

Danesi, M. (2003). *Second language teaching: A view from the right side of the brain.* Dordrecht, The Netherlands: Kluwer Academic.

Dapretto, M., & Bjork, E. L. (2000). The development of word retrieval abilities in the second year and its relation to early vocabulary growth. *Child Development, 71*, 635–648.

Dawson, P. W., Blamey, P. J., Dettman, S. J., Barker, E. J., & Clark, G. M. (1995). A clinical report on receptive vocabulary skills in cochlear implant users. *Ear & Hearing, 16*, 287–294.

Deacon, T. W. (1997). *The symbolic species.* New York: Norton.

Deák, G. O., & Maratsos, M. (1998). On having complex representations of things: Preschoolers use multiple words for objects and people. *Developmental Psychology, 34*, 224–240.

DeLoache, J. S. (1984). What's this? Maternal questions in joint picture book reading with toddlers. *Quarterly Newsletter of the Laboratory of Comparative Human Cognition, 6*, 87–95.

Demuth, K. (1996). Collecting spontaneous production data. In D. McDaniel, C. McKee, & H. Smith (Eds.), *Methods for assessing children's syntax* (pp. 3–22). Cambridge: MIT Press.

DeNavas-Walt, C., Proctor, B. D., & Lee, C. H. (2005). *Income, poverty, and health insurance coverage in the United States: 2004.* Washington, DC: U.S. Census Bureau.

Dixon, J. A., & Foster, D. H. (1997). Gender and hedging: From sex differences to situated practice. *Journal of Psycholinguistic Research, 26*, 89–107.

Dollaghan, C. A., Campbell, T. F., Paradise, J. L., Feldman, H. M., Janosky, J. E., Pitcairn, D. N., et al. (1999, December). Maternal education and measures of early speech and language development. *Journal of Speech, Language, and Hearing Research, 42*, 1432–1443.

Duffy, J. R. (1995). *Motor speech disorders: Substrates, differential diagnosis, and management.* St. Louis, MO: Mosby.

Dunbar, R. I. M., & Aiello, L. C. (1993). Neocortex size, group size, and the evolution of language. *Current Anthropology, 34*, 184–193.

Dunbar, R. I. M., Duncan, N. D., & Nettle, D. (1994). Size and structure of freely forming conversational groups. *Human Nature, 6*, 67–78.

Dunn, L., & Dunn, L. (1981). *Peabody Picture Vocabulary Test—Revised.* Circle Pines, MN: American Guidance Service.

Dunn, L. M., & Dunn, L. M. (1997). *Peabody Picture Vocabulary Test* (3rd ed.). Circle Pines, MN: American Guidance Service.

Dunn, L., & Dunn, L. (2006). *Peabody Picture Vocabulary Test* (4th ed.). Bloomington, MN: Pearson Assessments.

Eastwood, J., & Mackin, R. (1982). *A basic English grammar.* Oxford, England: Oxford University Press.

Edwards, C. P. (1984). The age group labels and categories of preschool children. *Child Development, 55*, 440–452.

Ehlers, S., & Gillberg, C. (1993). The epidemiology of Asperger syndrome: A total population study. *Journal of Child Psychology and Psychiatry, 34*, 1327–1350.

Ehrenreich, B. (1981). The politics of talking in couples. *Ms., 5*, 43–45, 86–89.

Eisenberg, S. (2006). Grammar: How can I say that better? In T. Ukrainetz (Ed.), *Contextualized language intervention* (pp. 145–194). Eau Claire, WI: Thinking.

Ellis Weismer, S., Murray-Branch, J., & Miller, J. F. (1994). A prospective longitudinal study of language development in late talkers. *Journal of Speech and Hearing Research, 37*, 852–867.

Elman, J. L., Bates, E. A., Johnson, M. H., Parisi, D., & Plunkett, K. (1996). *Rethinking innateness: A connectionist perspective on development.* Cambridge: MIT Press.

Ely, R., Berko Gleason, J., & McCabe, A. (1996). Why didn't you talk to your mommy, honey? Gender differences in talk about past talk. *Research on Language in Social Interaction, 29*, 7–25.

Ertmer, D. J. (2002). Prologue: Challenges in optimizing oral communication in children with cochlear implants. *Language, Speech, and Hearing Services in Schools, 33*, 149–152.

Ertmer, D. J., Strong, L., & Sadagopan, N. (2003). Beginning to communicate after cochlear implantation: Oral language development in a young child. *Journal of Speech, Language, and Hearing Research, 46,* 328–340.

Evans, M. A. (1996). Reticent primary grade children and their more talkative peers: Verbal, nonverbal, and self-concept characteristics. *Journal of Educational Psychology, 88*, 739–749.

Ezell, H. K., & Goldstein, H. (1991). Observational learning of comprehension monitoring skills in children who exhibit mental retardation. *Journal of Speech and Hearing Research, 34*, 141–154.

Ezell, H. K., & Justice, L. M. (2000). Increasing the print focus of shared reading through observational learning. *American Journal of Speech–Language Pathology, 9*, 36–47.

Farber, J. G., & Klein, E. R. (1999). Classroom-based assessment of a collaborative intervention program with kindergarten and first-grade students. *Language, Speech, and Hearing Services in Schools, 30*, 83–91.

Fazio, B. B., Naremore, R. C., & Connell, P. J. (1996). Tracking children from poverty at risk for specific language impairment: A 3-year longitudinal study. *Journal of Speech and Hearing Research, 39*, 611–624.

Fenson, L., Bates, E., Dale, P., Goodman, J., Reznick, J. S., & Thal, D. (2000). Measuring variability in early child language: Don't shoot the messenger. *Child Development, 71*, 323–328.

Fenson, L., Dale, P. S., Reznick, J. S., Bates, E., & Thal, D. (1994). Variability in early communicative development. *Monographs of the Society for Research in Child Development, 59*(5), 1–185.

Fenson, L., Dale, P. S., Reznick, J. S., Thal, D., Bates, E., Hartung, J., et al. (1993). *The MacArthur Communicative Development Inventories.* San Diego: Singular.

Fenson, L., Dale, P. S., Reznick, J. S., Thal, D., Bates, E., Hartung, J. P., et al. (2003). *MacArthur–Bates Communicative Development Inventories.* Baltimore: Brookes.

Fenson, L., Pethick, S., Renda, C., Cox, J. L., Dale, P. S., & Reznick, J. S. (2000). Short form versions of the MacArthur Communicative Development Inventories. *Applied Psycholinguistics, 21*, 95–116.

Fernald, A. (1989). Intonation and communicative intent in mothers' speech to infants: Is the melody the message? *Child Development, 60*, 1497–1510.

Fernald, A. (2000). Speech to infants as hyper-speech: Knowledge-driven processes in early word recognition. *Phonetica, 57*, 242–254.

Fernald, A., & Kuhl, P. (1987). Acoustic determinants of infant preference for motherese speech. *Infant Behavior and Development, 10*, 279–293.

Fernald, A., & Mazzie, C. (1991). Prosody and focus in speech to infants and adults. *Developmental Psychology, 27*, 209–221.

Fernald, A., & Simon, T. (1984). Expanded intonation contours in mothers' speech to newborns. *Developmental Psychology, 20*, 104–113.

Fernald, A., Swingley, D., & Pinto, J. P. (2001). When half a word is enough: Infants can recognize spoken words using partial phonetic information. *Child Development, 72*, 1003–1015.

Fernald, A., Taeschner, T., Dunn, J., Papousek, M., de Doyson-Baries, B., & Fukui, I. (1989). A cross-linguistic study of prosodic modifications in mothers' and fathers' speech to preverbal infants. *Journal of Child Language, 16*, 477–501.

Fernandez-Duque, D., Baird, J., & Posner, M. (2000). Executive attention and metacognitive regulation. *Consciousness and Cognition, 9*, 288–307.

Fey, M. E. (1986). *Language intervention with young children.* Boston: Allyn & Bacon.

Fey, M. E., Cleave, P. L., Long, S. H., & Hughes, D. L. (1993). Two approaches to the facilitation of grammar in children with language impairment: An experimental evaluation. *Journal of Speech and Hearing Research, 36*, 141–157.

Fey, M. E., & Frome Loeb, D. (2002). An evaluation of the facilitative effects of inverted yes–no questions on the acquisition of auxiliary verbs. *Journal of Speech, Language, and Hearing, 45*, 160–174.

Fey, M. E., Long, S. H., & Finestack, L. M. (2003). Ten principles of grammar facilitation for children with specific language impairments. *American Journal of Speech–Language Pathology, 12*, 3–15.

Fisher, C. (2002). Structural limits on verb mapping: The role of abstract structure in 2.5-year-old's interpretations of novel verbs. *Developmental Science, 5*, 55–64.

Fisher, C., & Tokura, H. (1996). Acoustic cues to grammatical structure in infant-directed speech: Cross-linguistic evidence. *Child Development, 67*, 3192–3218.

Fitch, R. H., Miller, S., & Tallal, P. (1997). Neurobiology of speech perception. *Annual Reviews of Neuroscience, 20*, 331–353.

Fitzpatrick, J. (2006). Beantown babble (Boston, MA). In W. Wolfram & B. Ward (Eds.), *American voices: How dialects differ from coast to coast* (pp. 63–69). Malden, MA: Blackwell.

Fletcher, P. (1992). Subgroups in school-age language-impaired children. In P. Fletcher & D. Hall (Eds.), *Specific speech and language disorders in children: Correlates, characteristics, and outcomes* (pp. 152–165). London: Whurr.

Flexer, C. (1994). *Facilitating hearing and listening in young children*. San Diego, CA: Singular.

Fodor, J. (1983). *The modularity of mind*. Cambridge: MIT Press.

Frackowiak, R. S. J., Friston, K. J., Frith, C. D., Dolan, R. J., Price, C. J., Zeki, S., et al. (2004). *Human brain function* (2nd ed.). San Diego: Academic Press.

Fraser, C., Bellugi, U., & Brown, R. (1963). Control of grammar in imitation, comprehension, and production. *Journal of Verbal Learning and Verbal Behavior, 2*, 121–135.

Frazer, T. C. (1996). Chicano English and Spanish interference in midwestern United States. *American Speech, 71*, 72–85.

Friederici, A. D., Opitz, B., & von Cramon, D. (2000). Segregating semantic and syntactic aspects of processing in the human brain: An fMRI investigation of different word types. *Cerebral Cortex, 10*, 698–705.

Fujiki, M., Brinton, B., Morgan, M., & Hart, C. H. (1999). Withdrawn and sociable behavior of children with language impairment. *Language, Speech, and Hearing Services in Schools, 30*, 183–195.

Fujiki, M., Brinton, B., & Todd, C. M. (1996). Social skills of children with specific language impairment. *Language, Speech, and Hearing Services in Schools, 27*, 195–201.

Fujiura, G. T., & Yamaki, K. (1997). Analysis of ethnic variations in developmental disability prevalence and household economic status. *Mental Retardation, 35*, 286–294.

Functional MRI Research Center, Columbia University. (2005). *About functional MRI*. Retrieved December 30, 2005, from http://www.fmri.org/fmri.htm

Gallagher, A., Frith, U., & Snowling, M. J. (2000). Precursors of literacy delay among children at genetic risk for dyslexia. *Journal of Child Psychology and Psychiatry, 41*, 203–213.

Gallaudet Research Institute. (2001, January). *Regional and national summary report of data from the 1999–2000 Annual Survey of Deaf and Hard of Hearing Children and Youth*. Washington, DC: Gallaudet University.

Ganger, J., & Brent, M. R. (2004). Reexamining the vocabulary spurt. *Developmental Psychology, 40*, 621–632.

Gard, A., Gilman, L., & Gorman, J. (1993). *Speech and language development chart*. Austin, TX: PRO-ED.

Gardner, M. (1979). *Expressive One-Word Picture Vocabulary Test*. Novato, CA: Academic Therapy.

Gardner, M. (1990). *Receptive One-Word Picture Vocabulary Test—Revised*. Novato, CA: Academic Therapy.

Gass, S. M., & Selinker, L. (2001). *Second language acquisition: An introductory course*. Mahwah, NJ: Erlbaum.

Gauger, L. M., Lombardino, L. J., & Leonard, C. M. (1997). Brain morphology in children with specific language impairment. *Journal of Speech, Language, and Hearing Research, 40*, 1272–1284.

Genesee, F. (1989). Early bilingual development: One language or two? *Journal of Child Language, 16*, 171–179.

Genesee, F., Nicoladis, E., & Paradis, J. (1995). Language differentiation in early bilingual development. *Journal of Child Language, 22*, 611–631.

Genesee, F., Paradis, J., & Crago, M. B. (2004). *Dual language development and disorders: A handbook on bilingualism & second language learning*. Baltimore: Brookes.

Gerken, L., & Aslin, R. N. (2005). Thirty years of research on infant speech perception: The legacy of Peter W. Jusczyk. *Language Learning and Development, 1*, 5–21.

Gerken, L., & Shady, M. E. (1996). The picture selection task. In D. McDaniel, C. McKee, & H. Smith (Eds.), *Methods for assessing children's syntax* (pp. 125–145). Cambridge: MIT Press.

Gershkoff-Stowe, L. (2001). The course of children's naming errors in early word learning. *Journal of Cognition and Development, 2*, 131–155.

Gibbs, R. (1987). Linguistic factors in children's understanding of idioms. *Journal of Child Language, 14*, 569–586.

Gindis, B. (1999). Language-related issues for international adoptees and adoptive families. In T. Tepper, L. Hannon, & D. Sandstrom (Eds.), *International adoption: Challenges and opportunities* (pp. 98–107). Meadowlands, PA: First Edition.

Girolametto, L., Pearce, P. S., & Weitzman, E. (1996). Interactive focused stimulation for toddlers with expressive vocabulary delays. *Journal of Speech and Hearing Research, 39*, 1274–1283.

Girolametto, L., & Weitzman, E. (2002). Responsiveness of child care providers in interactions with toddlers and preschoolers. *Language, Speech and Hearing Services in Schools, 33*, 268–281.

Girolametto, L., Weitzman, E., & Greenberg, J. (2003). Training day care staff to facilitate children's language. *American Journal of Speech–Language Pathology, 12*, 299–311.

Gleitman, L. (1990). The structural sources of verb meanings. *Language Acquisition, 1*, 3–55.

Gleitman, L. R., Cassidy, K., Nappa, R., Papafragou, A., & Trueswell, J. C. (2005). Hard words. *Language Learning and Development, 1*, 23–64.

Glennen, S. (2002). Language development and delay in internationally adopted infants and toddlers: A review. *American Journal of Speech–Language Pathology, 11*, 333–339.

Glennen, S., & Masters, M. G. (2002). Typical and atypical language development in infants and toddlers adopted from Eastern Europe. *American Journal of Speech–Language Pathology, 11*, 417–433.

Glezerman, T. B., & Balkoski, V. (1999). *Language, thought, and the brain*. New York: Kluwer Academic.

Goldin-Meadow, S. (2000). Beyond words: The importance of gesture to researchers and learners. *Child Development, 71*, 231–239.

Goldman, R., & Fristoe, M. (2000). *Goldman–Fristoe Test of Articulation* (2nd ed.). Circle Pines, MN: American Guidance Services.

Goldstein, B., & Iglesias, A. (2004). Language and dialectal variations. In J. E. Bernthal & N. W. Bankson (Eds.), *Articulation and phonological disorders* (5th ed., pp. 348–375). Boston: Allyn & Bacon.

Golinkoff, R. M., & Alioto, A. (1995). Infant-directed speech facilitates lexical learning in adults hearing Chinese: Implications for language acquisition. *Journal of Child Language, 22*, 703–726.

Golinkoff, R. M., & Hirsh-Pasek, K. (1999). *How babies talk: The magic and mystery of language in the first three years of life*. New York: Dutton.

Golinkoff, R. M., Hirsh-Pasek, K., Cauley, K. M., & Gordon, L. (1987). The eyes have it: Lexical and syntactic comprehension in a new paradigm. *Journal of Child Language, 14*, 23–45.

Golinkoff, R. M., Mervis, C. V., & Hirsh-Pasek, K. (1994). Early object labels: The case for a developmental lexical principles framework. *Journal of Child Language, 21*, 125–155.

Golinkoff, R. M., Shuff-Bailey, M., Olguin, R., & Ruan, W. (1995). Young children extend novel words at the basic level: Evidence for the principle of categorical scope. *Developmental Psychology, 31*, 494–505.

Goodman, R., & Yude, C. (1996). IQ and its predictors in childhood hemiplegia. *Developmental Medicine and Child Neurology, 38*, 881–890.

Gopnik, A., & Meltzoff, A. N. (1997). *Words, thoughts, and theories*. Cambridge: MIT Press.

Gordon, M. J. (2006). Straight talking from the heartland (Midwest). In W. Wolfram & B. Ward (Eds.), *American voices: How dialects differ from coast to coast* (pp. 106–111). Malden, MA: Blackwell.

Goswami, U. (1990). A special link between rhyming skills and the use of orthographic analogies by beginning readers. *Journal of Child Psychology and Psychiatry, 31*, 301–311.

Goswami, U. (1991). Learning about spelling sequences: The role of onsets and rimes in analogies in reading. *Child Development, 62*, 1110–1123.

Goswami, U., & Mead, F. (1992). Onset and rime awareness and analogies in reading. *Reading Research Quarterly, 27*, 152–162.

Grabe, W. (2002). Applied linguistics: An emerging discipline for the twenty-first century. In R. A. Kaplan (Ed.), *The Oxford handbook of applied linguistics* (pp. 3–12). New York: Oxford University Press.

Gray, J. (1993). *Men are from Mars, Women are from Venus: A practical guide for improving communication and getting what you want in your relationships*. New York: HarperCollins.

Gray, S. (2003). Word learning by preschoolers with specific language impairment: Predictors and poor learners. *Journal of Speech, Language, and Hearing Research, 47*, 1117–1132.

Grela, B., Rashiti, L., & Soares, M. (2004). Dative prepositions in children with specific language impairment. *Applied Psycholinguistics, 25*, 467–480.

Grief, E., & Berko Gleason, J. B. (1980). Hi, thanks, and goodbye: More routine information. *Language in Society, 9*, 159–167.

Grodzinsky, Y. (1990). *Theoretical perspectives on linguistic deficits*. Cambridge: MIT Press.

Gross, T. (2005, December 12). Getting the shmootz on Yiddish [Interview with Michael Wex]. *In Fresh Air from WHYY*. Washington, DC: National Public Radio. Available from http://www.npr.org/templates/story/story.php?storyId=5048943

Grunwell, P. (1997). Developmental phonological disability: Order in disorder. In B. W. Hodson & M. L. Edwards (Eds.), *Perspectives in applied phonology* (pp. 61–104). Gaithersburg, MD: Aspect.

Gutiérrez-Clellen, V. F., Restrepo, M. A., Bedore, L., Peña, E., & Anderson, R. (2000). Language sample analysis in Spanish-speaking children: Methodological considerations. *Language, Speech, and Hearing Services in Schools, 31*, 88–98.

Haelsig, P. C., & Madison, C. L. (1986). A study of phonological processes exhibited by 3-, 4-, and 5-year-old children. *Language, Speech, and Hearing Services in Schools, 17*, 107–114.

Hakuta, K. (2001). A critical period of second language acquisition? In D. Bailey, J. T. Bauer, F. J. Symons, & J. W. Lichtman (Eds.), *Critical thinking about critical periods* (pp. 193–208). Baltimore: Brookes.

Hall, D. G. (1996). Preschoolers' default assumptions about word meaning: Proper names designate unique individuals. *Developmental Psychology, 32*, 177–186.

Hall, D. G., Burns, T. C., & Pawluski, J. L. (2003). Input and word learning: Caregivers' sensitivity to lexical category distinctions. *Journal of Child Language, 30*, 711–729.

Halliday, M. A. K. (1975). *Learning how to mean: Exploration in the development of language*. London: Edward Arnold.

Halliday, M. A. K. (1977). *Exploration in the functions of language*. New York: Elsevier North-Holland.

Halliday, M. A. K. (1978). *Language as a social semiotic: The social interpretation of language and meaning.* Baltimore: University Park Press.

Halliday, M. A. K., & Hasan, R. (1985). *Language, context, and text: Aspects of language in a social-semiotic perspective.* Oxford, England: Oxford University Press.

Hammill, D. D., & Newcomer, P. L. (1997). *Test of Language Development—Primary* (3rd ed.). Austin, TX: PRO-ED.

Hannah, A., & Murachver, T. (1999). Gender and conversational style as predictors of conversational behavior. *Journal of Language and Social Psychology, 18,* 153–174.

Harley, T. (2001). *The psychology of language: From data to theory* (2nd ed.). New York: Taylor & Francis.

Hart, B., & Risley, T. (1995). *Meaningful differences in the everyday experiences of young American children.* Baltimore: Brookes.

Hart, B., & Risley, T. R. (1999). *The social world of children learning to talk.* Baltimore: Brookes.

Haviland, S. E., & Clark, E. V. (1974). This man's father is my father's son: A study of the acquisition of English kin terms. *Journal of Child Language, 1,* 23–47.

Hecker, D. E. (2001). Occupational employment projections to 2010. *Monthly Labor Review Online, 124*(11), 57–84.

Hedrick, D., Prather, E., & Tobin, A. (1984). *Sequenced Inventory of Communication Development* (Rev.). Los Angeles, CA: Western Psychological Services.

Heflin, L. J., & Simpson, R. L. (1998). Interventions for children and youth with autism: Prudent choices in a world of exaggerated claims and empty promises. Part 1: Intervention and treatment option review. *Focus on Autism and Other Developmental Disabilities, 13,* 194–211.

Heward, W. L. (2003). *Exceptional children: An introduction to special education* (7th ed.). Upper Saddle River, NJ: Merrill/Prentice Hall.

Hirsh-Pasek, K., & Golinkoff, R. M. (1996). *The origins of grammar: Evidence from early language comprehension.* Cambridge: MIT Press.

Hirsh-Pasek, K., & Golinkoff, R. M. (2003). *Einstein never used flashcards.* New York: Rodale.

Hirsh-Pasek, K., Golinkoff, R. M., & Hollich, G. (2000). An emergentist coalition model for word learning: Mapping words to objects is a product of the interaction of multiple cues. In R. M. Golinkoff, K. Hirsh-Pasek, L. Bloom, L. B. Smith, A. L. Woodward, N. Akhtar, et al. (Eds.), *Becoming a word learner: A debate on lexical acquisition* (pp. 136–164). New York: Oxford University Press.

Hoff, E. (2003). The specificity of environmental influence: Socioeconomic status affects early vocabulary development via maternal speech. *Child Development, 74,* 1368–1378.

Hoff, E. (2004). Progress, but not a full solution to the logical problem of language acquisition. *Journal of Child Language, 31,* 923–926.

Hoff-Ginsberg, E. (1997). *Language development.* Pacific Grove, CA: Brooks/Cole.

Hoff-Ginsberg, E. (1998). The relation of birth order and socioeconomic status to children's language experience and language development. *Applied Psycholinguistics, 19,* 603–629.

Hollich, G., Hirsh-Pasek, K., & Golinkoff, R. M. (2000). Breaking the language barrier: An emergentist coalition model of the origins of word learning. *Monographs of the Society for Research in Child Development, 65*(3), v–137.

Hollich, G., Newman, R. S., & Jusczyk, P. W. (2005). Infants' use of synchronized visual information to separate streams of speech. *Child Development, 76,* 598–613.

Hollich, G., Rocroi, C., Hirsh-Pasek, K., & Golinkoff, R. (1999, April). *Testing language comprehension in infants: Introducing the split-screen preferential looking paradigm.* Poster session presented at the Society for Research in Child Development, Albuquerque, NM.

Horton-Ikard, R., & Ellis Weismer, S. (2005). *A preliminary examination of vocabulary and word learning in African-American toddlers from low and middle SES homes.* Poster session presented at the 2005 Symposium on Research in Child Language Disorders, Madison, WI.

Hsu, H. (2001). Infant vocal development in a dynamic mother–infant communication system. *Infancy, 2,* 87–109.

Hubel, D. H., & Wiesel, T. N. (1970). The period of susceptibility to the physiological effects of unilateral eye closure in kittens. *Journal of Physiology, 206,* 419–436.

Hutchison, J. K. (2001). Telephone communications enhance children's narratives. *Dissertation Abstracts International.* (UMI No. AAT NQ72449)

Huttenlocher, J., Haight, W., Bryk, A., Seltzer, M., & Lyons, T. (1991). Early vocabulary growth: Relation to language input and gender. *Developmental Psychology, 27,* 236–248.

Huttenlocher, J., Vasilyeva, M., Cymerman, E., & Levine, S. (2002). Language input and child syntax. *Child Psychology, 45,* 337–374.

Huttenlocher, P. R. (2002). *Neural plasticity: The effects of environment on the development of the cerebral cortex.* Cambridge, MA: Harvard University Press.

Ilari, B., Polka, L., & Costa-Giomi, E. (2002, June). *Babies can un-ravel complex music.* Paper presented at the 143rd meeting of the Acoustical Society of America, Pittsburgh, PA. Retrieved from http://www.acoustics. org/press/143rd/Ilari.html

Imai, M., Haryu, E., & Okada, H. (2002). Is verb learning easier than noun learning for Japanese children? 3-year-old Japanese children's knowledge about object names and action names. In B. Skarabela, S. Fish, & A. H. J. Do (Eds.), *Proceedings of the 26th annual Boston University Conference on Language Development* (Vol. 1, pp. 324–335). Somerville, MA: Cascadilla Press.

Individuals with Disabilities Education Act Data. (2003). *Annual report tables.* Retrieved from http://www.ideadata.org/AnnualTables.asp

Individuals with Disabilities Education Improvement Act of 2004, Pub. L. No. 108–446, 118 Stat. 2647 (2004).

Ingram, D. (1986). Phonological development: Production. In P. Fletcher & M. Garman (Eds.), *Language acquisition* (2nd ed., pp. 223–239). New York: Cambridge University Press.

Ingram, D. (1989). *First language acquisition: Method, description, and explanation.* Cambridge, MA: Cambridge University Press.

Ingram, D. (1997). The categorization of phonological development. In B. W. Hodson & M. L. Edwards (Eds.), *Perspectives in applied phonology* (pp. 19–42). Gaithersburg, MD: Aspect.

Inhelder, B., & Piaget, J. (1958). *The growth of logical thinking from childhood to adolescence.* New York: Basic Books.

International Phonetic Association. (1996). *The International Phonetic Alphabet (revised to 1993, updated 1996).* Thessaloniki, Greece: Author. Retrieved from http://www.arts.gla.ac.uk/IPA/ipa.html

Invernizzi, M., Sullivan, A., Meier, J., & Swank, L. (2004). *Phonological Awareness Literacy Screening—PreK.* Charlottesville: University of Virginia.

Irwin, J. R. (2003). Parent and nonparent perception of the multimodal infant cry. *Infancy, 4,* 503–516.

Iverson, J. M., Longobardi, E., & Caselli, M. C. (2003). Relationship between gestures and words in children with Down's syndrome and typically developing children in the early stages of communicative development. *International Journal of Language and Communication Disorders, 38,* 179–197.

Jacobs, R. A. (1995). *English syntax: A grammar for English language professionals.* Oxford, England: Oxford University Press.

Jaswal, V. K., & Markman, E. M. (2001a). Learning proper and common names in inferential versus ostensive contexts. *Child Development, 72,* 768–786.

Jaswal, V. K., & Markman, E. M. (2001b). The relative strengths of indirect and direct word learning. *Developmental Psychology, 39,* 745–760.

Jia, G. (2003). The acquisition of the English plural morpheme by native Mandarin Chinese–speaking children. *Journal of Speech, Language, and Hearing Research, 46,* 1297–1311.

Jia, G., Aaronson, D., & Wu, Y. H. (2002). Long-term language attainment of bilingual immigrants: Predictive factors and language group differences. *Applied Psycholinguistics, 23,* 599–621.

Johnson, C. J., Beitchman, J. H., Young, A., Escobar, M., Atkinson, L., Wilson, B., et al. (1999). Fourteen-year follow-up of children with and without speech/language impairments: Speech/language stability and outcomes. *Journal of Speech, Language, and Hearing Research, 42,* 744–760.

Johnson, J. S., & Newport, E. L. (1989). Critical period effects in second language learning: The influence of maturational state on the acquisition of English as a second language. *Cognitive Psychology, 21,* 60–99.

Joint Committee on Infant Hearing. (1991). 1990 Position statement. *ASHA, 33*(Suppl. 5), 3–6.

Junker, D. A., & Stockman, I. J. (2002). Expressive vocabulary of German–English bilingual toddlers. *American Journal of Speech–Language Pathology, 11,* 381–394.

Jusczyk, P. W. (1993). From general to language-specific capacities: The WRAPSA model of how speech perception develops. *Journal of Phonetics, 21,* 3–28.

Jusczyk, P. W. (2003). Chunking language input to find patterns. In D. H. Rakison & L. M. Oakes (Eds.), *Early category and concept development: Making sense of the blooming, buzzing confusion* (pp. 27–49). New York: Oxford University Press.

Jusczyk, P. W., & Aslin, R. N. (1995). Infants' detection of sound patterns of words in fluent speech. *Cognitive Psychology, 29,* 1–23.

Jusczyk, P. W., Cutler, A., & Redanz, N. J. (1993). Infants' preference for the predominant stress patterns of English words. *Child Development, 64,* 675–687.

Jusczyk, P. W., Friederici, A. D., Wessels, J. M., Svenkerud, V. Y., & Jusczyk, A. M. (1993). Infants' sensitivity to the sound patterns of native language words. *Journal of Memory and Language, 32,* 402–420.

Jusczyk, P. W., Hirsh-Pasek, K., Kemler Nelson, D. G., Kennedy, L. J., Woodward, A., & Piwoz, J. (1992). Perception of acoustic correlates of major phrasal units by young infants. *Cognitive Psychology, 24,* 252–293.

Jusczyk, P. W., Jusczyk, A. M., Kennedy, L. J., Schomberg, T., & Koenig, N. (1995). Young infants' retention of information about bisyllabic utterances. *Journal of Experimental Psychology: Human Perception and Performance, 21,* 822–836.

Jusczyk, P. W., Kennedy, L. J., & Jusczyk, A. M. (1995). Young infants' retention of information about syllables. *Infant Behavior and Development, 18,* 27–42.

Jusczyk, P. W., & Luce, P. A. (1994). Infant's sensitivity to phonotactic patterns in the native language. *Journal of Memory and Language, 33,* 630–645.

Jusczyk, P. W., Luce, P. A., & Charles-Luce, J. (1994). Infants' sensitivity to phonotactic patterns in the native language. *Journal of Memory and Language, 33,* 630–645.

Jusczyk, P. W., Pisoni, D. B., & Mullennix, J. (1992). Some consequences of stimulus variability on speech processing by 2-month-old infants. *Cognition, 43,* 253–291.

Justice, L. M. (2006). *Communication sciences and disorders: An introduction.* Upper Saddle River, NJ: Merrill/Prentice Hall.

Justice, L. M., Bowles, R., Kaderavek, J., Ukrainetz, T., Eisenberg, S., & Gillam, R. (2006). The index of narrative micro-structure (INMIS): A clinical tool for analyzing school-age children's narrative performance. *American Journal of Speech–Language Pathology, 15,* 1–15.

Justice, L. M., & Ezell, H. K. (2002a). *The syntax handbook.* Eau Claire, WI: Thinking.

Justice, L. M., & Ezell, H. K. (2002b). Use of storybook reading to increase print awareness in at-risk children. *American Journal of Speech–Language Pathology, 11*, 17–29.

Justice, L. M., & Ezell, H. K. (2004). Print referencing: An emergent literacy enhancement technique and its clinical applications. *Language, Speech, and Hearing Services in Schools, 35*, 185–193.

Justice, L. M., & Kaderavek, J. N. (2003). Topic control during shared storybook reading: Mothers and their children with language impairments. *Topics in Early Childhood Special Education, 23*, 137–150.

Justice, L. M., Pence, K., Bowles, R., & Wiggins, A. (2006). An investigation of four hypotheses concerning the order by which 4-year-old children learn the alphabet letters. *Early Childhood Research Quarterly, 21*, 374–389.

Justice, L. M., & Pullen, P. (2003). Promising interventions for promoting emergent literacy skills: Three evidence-based approaches. *Topics in Early Childhood Special Education, 23*, 99–113.

Justice, L. M., & Schuele, C. M. (2004). Phonological awareness: Description, assessment, and intervention. In J. E. Bernthal & N. W. Bankson (Eds.), *Articulation and phonological disorders* (5th ed., pp. 376–406). New York: Allyn & Bacon.

Kaderavek, J. N., & Justice, L. M. (2004). Embedded-explicit emergent literacy. II: Goal selection and implementation in the early childhood classroom. *Language, Speech, and Hearing Services in Schools, 35*, 212–228.

Kaderavek, J. N., & Sulzby, E. (2000). Narrative productions by children with and without specific language impairment: Oral narratives and emergent readings. *Journal of Speech, Language, and Hearing Research, 43*, 34–49.

Kagan, J., & Snidman, N. (2004). *The long shadow of temperament*. Cambridge, MA: Harvard University Press.

Kail, R. (1994). A method of studying the generalized slowing hypothesis in children with specific language impairment. *Journal of Speech and Hearing Research, 37*, 418–421.

Karmiloff, K., & Karmiloff-Smith, A. (2001). *Pathways to language from fetus to adolescent*. Cambridge, MA: Harvard University Press.

Karrass, J., Braungart-Rieker, J. M., Mullins, J., & Lefever, J. B. (2002). Processes in language acquisition: The roles of gender, attention, and maternal encouragement of attention over time. *Journal of Child Language, 29*, 519–543.

Kelly, S. D. (2001). Broadening the units of analysis in communication: Speech and nonverbal behaviors in pragmatic comprehension. *Journal of Child Language, 28*, 325–349.

Kemler Nelson, D. G., Herron, L., & Holt, M. B. (2003). The sources of young children's name innovations for novel artifacts. *Journal of Child Language, 30*, 823–843.

Kenneally, S. M., Bruck, G. E., Frank, E. M., & Nalty, L. (1998). Language intervention after thirty years of isolation: A case study of a feral child. *Education and Training in Mental Retardation and Developmental Disabilities, 33*, 13–23.

Kent, R. D. (1994). *Reference manual for communicative sciences and disorders: Speech and language*. Austin, TX: PRO-ED.

Keogh, B. K. (2003). *Temperament in the classroom*. Baltimore: Brookes.

Kita, S., & Özyürek, A. (2003). What does cross-linguistics variation in semantic coordination of speech and gesture reveal? Evidence for an interface representation of spatial thinking and speaking. *Journal of Memory and Language, 48*, 16–32.

Koike, D. A. (1986). Differences and similarities in men's and women's directives in Carioca Brazilian Portuguese. *Hispania, 69*, 387–394.

Kovas, Y., Hayious-Thomas, M. E., Oliver, B., Bishop, D. V. M., Dale, P. S., & Plomin, R. (2005). Genetic influences in different aspects of language development: The etiology of language skills in 4.5-year-old twins. *Child Development, 76*, 632–651.

Krashen, S. (1985). *The input hypothesis: Issues and implications*. London: Longman.

Kristal, J. (2005). *The temperament perspective: Working with children's behavioral styles*. Baltimore: Brookes.

Kuder, S. (1997). *Teaching students with language and communication disabilities*. Boston: Allyn & Bacon.

Kuhl, P., Andruski, J., Chistovich, I., Chistovich, L., Kozhevnikova, E., Ryskina, V., et al. (1997). Cross-language analysis of phonetic units in language addressed to infants. *Science, 277*, 684–686.

Kuhl, P. K., & Meltzoff, A. N. (1982). The bimodal perception of speech in infancy. *Science, 218*, 1138–1141.

Labov, T. G. (1998). English acquisition by immigrants to the United States at the beginning of the twentieth century. *American Speech, 73*, 368–398.

Labov, W. (1972). *Language in the inner city: Studies in the Black English Vernacular*. Philadelphia: University of Pennsylvania Press.

Labov, W. (1998). Coexistent systems in African-American English. In S. Mufwene, J. Rickford, J. Baugh, & G. Bailey (Eds.), *The structure of African-American English* (pp. 110–153). London: Routledge.

Labov, W., Ash, S., & Boberg, C. (2005). *The atlas of North American English*. New York: Mouton/de Gruyter.

Lahey, M. (1988). *Language disorders and language development*. New York: Macmillan.

Lai, C. S., Fisher, S. E., Hurst, J. A., Vargha-Khadem, F., & Monaco, A. P. (2001). A forkhead-domain gene is mutated in severe speech and language disorder. *Nature, 413*, 519–523.

Lakoff, R. (1975). *Language and woman's place*. New York: Harper & Row.

Lalonde, C. E., & Werker, J. F. (1995). Cognitive influences on cross-language speech perception in infancy. *Infant Behavior and Development, 18*, 459–475.

Landau, B., & Gleitman, L. R. (1985). *Language and experience: Evidence from the blind child.* Cambridge, MA: Harvard University Press.

Landau, B., Smith, L., & Jones, S. (1998). Object shape, object function, and object name. *Journal of Memory and Language, 38*, 1–27.

Landry, S. H., Miller-Loncar, C. L., Smith, K. E., & Swank, P. R. (1997). Predicting cognitive-language and social growth curves from early maternal behaviors in children at varying degrees of biological risk. *Developmental Psychology, 33*, 1040–1053.

Larsen-Freeman, D., & Long, M. H. (1991). *An introduction to second language acquisition research.* New York: Longman.

Laucht, M., Esser, G., & Schmidt, M. H. (1995). Contrasting infant predictors of later cognitive functioning. *Journal of Child Psychology and Psychology and Applied Disciplines, 35*, 649–662.

Laws, G., & Bishop, D. V. M. (2003). A comparison of language abilities in adolescents with Down syndrome and children with specific language impairment. *Journal of Speech, Language, and Hearing Research, 46*, 1324–1339.

Leavens, D. A., Russell, J. L., & Hopkins, W. D. (2005). Intentionality as measured in the persistence and elaboration of communication by chimpanzees *(Pan troglodytes). Child Development, 76*, 291–306.

Lederberg, A. R., Prezbindowski, A. K., & Spencer, P. E. (2000). Word-learning skills of Deaf preschoolers: The development of novel mapping and rapid word-learning. *Child Development, 71*, 1571–1585.

Lee, L. L. (1974). *Developmental sentence analysis: A grammatical assessment procedure for speech and language clinicians.* Evanston, IL: Northwestern University Press.

Lenneberg, E. H. (1967). *Biological foundations of language.* New York: Wiley.

Leonard, L. B. (2000). *Children with specific language impairment.* Cambridge: MIT Press.

Lessow-Hurley, J. (1990). *The foundations of dual language instruction.* White Plains, NY: Longman.

Levorato, M. C., Nesi, B., & Cacciari, C. (2004). Reading comprehension and understanding idiomatic expressions: A developmental study. *Brain and Language, 91*, 303–314.

Liberman, A. M. (1999). When theories of speech meet the real world. *Journal of Psycholinguistic Research, 27*, 111–122.

Lieberman, P. (1991). *Uniquely human: The evolution of speech, thought, and selfless behavior.* Cambridge, MA: Harvard University Press.

Liiva, C. A., & Cleave, P. L. (2005). Roles of initiation and responsiveness in access and participation for children with specific language impairment. *Journal of Speech, Language, and Hearing Research, 48*, 868–883.

Liu, J., Golinkoff, R. M., & Sak, K. (2001). One cow does not an animal make: Young children can extend novel words at the superordinate level. *Child Development, 72*, 1674–1694.

Locke, J. L. (1983). *Phonological acquisition and change.* New York: Academic Press.

Lonigan, C. J., & Whitehurst, G. J. (1998). Relative efficacy of parent and teacher involvement in a shared-reading intervention for preschool children from low-income backgrounds. *Early Childhood Research Quarterly, 13*, 263–290.

Lord, C., & Risi, S. (2000). Diagnosis of autism spectrum disorders in young children. In A. M. Wetherby & B. M. Prizant (Eds.), *Autism spectrum disorders: A transactional developmental perspective* (pp. 11–30). Baltimore: Brookes.

Lovaas, O. I. (1987). Behavioral treatment and normal educational and intellectual functioning in young autistic children. *Journal of Consulting and Clinical Psychology, 55*, 3–9.

Lozanov, G. (1979). *Suggestology and outlines of suggestopedy.* New York: Gordon and Breach Science.

Lucy, J. A. (1992). *Language diversity and thought: A reformulation of the linguistic relativity hypothesis.* New York: Cambridge University Press.

Lund, N. J., & Duchan, J. F. (1993). *Assessing children's language in naturalistic contexts* (3rd ed.). Upper Saddle River, NJ: Prentice Hall.

Lust, B., Flynn, S., & Foley, C. (1996). What children know about what they say: Elicited imitation as a research method for assessing children's syntax. In D. McDaniel, C. McKee, & H. Smith (Eds.), *Methods for assessing children's syntax* (pp. 55–76). Cambridge: MIT Press.

MacWhinney, B. (1987). The competition model. In B. MacWhinney (Ed.), *Mechanisms of language acquisition* (pp. 249–308). Hillsdale, NJ: Erlbaum.

Maguire, M. J. (2004, September). Children's use of universal and language-specific cues in verb learning. *Dissertation Abstracts International, 65* (03), 1579. (UMI No. 9315947)

Mandler, J. (2000). Perceptual and conceptual processes in infancy. *Journal of Cognition and Development, 1*, 3–36.

Markman, E. M. (1989). *Categorization and naming in children: Problems of induction.* Cambridge: MIT Press.

Markman, E. M. (1990). Constraints children place on word meanings. *Cognitive Science, 14*, 57–77.

Markman, E. M. (1991). The whole-object, taxonomic, and mutual exclusivity assumptions as initial constraints on word meanings. In S. A. Gelman & J. P. Byrnes (Eds.), *Perspectives on language and thought: Interrelations in development* (pp. 72–106). New York: Cambridge University Press.

Markman, E. M., & Hutchinson, J. E. (1984). Children's sensitivity to constraints on word meaning: Taxonomic vs. thematic relations. *Cognitive Psychology, 16*, 1–27.

Markson, L., & Bloom, P. (1997). Evidence against a dedicated system for word learning in children. *Nature, 385*, 813–815.

Martin, F. (1994). *Introduction to audiology* (5th ed.). Upper Saddle River, NJ: Prentice Hall.

Martin, F., & Greer Clark, J. (2002). *Introduction to audiology* (8th ed.). Boston: Allyn & Bacon.

Mattingly, I. G., & Liberman, A. M. (1988). Specialized perceiving systems for speech and other biologically significant sounds. In G. M. Edelman, W. E. Gall, & W. M. Cowan (Eds.), *Functions of the auditory system* (pp. 775–793). New York: Wiley.

Mattys, S. L., & Jusczyk, P. W. (2001). Phonotactic cues for segmentation of fluent speech by infants. *Cognition, 78*, 91–121.

Mattys, S. L., Jusczyk, P. W., Luce, P. A., & Morgan, J. L. (1999). Word segmentation in infants: How phonotactics and prosody combine. *Cognitive Psychology, 38*, 465–494.

McBride-Chang, C. (1999). The ABCs of the ABCs: The development of letter–name and letter–sound knowledge. *Merrill–Palmer Quarterly, 45*, 285–308.

McClelland, J. L., Rumelhart, D. E., & Hinton, G. E. (1986). The appeal of parallel distributed processing. In D. Rumelhart, J. McClelland, & the PDP Group (Eds.), *Parallel distributed processing* (Vol. 1, pp. 3–44). Cambridge: MIT Press.

McConchie, A. (n.d.). *The great pop vs. soda controversy.* Retrieved from http://www.popvssoda.com

McCune, L., & Vihman, M. M. (2001). Early phonetic and lexical development: A productivity approach. *Journal of Speech, Language, and Hearing Research, 44*, 670–684.

McDaniel, D., McKee, C., & Smith, H. (1996). *Methods for assessing children's syntax.* Cambridge: MIT Press.

McDaniel, D., & Smith Cairns, H. (1998). Eliciting judgments of grammaticality and reference. In D. McDaniel, C. McKee, & H. Smith Cairns (Eds.), *Methods for assessing children's syntax* (pp. 233–254). Boston: MIT Press.

McEachern, D., & Haynes, W. O. (2004). Gesture–speech combinations as a transition to multiword utterances. *American Journal of Speech–Language Pathology, 13*, 227–235.

McEachin, J. J., Smith, T., & Lovaas, O. I. (1993). Long-term outcome for children with autism who received early intensive behavioral treatment. *American Journal on Mental Retardation, 97*, 359–372.

McGregor, K. K. (1997). The nature of word-finding errors of preschoolers with and without word-finding deficits. *Journal of Speech and Hearing Research, 40*, 1232–1244.

McGregor, K. K., Friedman, R. M., Reilly, R. M., & Newman, R. M. (2002). Semantic representation and naming in young children. *Journal of Speech, Language, and Hearing Research, 45*, 332–346.

McGregor, K. K., & Leonard, L. B. (1995). Intervention for word-finding deficits in children. In M. Fey, J. Windsor, & S. Warren (Eds.), *Language intervention: Preschool through the elementary years* (pp. 85–105). Baltimore: Brookes.

Meadows, D., Elias, G., & Bain, J. (2000). Mothers' ability to identify infants' communicative acts consistently. *Journal of Child Language, 27*, 393–406.

Mehler, J., Jusczyk, P. W., Lambetz, G., Halsted, N., Bertoncini, J., & Amiel-Tison, C. (1988). A precursor of language acquisition in young infants. *Cognition, 29*, 144–178.

Menyuk, P. (1999). *Reading and linguistic development.* Cambridge, MA: Brookline Books.

Mercer, C. (1997). *Students with learning disabilities* (5th ed.). Upper Saddle River, NJ: Prentice Hall.

Merriman, W. E., & Bowman, L. (1989). The mutual exclusivity bias in children's early word learning. *Monographs of the Society for Research in Child Development, 54*(3–4), 1–129.

Mervis, C. B. (1987). Child–basic object categories and early development. In U. Neisser (Ed.), *Concepts and conceptual development: Ecological and intellectual factors in categorization* (pp. 201–233). New York: Cambridge University Press.

Mervis, C. B., & Crisafi, M. A. (1982). Order of acquisition of subordinate, basic, and superordinate categories. *Child Development, 53*, 258–266.

Meyer, M., Leonard, S., Hirsh-Pasek, K., Imai, E., Haryu, E., Pulverman, R., et al. (2003, November). *Making a convincing argument: A crosslinguistic comparison of noun and verb learning in Japanese and English.* Boston: Boston University Conference on Language Development.

Meyer, T. A., Svirsky, M. A., Kirk, K. I., & Miyamoto, R. T. (1998). Improvements in speech perception by children with profound prelingual hearing loss: Effects of device, communication mode, and chronological age. *Journal of Speech, Language, and Hearing Research, 41*, 846–858.

Miller, C. L. (1988). Parents' perceptions and attributions of infant vocal behaviour and development. *First Language, 8*, 125–141.

Miller, E. K. (1999). The prefrontal cortex: Complex neural properties for complex behavior. *Neuron, 22*, 15–17.

Miller, J. (1981). *Assessing language production in children: Experimental procedures.* Baltimore: University Park Press.

Miller, J., & Chapman, R. (1981). The relationship between age and mean length of utterance in morphemes. *Journal of Speech and Hearing Research, 24*, 154–161.

Miller, J., & Chapman, R. (2000). *SALT: Systematic Analysis of Language Transcripts.* Madison: Language Analysis Laboratory, Waisman Center, University of Wisconsin—Madison.

Miller, J., & Iglesias, A. (2006). *A systematic analysis of language transcripts* (SALT; English & Spanish, Version 9).

Madison: Language Analysis Lab, University of Wisconsin—Madison.

Mistry, R. S., Biesanz, J. C., Taylor, L. C., Burchinal, M., & Cox, M. J. (2004). Family income and its relation to preschool children's adjustment for families in the NICHD study of early child care. *Developmental Psychology, 40*, 727–745.

Molfese, D. L. (1990). Auditory evoked responses recorded from 16-month-old human infants to words they did and did not know. *Brain and Language, 38*, 345–363.

Moore, J. A., & Teagle, H. F. B. (2002). An introduction to cochlear implant technology, activation, and programming. *Language, Speech, and Hearing Services in Schools, 33*, 153–161.

Morales, M., Mundy, P., & Rojas, J. (1998). Following the direction of gaze and language development in 6-month-olds. *Infant Behavior and Development, 21*, 373–377.

Muñoz, M. L., Gillam, R. B., Peña, E. B., & Gulley-Faehnle, A. (2003). Measures of language development in fictional narratives of Latino children. *Language, Speech, and Hearing Services in Schools, 34*, 332–342.

Naigles, L., & Kako, E. (1993). First contact in verb acquisition: Defining a role for syntax. *Child Development, 64*, 1665–1687.

Naremore, R. C., Densmore, A. E., & Harman, D. R. (1995). *Language intervention with school-aged children: Conversation, narrative, and text.* San Diego, CA: Singular.

Nash, M., & Donaldson, M. L. (2005). Word learning in children with vocabulary deficits. *Journal of Speech, Language, and Hearing Research, 48*, 439–458.

Nathani, S. R., Ertmer, D. J., & Stark, R. E. (2000). *Stark Assessment of Early Vocal Development.* Unpublished manuscript, Purdue University, West Lafayette, IN.

National Institute of Child Health and Human Development (NICHD). (n.d.). *The NICHD Study of Early Child Care and Youth Development.* Rockville, MD: Author. Retrieved September 5, 2006, from http://secc.rti.org/

National Institute of Child Health and Human Development (NICHD) Early Child Care Research Network. (1996). Characteristics of infant child care: Factors contributing to positive caregiving. *Early Childhood Research Quarterly, 11*, 269–306.

National Institute of Child Health and Human Development (NICHD) Early Child Care Research Network. (1997). Familial factors associated with the characteristics of nonmaternal care for infants. *Journal of Marriage and the Family, 59*, 389–408.

National Institute of Child Health and Human Development (NICHD) Early Child Care Research Network. (2000). The relation of child care to cognitive and language development. *Child Development, 71*, 960–980.

National Institute on Deafness and Other Communication Disorders. (n.d.). *Milestones in your child's speech and language development.* Bethesda, MD: Author. Retrieved September 5, 2006, from http://www.nidcd.nih.gov/health/voice/thebasics_speechandlanguage.asp

National Institute on Deafness and Other Communication Disorders. (2003). *Traumatic brain injury: Cognitive and communication disorders.* Bethesda, MD: Author. Retrieved July 9, 2006, from http://www.nidcd.nih.gov/health/voice/tbrain.htm

Nelson, K. (1973). Structure and strategy in learning to talk. *Monographs of the Society of Research in Child Development, 38*(1–2), 1–135.

Nelson, N. W. (1998). *Childhood language disorders in context.* Boston: Allyn & Bacon.

Neuman, S. (2006). The knowledge gap: Implications for early education. In D. Dickinson & S. Neuman (Eds.), *Handbook of early literacy research* (Vol. 2, pp. 29–40). New York: Guilford Press.

Newman, M. (2006). New York tawk (New York City). In W. Wolfram & B. Ward (Eds.), *American voices: How dialects differ from coast to coast* (pp. 82–87). Malden, MA: Blackwell.

Newport, E. (1990). Maturational constraints on language learning. *Cognitive Science, 14*, 11–28.

Nicely, P., Tamis-LeMonda, C. S., & Bornstein, M. H. (1999). Mothers' attuned responses to infant affect expressivity promote earlier achievement of language milestones. *Infant Behavior and Development, 22*, 557–568.

Nicholas, J. G., & Geers, A. E. (1997). Communication of oral Deaf and normally hearing children at 36 months of age. *Journal of Speech, Language, and Hearing Research, 40*, 1314–1327.

Ninio, A., & Bruner, J. (1978). The achievement and antecedents of labeling. *Journal of Child Language, 5*, 1–15.

Nippold, M. A. (1998). *Later language development: The school-age and adolescent years* (2nd ed.). Austin, TX: PRO-ED.

Nippold, M. A. (2000). Language development during the adolescent years: Aspects of pragmatics, syntax, and semantics. *Topics in Language Disorders, 20*, 1528.

Nippold, M. A., Ward-Lonergan, J. M., & Fanning, J. L. (2005). Persuasive writing in children, adolescents, and adults: A study of syntactic, semantic, and pragmatic development. *Language, Speech, and Hearing Services in Schools, 36*, 125–138.

Nittrouer, S. (1996). The relation between speech perception and phonemic awareness: Evidence from low-SES children and children with chronic OM. *Journal of Speech and Hearing Research, 39*, 1059–1070.

Noback, C. R., Strominger, N. L., Demarest, R. J., & Ruggiero, D. A. (2005). *The human nervous system: Structure and function* (6th ed.). Totowa, NJ: Humana Press.

O'Connor, R. E., & Jenkins, J. R. (1999). Prediction of reading disabilities in kindergarten and first grade. *Scientific Studies of Reading, 3*, 159–197.

Office of the Federal Register. (1990). *Presidential Proclamation 6158.* Retrieved December 30, 2005, from http://www.loc.gov/loc/brain/proclaim.html

O'Grady, W. (1997). Semantics: The analysis of meaning. In W. O'Grady, M. Dobrovolsky, & M. Arnoff (Eds.),

Contemporary linguistics (3rd ed., pp. 245–287). Boston: Bedford/St. Martin's.

O'Grady, W., Dobrovolsky, M., & Arnoff, M. (Eds.). (1997). *Contemporary linguistics* (3rd ed.). Boston: Bedford/St. Martin's.

Oliver, B. R., Dale, P. S., & Plomin, R. (2005). Predicting literacy at age 7 from preliteracy at age 4: A longitudinal genetic analysis. *Psychological Science, 16*, 861–865.

Oller, D. K., Eilers, R. E., Urbano, R., & Cobo-Lewis, A. B. (1997). Development of precursors to speech in infants exposed to two languages. *Journal of Child Language, 24*, 407–425.

Owens, R. (1996). *Language development: An introduction* (4th ed.). New York: Allyn & Bacon.

Owens, R. E. (2001). *Language development: An introduction* (5th ed.). Needham Heights, MA: Allyn & Bacon.

Owens, R. E. (2005). *Language development: An introduction* (6th ed.). Boston: Allyn & Bacon.

Pakulski, L. (2006). Pediatric hearing loss. In L. Justice (Ed.), *Communication sciences and disorders: An introduction* (pp. 428–467). Upper Saddle River, NJ: Merrill/Prentice Hall.

Pallier, C., Dehaene, S., Poline, J. B., LeBihan, D., Argenti, A. M., Dupoux, E., et al. (2003). Brain imaging of language plasticity in adopted adults: Can a second language replace the first? *Cerebral Cortex, 13*, 155–161.

Papousek, M., Papousek, H., & Symmes, D. (1991). The meanings of melodies in motherese in tone and stress languages. *Infant Behavior and Development, 14*, 415–440.

Paradis, J. (2005). Grammatical morphology in children learning English as a second language: Implications of similarities with specific language impairment. *Language, Speech, and Hearing Services in Schools, 36*, 172–187.

Paul, R. (1995). *Language disorders from infancy through adolescence: Assessment and intervention.* St. Louis, MO: Mosby–Year Book.

Paul, R. (2001). *Language disorders from infancy through adolescence: Assessment and intervention* (2nd ed.). St. Louis, MO: Mosby.

Paul, R., & Smith, R. L. (1993). Narrative skills in 4-year-olds with normal, impaired, and late developing language. *Journal of Speech and Hearing Research, 36*, 592–598.

Paul, R., Spangle-Looney, S., & Dahm, P. S. (1991). Communication and socialization skills at ages 2 and 3 in "late talking" young children. *Journal of Speech and Hearing Research, 34*, 858–865.

Pence, K., Skibbe, L. E., Justice, L. M., Bowles, R., & Beckman, A. (2006). *Chronicity and timing of early childhood impairment and adjustment to kindergarten.* Manuscript under review.

Peterson, C. (1990). The who, when, and where of early narratives. *Journal of Child Language, 17*, 433–455.

Peterson, C., Jesso, B., & McCabe, A. (1999). Encouraging narratives in preschoolers: An intervention study. *Journal of Child Language, 26*, 49–67.

Petitto, L.-A., Holowka, S., Sergio, L. E., & Ostry, S. (2001). Language rhythms in baby hand movements. *Nature, 413*, 35–36.

Petitto, L.-A., Katerelos, M., Levy, B. G., Gauna, K., Tétreault, K., & Ferraro, V. (2001). Bilingual signed and spoken language acquisition from birth: Implications for the mechanisms underlying early bilingual language acquisition. *Journal of Child Language, 28*, 453–496.

Phillips, C. (2001). Levels of representation in the electrophysiology of speech perception. *Cognitive Science, 25*, 711–731.

Piaget, J. (1923). *The language and thought of the child.* London: Kegan Paul.

Piaget, J. (1970). *Structuralism.* New York: Basic Books.

Pinker, S. (1984). *Language learnability and language development.* Cambridge, MA: Harvard University Press.

Pinker, S. (1994). *The language instinct: How the mind creates language.* New York: Morrow.

Pinker, S. (1999). *Words and rules.* New York: Basic Books.

Pisoni, D., Cleary, M., Geers, A., & Tobey, E. (2000). Individual differences in effectiveness of cochlear implants in children who are prelingually Deaf: New process measures of performance. *Volta Review, 10*, 111–164.

Poole, I. (1934). Genetic development of consonant sounds in speech. *Elementary English Review, 11*, 159–161.

Poplack, S. (1978). Dialectical acquisition among Puerto Rican bilinguals. *Language in Society, 7*, 89–103.

Prather, E. M., Hedrick, E. L., & Kerin, C. A. (1975). Articulation development in children aged two to four years. *Journal of Speech and Hearing Disorders, 40*, 179–191.

Pulverman, R., & Golinkoff, R. M. (2004). *Seven-month-olds' attention to potential verb referents in nonlinguistic events.* Paper presented at the 28th annual Boston University Conference on Language Development, Boston, MA.

Purnell, T., Idsardi, W., & Baugh, J. (1999). Perceptual and phonetic experiments on American English dialect identification. *Journal of Language and Social Psychology, 18*, 10–30.

Pye, C. (1992). The acquisition of K'iche' Maya. In D. Slobin (Ed.), *The crosslinguistic study of language acquisition* (Vol. 3, pp. 221–308). Hillsdale, NJ: Erlbaum.

Quinn, P. C., Eimas, P. D., & Rosenkrantz, S. L. (1993). Evidence for representations of perceptually similar natural categories by 3-month-old and 4-month-old infants. *Perception, 22*, 463–475.

Radford, A., & Ploennig-Pacheco, I. (1995). The morphosyntax of subjects and verbs in child Spanish: A case study. *Essex Research Reports in Linguistics, 5*, 23–67.

Ramus, F. (n.d.). *Non-nutritive sucking at birth.* Paris: Laboratoire de Sciences Cognitives et Psycholinguistique Ecole Normale Supérieure.

Rapin, I., & Allen, D. A. (1987). Developmental dysphasia and autism in pre-school children: Characteristics and subtypes. In J. Martin, P. Fletcher, P. Grunwell, & D. Hall (Eds.), *Proceedings of the First International Symposium on Specific Speech and Language Disorders in*

Children (pp. 20–35). London: Association for All Speech-Impaired Children (AFASIC).

Ratner, V. L., & Harris, L. R. (1994). *Understanding language disorders: The impact on learning.* Eau Claire, WI: Thinking.

Redmond, S., & Rice, M. L. (1998). The socioemotional behaviors of children with SLI: Social adaptation or social deviance? *Journal of Speech, Language, and Hearing Research, 41,* 688–700.

Reid, D. K. (2000). Ebonics and Hispanic, Asian, and Native American dialects of English. In K. R. Fahey & D. K. Reid (Eds.), *Language development, differences, and disorders* (pp. 219–246). Austin, TX: PRO-ED.

Reid, D. K., Hresko, W., & Hammill, D. (2002). *Test of Early Reading Ability* (3rd ed.). Austin, TX: PRO-ED.

Rescorla, L. (1980). Overextension in early language development. *Journal of Child Language, 7,* 321–335.

Rescorla, L. (1993a). Language Development Survey (LDS): The use of parental report in the identification of communicatively delayed toddlers. *Seminars in Speech and Language, 14,* 264–277.

Rescorla, L. A. (1993b, March). *Outcomes of toddlers with specific expressive language delay (SELD) at ages 3, 4, 5, 6, 7, and 8.* Paper presented at the biennial meeting of the Society for Research in Child Development, New Orleans, LA.

Rescorla, L., Roberts, J., & Dahlsgaard, K. (1997). Late talkers at 2: Outcome at age 3. *Journal of Speech, Language, and Hearing Research, 40,* 556–566.

Rescorla, L., & Schwartz, E. (1990). Outcome of toddlers with specific expressive language delay. *Applied Psycholinguistics, 11,* 393–407.

Reznick, J. S., & Goldfield, B. A. (1992). Rapid change in lexical development in comprehension and production. *Developmental Psychology, 28,* 406–413.

Rice, M. L. (1996). *Toward a genetics of language.* Mahwah, NJ: Erlbaum.

Rice, M. L., Haney, K. R., & Wexler, K. (1998). Family histories of children with SLI who show extended optional infinitives. *Journal of Speech, Language, and Hearing Research, 41,* 419–432.

Rice, M. L., & Wexler, K. (1996). Toward tense as a clinical marker of specific language impairment in English-speaking children. *Journal of Speech and Hearing Research, 39,* 1239–1257.

Rice, M. L., Wexler, K., & Cleave, P. L. (1995). Specific language impairment as a period of extended optional infinitive. *Journal of Speech and Hearing Research, 38,* 850–863.

Richards, B. J. (1990). *Language development and individual differences: A study of auxiliary verb learning.* Cambridge, England: Cambridge University Press.

Rizzolatti, G., & Craighero, L. (2004). The mirror-neuron system. *Annual Review of Neuroscience, 27,* 169–192.

Robbins, C., & Ehri, L. C. (1994). Reading storybooks to kindergartners helps them learn new vocabulary words. *Journal of Education Psychology, 86,* 54–64.

Roberts, J., Nagy, N., & Boberg, C. (2006). Yakking with the Yankees (New England). In W. Wolfram & B. Ward (Eds.), *American voices: How dialects differ from coast to coast* (pp. 57–62). Malden, MA: Blackwell.

Roberts, J. A., Pollock, K. E., Krakow, R., Price, J., Fulmer, K., & Wang, P. P. (2005). Language development in preschool-age children adopted from China. *Journal of Speech, Language, and Hearing Research, 48,* 93–107.

Robertson, K., & Murachver, T. (2003). Children's speech accommodation to gendered language styles. *Journal of Language and Social Psychology, 22,* 321–333.

Robinson, N. M., Dale, P. S., & Landesman, S. (1990). Validity of Stanford–Binet IV with linguistically precocious toddlers. *Intelligence, 14,* 173–186.

Rosenberg, S., & Abbeduto, L. (1993). *Language and communication in mental retardation.* Hillsdale, NJ: Erlbaum.

Rossetti, L. (1990). *Infant–Toddler Language Scale.* East Moline, IL: LinguiSystems.

Rumelhart, D. E. (1980). Schemata: The building blocks of cognition. In R. J. Spiro, B. C. Bruce, & W. F. Brewer (Eds.), *Theoretical issues in reading* (pp. 34–58). Hillsdale, NJ: Erlbaum.

Rumelhart, D. E., & McClelland, J. L. (1986). On learning the past tenses of English verbs. In D. E. Rumelhart & J. L. McClelland (Eds.), *Parallel distributed processing: Explorations in the microstructure of cognition: Vol. 2. Psychological and biological models* (pp. 216–271). Cambridge: MIT Press.

Rush, K. L. (1999). Caregiver–child interactions and early literacy development of preschool children from low-income environments. *Topics in Early Childhood Special Education, 19,* 3–14.

Russell, N. K. (1993). Educational considerations in traumatic brain injury: The role of the speech–language pathologist. *Language, Speech, and Hearing Services in Schools, 24,* 67–75.

Safran, S. P., Safran, J. S., & Ellis, K. (2003). Intervention ABCs for children with Asperger syndrome. *Topics in Language Disorders, 23,* 154–165.

Salvucci, C. (2006). Expressions of brotherly love (Philadelphia, PA). In W. Wolfram & B. Ward (Eds.), *American voices: How dialects differ from coast to coast* (pp. 88–92). Malden, MA: Blackwell.

Sander, E. K. (1972). When are speech sounds learned? *Journal of Speech and Hearing Disorders, 37,* 55–63.

Sapir, E. (1921). *Language: An introduction to the study of speech.* New York: Harcourt, Brace.

Saylor, M. M., & Sabbagh, M. A. (2004). Different kinds of information affect word learning in the preschool years: The case of part-term learning. *Child Development, 75,* 395–408.

Scarborough, H. (1990). Very early language deficits in dyslexic children. *Child Development, 61,* 1728–1743.

Scarborough, H. S. (2001). Connecting early language and literacy to later reading (dis)abilities: Evidence, theory, and practice. In S. B. Neuman & D. K. Dickinson (Eds.),

Handbook of early literacy research (pp. 97–110). New York: Guilford Press.

Schieffelin, B. B., & Ochs, E. (1986). Language socialization. *Annual Review of Anthropology, 15*, 163–191.

Schull, W. J. (1998). The Japanese experience, 1947–1997. *Proceedings of the National Academy of Science, 95*, 5437–5441.

Semel, E., Wiig, E. H., & Secord, W. H. (2004). *Clinical Evaluation of Language Fundamentals—Preschool* (2nd ed.). San Antonio, TX: Harcourt Assessment.

Sénéchal, M. (1997). The differential effect of storybook reading on preschoolers' acquisition of expressive and receptive vocabulary. *Journal of Child Language, 24*, 123–138.

Sénéchal, M., Thomas, E., & Monker, J. (1995). Individual differences in 4-year-old children's acquisition of vocabulary during storybook reading. *Journal of Educational Psychology, 87*, 218–229.

Senghas, A., & Coppola, M. (2001). Children creating language: How Nicaraguan Sign Language acquired a spatial grammar. *Psychological Science, 12*, 323–328.

Shatz, M., Hoff-Ginsberg, E., & MacIver, D. (1989). Induction and the acquisition of English auxiliaries: The effects of differentially enriched input. *Journal of Child Language, 12*, 199–207.

Shavelson, R. J., & Towne, L. (Eds.). (2002). *Scientific research in education.* Washington, DC: National Academy Press.

Shaywitz, B. A., Shaywitz, S. E., Pugh, K. R., Constable, R. T., Skudlarski, P., Fulbright, R. K., et al. (1995). Sex differences in the functional organization of the brain for language. *Nature, 373*, 607–609.

Shonkoff, J. P., & Phillips, D. A. (Eds.). (2000). *From neurons to neighborhoods: The science of early childhood development.* Washington, DC: National Academy Press.

Shriberg, L. D., Friel-Patti, S., Flipsen, P., Jr., & Brown, R. L. (2000). Otitis media, fluctuant hearing loss and speech–language delay: A preliminary structural equation model. *Journal of Speech, Language, and Hearing Research, 43*, 100–120.

Simon, C., & Holway, C. L. (1991). Presentation of communication evaluation information. In C. Simon (Ed.), *Communication skills and classroom success* (pp. 151–199). Eau Claire, WI: Thinking.

Sinclair-de-Zwart, H. (1973). Language acquisition and cognitive development. In T. E. Moore (Ed.), *Cognitive development and the acquisition of language* (pp. 9–26). New York: Academic Press.

Skinner, B. F. (1957). *Verbal behavior.* New York: Appleton Century Crofts.

Sloutsky, V. M., & Napolitano, A. C. (2003). Is a picture worth a thousand words? Preference for auditory modality in young children. *Child Development, 74*, 822–833.

Smiley, P., & Huttenlocher, J. (1995). Conceptual development and the child's early words for events, objects and persons. In M. Tomasello & W. Merriman (Eds.), *Beyond names for things: Young children's acquisition of verbs* (pp. 21–61). Hillsdale, NJ: Erlbaum.

Smith, L. B., Jones, S. S., & Landau, B. (1992). Count nouns, adjectives, and perceptual properties in children's novel word interpretations. *Developmental Psychology, 28*, 273–286.

Smith-Hefner, N. (1988). The linguistic socialization of Javanese children in two communities. *Anthropological Linguistics, 30*, 166–198.

Snow, C. E. (1972). Mothers' speech to children learning language. *Child Development, 43*, 549–565.

Snow, C. E., & Ferguson, C. A. (1977). *Talking to children: Language input and acquisition.* New York: Cambridge University Press.

Sorsby, A. J., & Martlew, M. (1991). Representational demands in mothers' talk to preschool children in two contexts: Picture book reading and a modeling task. *Journal of Child Language, 18*, 373–395.

Southerland, R. H. (1997). Language in social contexts. In W. O'Grady, M. Dobrovolsky, & M. Arnoff (Eds.), *Contemporary linguistics: An introduction* (3rd ed., pp. 509–551). Boston: Bedford/St. Martin's.

Spaulding, T. J., Plante, E., & Farinella, K. A. (2006). Eligibility criteria for language impairment: Is the low end of normal always appropriate? *Language, Speech, and Hearing Services in Schools, 37*, 61–72.

Speece, D. L., Roth, F. P., Cooper, D. H., & De La Paz, S. (1999). The relevance of oral language skills to early literacy: A multivariate analysis. *Applied Psycholinguistics, 20*, 167–190.

Spelke, E. S. (1979). Exploring audible and visual events in infancy. In A. D. Pick (Ed.), *Perception and its development: A tribute to Eleanor J. Gibson* (pp. 221–233). Hillsdale, NJ: Erlbaum.

Spinath, F. M., Price, T. S., Dale, P. S., & Plomin, R. (2004). The genetic and environmental origins of language disability and ability. *Child Development, 75*, 445–454.

Stager, C. L., & Werker, J. F. (1997). Infants listen for more phonetic detail in speech perception than in word-learning tasks. *Nature, 388*, 381–382.

Stanovich, K. E. (2000). *Progress in understanding reading: Scientific foundations and new frontiers.* New York: Guilford Press.

Stein, N. (1982). What's in a story: Interpreting the interpretations of story grammars. *Discourse Processes, 5*, 319–335.

Stoel-Gammon, C., & Dunn, C. (1985). *Normal and disordered phonology in children.* Austin, TX: PRO-ED.

Stokes, D. E. (1997). *Pasteur's quadrant: Basic science and technological innovation.* Washington, DC: Brookings Institution Press.

Storkel, H. L. (2001). Learning new words. I: Phonotactic probability in language development. *Journal of Speech, Language, and Hearing Research, 44*, 1321–1337.

Stothard, S. E., Snowling, M. J., Bishop, D. V. M., Chipchase, B. B., & Kaplan, C. A. (1998). Language-impaired preschoolers: A follow-up into adolescence. *Journal of Speech, Language, and Hearing Research, 41*, 407–418.

Strommen, E. F., & Frome, F. S. (1993). Talking back to Big Bird: Preschool users and a simple speech recognition system. *Educational Technology Research and Development, 41,* 5–16.

Stromswold, K. (2001). The heritability of language: A review and metaanalysis of twin, adoption, and linkage studies. *Language, 77,* 647–723.

Tabors, P. O. (1997). *One child, two languages: A guide for preschool educators of children learning English as a second language.* Baltimore: Brookes.

Tamis-LeMonda, C. S., Bornstein, M. H., & Baumwell, L. (2001). Maternal responsiveness and children's achievement of language milestones. *Child Development, 72,* 748–757.

Tannen, D. (1991). *You just don't understand: Women and men in conversation.* New York: Ballantine Books.

Tannen, D. (1994). *Talking from 9 to 5: How women's and men's conversational styles affect who gets heard, who gets credit, and what gets done at work.* London: Virago.

Taylor, G. R. (2001). *Educational interventions and services for children with exceptionalities.* Springfield, IL: Charles C Thomas.

Templin, M. C. (1957). *Certain language skills in children* (Institute of Child Welfare Monograph Series 26). Minneapolis: University of Minnesota Press.

Terrell, T. D. (1977). A natural approach to second language acquisition and learning. *Modern Language Journal, 61,* 325–337.

Thal, D., & Tobias, S. (1992). Communicative gestures in children with delayed onset of oral expressive vocabulary. *Journal of Speech and Hearing Research, 35,* 1281–1289.

Thiessen, E. D., & Saffran, J. R. (2003). When cues collide: Use of stress and statistical cues to word boundaries by 7- to 9-month-old infants. *Developmental Psychology, 39,* 706–716.

Thompson, C. K., Shapiro, L. P., Kiran, S., & Sobecks, J. (2003). The role of syntactic complexity in treatment of sentence deficits in agrammatic aphasia: The complexity account of treatment efficacy (CATE). *Journal of Speech, Language, and Hearing Research, 46,* 591–607.

Throneburg, R. N., Calvert, L. K., Sturm, J. J., Paramboukas, A. A., & Paul, P. J. (2000). A comparison of service delivery models: Effects on curricular vocabulary skills in the school setting. *American Journal of Speech–Language Pathology, 9,* 10–20.

Tomasello, M. (1987). Learning to use prepositions: A case study. *Journal of Child Language, 14,* 79–98.

Tomasello, M. (1988). The role of joint attentional processes in early language development. *Language Sciences, 10,* 69–88.

Tomasello, M. (2003). *Constructing a language.* Cambridge, MA: Harvard University Press.

Tomasello, M., & Todd, J. (1983). Joint attention and lexical acquisition style. *First Language, 4,* 197–212.

Tomblin, J. B. (1989). Familial concentration of developmental language impairment. *Journal of Speech and Hearing Disorders, 54,* 287–295.

Tomblin, J. B., Records, N. L., Buckwalter, P., Zhang, X., Smith, E., & O'Brien, M. (1997). Prevalence of specific language impairment in kindergarten children. *Journal of Speech, Language, and Hearing Research, 40,* 1245–1260.

Tomblin, J. B., Zhang, X., Buckwalter, P., & O'Brien, M. (2003) The stability of primary language disorder: Fours years after kindergarten diagnosis. *Journal of Speech, Language, and Hearing Research, 46,* 1283–1296.

Trainor, L. J., & Desjardins, R. N. (2002). Pitch characteristics of infant-directed speech affect infants' ability to discriminate vowels. *Psychonomic Bulletin and Review, 9,* 335–340.

Treiman, R., & Broderick, V. (1998). What's in a name? Children's knowledge about the letters in their own names. *Journal of Experimental Child Psychology, 70,* 97–116.

Trouton, A., Spinath, F. M., & Plomin, R. (2002). Twins Early Development Study (TEDS): A multivariate, longitudinal genetic investigation of language, cognition, and behaviour problems in childhood. *Twin Research, 5,* 444–448.

Tsao, F. M., Liu, H. M., & Kuhl, P. K. (2004). Speech perception in infancy predicts language development in the second year of life: A longitudinal study. *Child Development, 75,* 1067–1084.

Tye-Murray, N. (2000). The child who has severe or profound hearing loss. In J. B. Tomblin, H. L. Morris, & D. C. Spriestersbach (Eds.), *Diagnosis in speech–language pathology* (2nd ed.). San Diego, CA: Singular.

Ukrainetz, T. A., Justice, L. M., Kaderavek, J. N., Eisenberg, S. L., Gillam, R. B., & Harm, H. M. (2005). The development of expressive elaboration in fictional narratives. *Journal of Speech, Language, and Hearing Research, 48,* 1363–1377.

U.S. Department of Education. (1999). Assistance to states for the education of children with disabilities and the early intervention program for infants and toddlers with disabilities: Final regulations. *Federal Register, 64*(48), CFR Parts 300 and 303.

U.S. Department of Education. (2001). *Twenty-third annual report to Congress on the implementation of the Individuals with Disabilities Education Act.* Washington, DC: Author.

U.S. Department of Education, National Center for Education Statistics. (2005). *Public elementary and secondary students, staff, schools, and school districts: School year 2002–03* (Rep. No. NCES 2005–314). Washington, DC: Author.

U.S. Department of Health and Human Services. (1999). *Traumatic brain injury in the United States: A report to Congress.* Washington, DC: Author.

U.S. Department of State. (2005). *Immigrant visas issued to orphans coming to the U.S.* Washington, DC: Author.

Retrieved December 30, 2005, from http://travel.state.gov/family/adoption/stats/stats_451.html

Valdez-Menchaca, M. C., Marta, C., & Whitehurst, G. J. (1992). Accelerating language development through picture book reading: A systematic extension to Mexican day care. *Developmental Psychology, 28*, 1106–1114.

van der Lely, H. K. J., & Stollwerck, L. (1996). A grammatical specific language impairment in children: An autosomal dominant inheritance? *Brain and Language, 52*, 484.

Van Hulle, C. A., Goldsmith, H. H., & Lemery, K. S. (2004). Genetic, environmental, and gender effects on individual differences in toddler expressive language. *Journal of Speech, Language, and Hearing Research, 47*, 904–912.

Vasilyeva, M., Huttenlocher, J., & Waterfall, H. (2006). Effects of language intervention on syntactic skill levels in preschoolers. *Developmental Psychology, 42*, 164–174.

Vaux, B. (2004). American dialects. In J. Todd (Ed.), *Let's go USA 2004*. New York: St. Martin's Press.

Volterra, V., Caselli, M. C., Capirci, O., & Pizzuto, E. (2005). Gesture and the emergence and development of language. In M. Tomasello & D. I. Slobin (Eds.), *Beyond nature–nurture: Essays in honor of Elizabeth Bates* (pp. 3–40). Mahwah, NJ: Erlbaum.

Volterra, V., & Taeschner, T. (1978). The acquisition and development of language by bilingual children. *Journal of Child Language, 5*, 311–326.

Vygotsky, L. S. (1978). *Mind in society: The development of higher psychological processes*. Cambridge, MA: Harvard University. (Edited by M. Cole, V. John-Steiner, S. Scribner, & E. Souberman)

Wallace, I. F., Roberts, J. E., & Lodder, D. E. (1998). Interactions of African American infants and their mothers: Relations with development at 1 year of age. *Journal of Speech, Language, and Hearing Research, 41*, 900–912.

Walley, A. C. (1993). The role of vocabulary development in children's spoken word recognition and segmentation ability. *Developmental Review, 13*, 286–350.

Wang, Q., & Leichtman, M. D. (2000). Same beginnings, different stories: A comparison of American and Chinese children's narratives. *Child Development, 71*, 1329–1346.

Washington, J., & Craig, H. (1994). Dialectal forms during discourse of poor, urban, African-American preschoolers. *Journal of Speech and Hearing Research, 37*, 816–823.

Wasik, B. A., Bond, M. A., & Hindman, A. (2006). The effects of a language and literacy intervention on Head Start children and teachers. *Journal of Educational Psychology, 98*, 63–74.

Watkins, R., & Rice, M. L. (Eds.). (1994). *Specific language impairments in children*. Baltimore: Brookes.

Watkins, R., Rice, M., & Molz, C. (1993). Verb use by language-impaired and normally developing children. *First Language, 37*, 133–143.

Waxman, S. R., & Booth, A. (2000). Principles that are involved in the acquisition of words, but not facts. *Cognition, 77*, B33–B43.

Waxman, S. R., & Booth, A. E. (2001). On the insufficiency of evidence for a domain-general account of word learning. *Cognition, 78*, 277–279.

Weijer, J., van de. (2001). Vowels in infant- and adult-directed speech. In A. Karlsson & J. van de Weijer (Eds.), *Papers from Fonetik 2001 held at Örenäs, May 30–June 1, 2001* (Working Paper 49, pp. 172–175). Lund, Sweden: Lund University.

Weismer, S. E., Plante, E., Jones, M., & Tomblin, J. B. (2005). A functional magnetic resonance imaging investigation of verbal working memory in adolescents with specific language impairment. *Journal of Speech, Language, and Hearing Research, 48*, 405–425.

Weismer, S. E., & Thordardottir, E. (2002). Cognition and language. In P. Accardo, B. Rogers, & A. Capute (Eds.), *Disorders of language development* (pp. 21–37). Timonium, MD: York Press.

Weiss, C. E., Gordon, M. E., & Lillywhite, H. S. (1987). *Clinical management of articulatory and phonologic disorders* (2nd ed.). Baltimore: Williams & Wilkins.

Weist, R. M. (2002). Temporal and spatial concepts in child language: Conventional and configurational. *Journal of Psycholinguistic Research, 31*, 195–210.

Weitzman, E., & Greenberg, J. (2002). *Learning language and loving it: A guide to promoting children's social, language, and literacy development in early childhood settings* (2nd ed.). Toronto, Ontario, Canada: The Hanen Centre.

Wellman, B., Case, I., Mengert, I., & Bradbury, D. (1931). Speech sounds of young children. *State University of Iowa Studies in Child Welfare, 5, 2*.

Werker, J. F. (1995). Age-related changes in cross-language speech perception. In W. Strange (Ed.), *Speech perception and linguistic experience: Issues in cross-language research* (pp. 155–169). Timonium, MD: York Press.

Werker, J. F., & Tees, R. C. (1992). The organization and reorganization of human speech perception. *Annual Reviews of Neuroscience, 15*, 377–402.

Westby, C. E. (1985). Learning to talk—Talking to learn: Oral-literate language differences. In C. S. Simon (Ed.), *Communication skills and classroom success: Therapy methodologies for language-learning disabled students* (pp. 181–218). San Diego, CA: College-Hill Press.

Westby, C. E. (1991). Learning to talk—Talking to learn: Oral-literate language differences. In C. S. Simon (Ed.), *Communication skills and classroom success: Assessment and therapy methodologies for language and learning disabled students* (Rev. ed., pp. 334–357). Eau Claire, WI: Thinking.

Westby, C. E. (1998). Communicative refinement in school age and adolescence. In W. O. Haynes & B. B. Shulman (Eds.), *Communication development: Foundations, processes, and clinical implications* (pp. 311–360). Baltimore: Williams & Wilkins.

White, T. G., Sowell, J., & Yanagihara, A. (1989). Teaching elementary students to use word-part clues. *Reading Teacher, 42*, 302–308.

Whitehurst, G. J. (1997). Language processes in context: Language learning in children reared in poverty. In L. B. Adamson & M. A. Romski (Eds.), *Communication and language acquisition: Discoveries from atypical development* (pp. 233–265). Baltimore: Brookes.

Whitehurst, G. J., Arnold, D. S., Epstein, J. N., Angell, A. L., Smith, M., & Fischel, J. E. (1994). A picture book reading intervention in day-care and home for children from low-income families. *Developmental Psychology, 30,* 679–689.

Whitehurst, G. J., Falco, F. L., Lonigan, C. J., Fischel, J. E., De-Baryshe, B. D., Valdez-Menchaca, M. C., et al. (1988). Accelerating language development through picture book reading. *Developmental Psychology, 24,* 552–559.

Whitehurst, G. J., & Lonigan, C. J. (1998). Child development and emergent literacy. *Child Development, 68,* 848–872.

Wiig, E. H., & Secord, W. (1989). *Test of Language Competence—Expanded.* San Antonio, TX: Psychological Corporation.

Wiig, E. H., & Secord, W. (1992). *Test of Word Knowledge.* San Antonio, TX: Psychological Corporation.

Wiig, E., Secord, W., & Semel, E. (1992). *Clinical Evaluation of Language Fundamentals—Preschool.* San Antonio, TX: Psychological Corporation.

Wolfram, W., & Schilling-Estes, N. (2006). Language evolution or dying traditions? The state of American dialects. In W. Wolfram & B. Ward (Eds.), *American voices: How dialects differ from coast to coast* (pp. 1–7). Malden, MA: Blackwell.

Woodward, A., & Hoyne, K. (1999). Infants' learning about words and sounds in relation to objects. *Child Development, 70,* 65–77.

World Health Organization. (2001). *International classification of diseases, disabilities, and handicaps.* Geneva: Author.

Yeargin-Allsopp, M., Rice, C., Karapurkar, T., Doernberg, N., Boyle, C., & Murphy, C. (2003). Prevalence of autism in a U.S. metropolitan area. *Journal of the American Medical Association, 289,* 49–55.

Yoder, P. J., & Kaiser, A. P. (1989). Alternative explanations for the relationship between maternal verbal interaction style and child language development. *Journal of Child Language, 16,* 141–160.

Zemlin, W. R. (1988). *Speech and hearing science: Anatomy and physiology* (3rd ed.). Upper Saddle River, NJ: Prentice Hall.

Zentella, A. C. (1997). *Growing up bilingual.* Malden, MA: Blackwell.

Zimmerman, I., Steiner, V., & Pond, R. (1992). *Preschool Language Scale—3.* San Antonio, TX: Psychological Corporation.

Zimmerman, I. L., Steiner, V. G., & Pond, R. E. (2002). *Preschool Language Scale* (4th ed.). San Antonio, TX: Psychological Corporation.

Name Index

SUBJECT INDEX